"In this compelling and masterful narrative, Andrea Tone documents America's love/hate relationship with tranquilizers; it is a must-read for those who consume the drugs and also for those who do not. Tone uses sources as diverse as consumer letters to the FDA, pharmaceutical company records, the scripts of Hollywood films, and transcripts of Senate hearings to help us understand why the Age of Anxiety has lasted for six decades, and why men as well as women, children as well as adults, physicians as well as patients are so likely to be popping pills—and so unwilling to stop."

—Ruth Schwartz Cowan, Janice and Julian Bers Professor, University of Pennsylvania; author of *Heredity and Hope*

"Extensively researched and convincingly argued, *The Age of Anxiety* sets the gold standard for histories of contemporary pharmacology. It is required reading for anyone interested in the ways in which psychiatric drugs become metabolized into the American popular imagination."

—Jonathan M. Metzl, author of *Prozac On the Couch*

"This gripping book is much more than a history of psychopharmaceutical invention; it is an account of our fears and fantasies about pills. . . . *The Age of Anxiety* is a remarkable window into modern America and the ways in which Americans choose to live their lives."

—Tanya Luhrmann, author of *Of Two Minds: An Anthropologist Looks at American Psychiatry*

THE AGE OF ANXIETY

ALSO BY ANDREA TONE

Medicating Modern America

Devices and Desires

The Business of Benevolence

Controlling Reproduction

The Age of Anxiety

A History of America's Turbulent Affair with Tranquilizers

ANDREA TONE

BASIC
BOOKS

A Member of the Perseus Books Group
New York

Published by Basic Books,
A Member of the Perseus Books Group

Books published by Basic Books are available at special discounts for bulk
purchases in the United States by corporations, institutions, and other
organizations. For more information, please contact the Special Markets
Department at the Perseus Books Group, 2300 Chestnut Street, Suite 200,
Philadelphia, PA 19103, or call (800) 810-4145, ext. 5000, or e-mail
special.markets@perseusbooks.com.

Designed by Brent Wilcox

Library of Congress Cataloging-in-Publication Data
Tone, Andrea, 1964–
    The age of anxiety : a history of America's turbulent affair with tranquilizers /
Andrea Tone.
        p.   cm.
    Includes bibliographical references.
    ISBN 978-0-465-08658-0 (alk. paper)
    1. Tranquilizing drugs—United States—History. 2. Antipsychotic drugs—
United States—History. I. Title.
    [DNLM: 1. Antipsychotic Agents—history—United States. 2. Anxiety
Disorders—drug therapy—United States. 3. Pharmaceutical Preparations—
history—United States. QV 11 AA1 T664a 2009]
    RM333.T66 2009
    615'.7882—dc22
                                                                2008032718

10 9 8 7 6 5 4 3 2 1

For Sophia

CONTENTS

PREFACE

Years ago, as I was researching the history of oral contraceptives in the 1960s and 1970s, I came across numerous references to the era's other great pill: the tranquilizer Valium. Approved by the FDA in 1963, the drug the Rolling Stones nicknamed "mother's little helper" was the most widely prescribed pill in the Western world from the late 1960s to the early 1980s. In 1978 alone, Valium's manufacturer, Hoffman-La Roche, sold nearly 2.3 billion tablets, enough to medicate half the globe.[1]

As a historian of medicine interested in how ordinary people experience technological and social change, I wanted to know more about this phenomenon. Many books had been published on other psychiatric medications, but the history of minor tranquilizers, I quickly discovered, had been largely ignored. Minor tranquilizers are referred to as "minor" to distinguish them from drugs such as Thorazine or reserpine, first called major tranquilizers and now more commonly classified as antipsychotics or neuroleptics. (To avoid confusion, I use "minor tranquilizers" and "tranquilizers" interchangeably throughout this book but refer to drugs such as Thorazine as major tranquilizers or antipsychotics.) Scholars, patients, clinicians, and critics have paid a staggering amount of attention to depression; one thinks, for example, of *Listening to Prozac, Talking Back to Prozac, Prozac Nation, The Noonday Demon, Let Them Eat Prozac,* and the late William Styron's eloquent *Darkness Visible.* Here then, I thought, was a book that needed to be written: a history of tranquilizers set in the context of the golden age of post–World War II pharmaceutical science, the changing dynamics of psychiatric thought and practice, and shifting cultural ideas surrounding consumer culture, convenience, drug use, and social roles.[2]

There was also a more personal reason behind my decision to write this book. My own brush with acute anxiety happened unexpectedly. It was a sunny morning in June 2001, and I was on a plane bound for New York City. Comfortably cruising (or so our stalwart pilot told us) at 30,000 feet, our plane hit a patch of unexpected turbulence. Almost immediately, I felt tremors of fear wrack my body. The passenger on my right, a hefty man perched awkwardly in his economy-size seat, was asleep. The woman to my left was reading *Bridget Jones's Diary*, an occasional giggle passing her lips. I, on the other hand, was a wreck. My palms were sticky. My body suddenly felt warm. I had flown hundreds of times before. What had transformed me from someone who once viewed plane travel as quiet time for reading into a tremulous passenger fearful that at any moment our airplane would hurl me and its contents to the ground?

I chalked it up to nerves. I had just published my book *Devices and Desires* on the history of contraceptives. My days in New York were packed with television shoots and radio interviews. Then there was Sophia, my seven-month-old daughter. It was my first separation from her and I hated it. As every hiccup of turbulence struck me as a prelude to a fiery death, I clutched her photo tighter, her big brown eyes staring back. That's when I started perspiring.

It was embarrassing. I felt anxious even as I felt silly for feeling anxious. The same brain that conjured up images of twisted metal engulfed in flames knew that air travel was the safest method of human transport in the world. My calm returned once the plane landed and I enjoyed a productive stay in Manhattan. But when this experience of anxiety failed to improve on the flight home, I made an appointment to see my doctor. My internist, a compassionate soul resistant to quick fixes, reassured me that it was not uncommon for new parents, particularly mothers, to develop a fear of flying when they first left their children. She promised it would get better and that it would improve the more I flew. Exposure therapy is what clinical therapists call it. The more we're exposed to what we fear—be it flying, public speaking, tall buildings, or spiders—the easier it becomes to vanquish that fear.

We discussed strategies for managing my anxiety. Clearly I had to keep flying. Cognitive behavioral therapy (also known as CBT), a form of psychotherapy in which trained therapists teach patients techniques to understand their reactions to events and to modify their behavior, has an excellent track record helping people overcome phobias. Unfortunately I was an academic at a university without maternity leave or day care, and fitting counseling sessions into an already overextended schedule would have been a challenge in its own right. In addition, my health insurance didn't include comprehensive counseling benefits. After a limited number of sessions, I would have to assume the full cost of therapy on my own. As my doctor and I weighed the pros and cons of different treatment options, we yielded to pharmaceutical pragmatism, as had countless Americans before me. Enthusiastic about CBT in principle, we regretted the obstacles that made it difficult, even for a full-time professional, to undertake it in practice. In contrast, there was something to be said for tranquilizers' convenience. Inexpensive and fast-acting, the drugs had an enviable efficacy record: for a majority of people, and especially for those who have not taken them before or take them only intermittently, a single dose will alleviate most anxiety symptoms within an hour. At the end of our consultation, she prescribed a short-acting tranquilizer, Ativan, to tame my nerves just enough to coax me aboard future flights. I already knew something about Ativan, the chemical cousin of the better-known Valium. Most of us know someone—a mother, an uncle, a neighbor, perhaps even ourselves—who has taken Valium, Ativan, Miltown, or one of the dozens of other tranquilizers available by prescription since the 1950s. Millions have, although they don't always admit it. I too chafed against the stigma, struggling with the implications of what it meant to need a tranquilizer to fly. But it worked. Several months later, I was back in the air. Soon I was flying drug-free.

The Age of Anxiety is not my history, although, as is true with all works of nonfiction, it is informed by personal experience. Indeed, after completing a book on contraceptives, I have often felt nostalgia for the obstetrician-gynecology conferences of my past, where it was rare to encounter medical practitioners, patients, or activists who questioned birth control's legitimacy. In contrast, studying the history of antianxiety drugs (also known as

anxiolytics) is a bit like walking into a political minefield. Discussing tranquilizers tends to raise a battery of disquieting questions: Are we more anxious now than we were in the past? Does the rising consumption of
tranquilizers since the 1950s reflect a higher prevalence of anxiety, better or at
least more respected treatments or, as some critics have charged, the pharmaceutical industry's growing power to pathologize the problems of everyday
life and expand the boundaries of diagnostic categories? Underlying these
questions is an equally thorny issue. Is anxiety socially constructed (largely a
by-product of a particular cultural milieu) or biologically driven?

My approach has been to consider anxiety as something at once real
and historically rooted: an actual experience inseparable from the constellation of ideas, individuals, and events that give it meaning.

In one sense, anxiety has always plagued us. History is replete with narratives of those who have suffered under its spell. "No Grand Inquisitor
has in readiness such terrible torture as has anxiety," wrote Danish
philosopher Søren Kierkegaard in 1844. Anxiety, he insisted, was a curse
that "every man has to affront if he would not go to perdition either by not
having known anxiety or by sinking under it." In 1902, philosopher and
psychologist William James recounted his own bout with the beast: "I
awoke morning after morning with a horrible dread at the pit of my stomach and with a sense of insecurity of life that I never knew before." Not
surprisingly, social commentators from different eras have resolutely insisted that theirs is the most anxious age. Viscount John Morley wrote of
a Victorian society beset by doubt. "Those who dwell in the tower of ancient faiths," he lamented in 1874, "look about them in constant apprehension, misgiving, and the hurried uneasy mien of people living amid
earthquakes. The air seems full of missiles, and all is doubt, hesitation, and
shivering expectancy." Decades later, in 1948, historian and scholar Arthur
M. Schlesinger Jr. could assert with equal resolve that "Western man in the
middle of the 20th century is tense, uncertain, adrift. . . . We look upon
our epoch as a time of troubles, an age of anxiety." Certainly many of
Schlesinger's contemporaries concurred that the late 1940s and early
1950s was America's quintessentially anxious age, an association cemented
by the 1947 publication of W. H. Auden's *The Age of Anxiety: A Baroque*

Eclogue, a six-part poem that garnered rave reviews, earned a Nobel Prize, and inspired a symphony of the same title by Leonard Bernstein.[3]

For each of these commentators, anxiety as an individual experience or collective malaise was *real,* a point I explore further in this book. Anxiety's expressions—worry, doubt, panic, fear—clearly existed. As such, anxiety's reality is confirmed by the place it has occupied in people's lives. Anxiety has shaped poets' prose, colored artists' visions, and haunted the words of the dying. It has followed soldiers onto the battlefield and clouded the minds of parents who wonder why their child is late from school, from a neighbor's, from a first date. As Kierkegaard suggested, being born human destines most of us to confront anxiety as an integral part of what it means be alive.[4]

But anxiety is not timeless. How it has been described, interpreted, and treated has varied across time and place. Consequently, we must resist the temptation to impose modern understandings of anxiety onto the past lest we flatten the chronological particularities that make history meaningful. William James's suffering may reference a feeling that echoes across generations, but it remains inseparable from James's particular worldview. Context matters.[5]

That is not to suggest that these contexts, at once familiar and particular, are beyond the historian's reach. Historians of illness and patient experience must walk a fine line. Acknowledging that another person's misery is too complex in its subjectivity to ever fully be known by another, they must not lose sight of the value of trying, as best as they are able, to understand it. Certainly this can be challenging. Virginia Woolf, no stranger to psychological suffering, explained the conundrum when she lamented the inadequacy of language to capture the essence of what it means to be ill. "English, which can express the thoughts of Hamlet and the tragedy of Lear, has no words for the shiver and the headache," she wrote with razor-sharp intelligence in 1926. "The merest schoolgirl, when she falls in love, has Shakespeare, Donne, Keats to speak her mind for her; but let a sufferer try to describe a pain in his head to a doctor and language at once runs dry. There is nothing made for him." As Woolf, who committed suicide in 1941, knew only too well, the fact that the experience of being ill often defies words does not negate the reality of physical and emotional distress. Indeed, one of the drawbacks of an approach that blames culture or the medical industry for manufacturing psychological problems is that it may unwittingly cause us to discount the gravity of suffering itself. If we blame outside forces for inventing problems, we run the risk of suggesting, ipso facto, that no problem exists. From the sufferer's perspective, the cause of one's anxiety may be less important than its unsettling visitation. Hence, a three-year-old's phobias of clowns or butterflies are no less terrifying to the three-year-old because we declare them to be socially constructed. Clowns and butterflies aren't known for their savage attacks on children, but the stricken toddler's tears, racing pulse, and abject panic are real.[6]

In addition, the tendency to regard mental illness as more of a cultural creation than a biological reality implies that the construction of disorders and therapies is a one-way process, as if society (or some powerful constituency within it) creates them out of thin air. Those so afflicted must simply accept or reject the disorder and its prescribed remedies. Of course, medical realities are far more complicated. Psychiatric disorders and the people who experience them are fluid and mutable. Changing psychiatric classifications, developments in medicinal chemistry, commercial agendas, people's interpretations of their health, and doctors' behavior are just some of the many variables that constantly revise ideas about disorders and treatments. Far from being a one-way street, the making of psychiatry and psychopharmacology has always involved multidirectional paths.[7]

In this book, I explore how these paths have converged in unexpected ways to create America's tranquilizer culture. My focus is less the subjective experience of anxiety than the related history of how people have tried to address and assuage it. Piecing together historical evidence—manufacturers' records, Food and Drug Administration (FDA) reports, personal letters, court cases, congressional investigations, interviews, and representations of popular culture—I ground the history of tranquilizers' development, popularity, and subsequent discrediting within the social, economic, and political contexts in which they came of age. Although we cannot say definitively that the post–World War II period was a more anxious era than any other, the fact that people in this era often perceived (and were encouraged to believe) that it was helped solidify a rationale and rhetoric that justified tranquilizers' use.

My book is not a political diatribe against the pharmaceutical industry or the psychiatric profession, a topic explored by other scholars. Instead, it is a history of the circumstances under which our contested and enduring relationship with tranquilizers took shape. It is a story of politics, passion, and people. It is a tale of success and addiction, of pharmaceutical revolution and political revulsion, and of people's long-standing desire to appear calm on the outside when they feel frazzled within.

The Age of Anxiety chronicles the history of a class of drugs that, over time, came to be regarded as intrinsic to psychiatry. Undoubtedly, the history of tranquilizers contains parallels to the histories of other psychiatric medications. Along with antidepressants and antipsychotics, for example, tranquilizers have been the focus of highly politicized debates over drug safety, efficacy, and consumers' rights. Critics sometimes (and understandably) have conflated tranquilizers with other classes of medications to argue that psychiatric medications have been overhyped, inadequately studied, and overused. While we can accept the validity of some complaints—such as the problems spawned by direct-to-consumer advertising or the concealment of negative clinical trial data—and seek to address these concerns, we cannot assume that what holds true for some drugs tells us "all we need to know" about every psychiatric medication. Tranquilizers have their own separate and culturally specific history. It is this unique story, with its points of convergence as well as divergence, that *The Age of Anxiety* tells.

My focus is the United States, where minor tranquilizers were developed and widely prescribed, and where they excited the popular imagination in a way they did not elsewhere. The availability of fast-acting, effective, and relatively cheap pills to tame quotidian distress carried special meaning to a cold war nation that championed political containment, economic efficiency, and consumer convenience, and that valorized homegrown innovations as a symbol of America's technological might. Along with England, the United States was also the country that experienced the most forceful backlash in the wake of the drugs' stigmatization as socially and medically hazardous; tranquilizers were, in the words of British psychiatrist Malcolm Lader, "the opium of the masses." Although a U.S. focus affords me the luxury of detailing the characteristics of America's encounter with tranquilizers, it is not

meant to discount the intellectual benefit that might come from telling this
history with a different geographic emphasis. Indeed, I hope that *The Age of
Anxiety* will help lay the groundwork for scholars to pursue other local,
transnational, or cross-cultural histories.[8]

Today, drugs for anxiety are a billion-dollar business in the United
States. Yet as recently as 1955, when Miltown, the first prescription minor
tranquilizer, became available, pharmaceutical executives at Carter-Wallace, its manufacturer, worried that there wouldn't be a market for anxiety
relief. Psychiatry departments throughout North America were enamored
with Freudian theories of neurosis. Talk therapy, not pharmacotherapy,
was the treatment of choice. Convinced that tranquilizers would never be
big money makers in Freud's America, the company's president kept the
drug shelved for years. When it was finally released, Miltown proved a
commercial sensation. Defying pundits' predictions, it became the first
psychotropic blockbuster and the fastest-selling drug in U.S. history. In a
way unimaginable in our current political environment, where many pharmaceutical "breakthroughs" are regarded with suspicion, people in the
1950s viewed tranquilizers with curiosity and excitement. In both big-city
and small-town America, patients who had read or heard about the new
doctor-sanctioned "emotional aspirins" and "peace pills" clamored for a
supply. By 1957, Americans had filled 36 million prescriptions for Miltown, more than a billion tablets had been manufactured, and tranquilizers accounted for a staggering one-third of all prescriptions.

What, I wondered, incited ordinary Americans to wait in line, sometimes for hours, to get their scripts filled? What enabled a pharmaceutical
firm with little experience in the competitive prescription drug market to
become the envy of established outfits? Why were the drugs nicknamed
Executive Excedrin in the 1950s and widely used by businessmen, male
talk show hosts and celebrities, when today we remember them as salves
for harried housewives? In short, what was it about the nature of anxiety
in 1950s America that made the mass consumption of tranquilizers both
astonishingly attractive and benignly banal?

Answering these questions involves deciphering this turning point in
the history of psychopharmacology on contemporaries' terms. In 1950s

American culture, anxiety was viewed less as a serious psychiatric disorder than as a badge of achievement: an emblem of struggle, but also of success. Anxiety was the predictable yet commendable offshoot of Americans' insatiable hunger to get ahead, their relentless determination to become new and improved. This can-do mentality also underlay the belief that Americans not only could accomplish anything but were entitled to do so with minimum discomfort and inconvenience. In this cultural tableau, tranquilizers were welcomed as a means of personal fulfillment with the same fervor as credit cards, electric refrigerators, television dinners, and cosmetics. Countless entertainers, writers, and sports stars in the 1950s, many of them men, boasted of their tranquilizer use. Their candor was not an admission of psychiatric problems but a celebration, of sorts, of their achievements and those of the nation as a whole.[9]

Americans' unexpected embrace of Miltown triggered consumer stampedes that emptied drugstores and inspired cocktails, jewelry, and television skits. The grassroots frenzy shaped psychiatric thinking and corporate strategizing from the bottom up. In many ways, middle-class Americans' responses to tranquilizers in the 1950s determined how successive generations interpreted anxiety as a disorder. In the 1950s and 1960s the everyday meanings of anxiety were defined less by committees of psychiatrists, diagnostic manuals, and corporate agendas than by Americans' exuberant response to antianxiety drugs. In 1955, there existed no clear-cut consensus that anxiety was a psychiatric disorder serious enough to require pharmaceutical care. Miltown's profitability and widespread cultural impact changed that, fomenting new perceptions of anxiety and its treatment and fueling the development of other psychiatric lifestyle drugs such as Valium and Prozac. Miltown's success as a consumer commodity that calmed nerves by altering the biochemical workings of the brain put pharmaceutical companies on alert and inspired research on the biological basis of anxiety. Around the world, firms caught off guard by Carter-Wallace's success (who would have predicted that a laxative company would hit the jackpot?) and eager to claim a slice of the fantastically profitable tranquilizer market ordered company scientists to invent a pill that would outsell the nation's mood-altering wonder drug. As reports about Miltown's habit-forming potential began to surface in the late 1950s, Hoffman-La Roche won FDA approval to market Librium in 1960, the first of a new class of tranquilizers known as the benzodiazepines. Valium followed in 1963. By then, the age of big-time psychopharmacology had begun. Years after Miltown took the country by storm, corporate and government-funded researchers in the emerging field of neuroscience began to identify the biochemical mechanisms that exacerbate and alleviate anxiety, findings that annealed scientific explanations to the positive testimonials of patients and doctors who had been insisting for years that "tranquilizers worked." As the tranquilizer bonanza continued, researchers' results cemented the belief that anxiety was a disorder of the brain amenable to pharmacotherapy, a view that is sacrosanct among many mental health experts today.[10]

The rise of a far-reaching tranquilizer culture and the medicalization of anxiety it galvanized were largely patient driven. For countless users, the decision to take tranquilizers was a seemingly cheap, fast (and, many thought, harmless) way to cope with suboptimal circumstances beyond one's immediate control. From the beginning, tranquilizers' low cost (especially relative to psychotherapy) and the American tendency to seek individual solutions, even when faced with problems largely social and political in character, gave tranquilizers a specific cultural cachet. Feminist researchers in the 1970s frequently blamed society's mistreatment of women for housewives' well-documented tranquilizer habit. The real problem, they averred, was the circumstances—isolated caregiving and unrealistically high expectations for women—that drove them to take pills to attenuate private pains. In a better world, universal day care and more egalitarian social arrangements might trump pharmaceutical solutions. In the here and now, though, tranquilizer use was understood to be a logical albeit regrettable response to the misfortunes and vicissitudes of life. Looking back, we need to understand the decision to take a "trank" as an individual act which, because it was made by millions of Americans, prompted widespread commentary and catalyzed long-lasting medical and political change.[11]

This important chapter in the history of psychopharmacology was thus at once a medical event as well as a social and political phenomenon. Many histories of medicine have given scientific theories or pioneering physicians the lion's share of attention. Yet the rise of America's tranquilizer culture cannot be understood apart from the political and cultural events that shaped it—events not always discussed in conventional histories of psychiatry. These include atomic anxiety and the rhetoric of containment and personal preparedness it spawned; a convenience mentality that prized quick, easy, and cheap fixes for social and personal problems; a long-standing tradition of barbiturate use that was reconfigured, through an act of Congress, into a prescription-only market; an almost evangelical faith in pharmaceutical innovation and the individual benefits of applied laboratory research; and the trendiness of Miltown itself, a drug that quickly became an affordable status symbol.

To confine the history of psychopharmacology to theory, medical institutions, or physicians ignores the social conditions that encouraged tranquilizers to flourish. The patients and pills that inaugurated our modern age of lifestyle drugs are best understood by studying the lifestyles of those who took them. Americans encountered Miltown during a time of prosperity and uncertainty. America was a land of suburban bomb shelters and duck-and-cover drills, of houses and lawns overflowing with toddler spit-up and baby buggies, and of Wall Street denizens scrambling to keep up with the Joneses. Connecting laboratory developments and medical debates with events at ground level, *The Age of Anxiety* roots this turning point in the rise of psychopharmacology firmly within history.

Indeed, the trials and tribulations of tranquilizers confirm that pharmaceutical drugs are pregnant with social meaning.[12] Once welcomed for their therapeutic potential, tranquilizers began to be vilified in the late 1960s and 1970s. The fact that the pharmacological properties of tranquilizers remained basically stable and that scientists had recognized their habit-forming potential years before their censure reminds us how the vagaries of politics can radically change perceptions of a drug's value.[13] In the end, the discrediting of tranquilizers in the age of pharmaceutical Calvinism tells us as much about the society that passed judgment on them as it does about the drugs' chemical properties. As anxiety became a legitimate mental illness, tranquilizers ceased to be regarded as the banal "peace pills" of the past. Their recasting as potent psychiatric medications at a moment in history when a disparate but vocal group of critics was able to draw attention to an alleged drug epidemic among middle-class Americans, especially women, elicited a reevaluation of tranquilizers' benefits and costs. Compounding concerns was incontrovertible evidence that thousands of Americans *had* developed a dependence on tranquilizers that made withdrawing from them difficult and medically dangerous, despite initial promises from jubilant journalists, doctors, government agencies, and pharmaceutical firms that antianxiety drugs were unlikely to induce harm. In media portrayals, lawsuits, and government hearings, the therapeutic miracles of yesteryears were somberly recast as America's newest drug addicts.

In the pages that follow, I explore the promises and perils of America's embrace of tranquilizers. It is a rich tapestry of events, ideas, and intriguing personalities: from the dogged determination of a refugee scientist to get his bosses at Carter-Wallace to take Miltown seriously, to the televised testimonials of celebrity devotees and, later, beleaguered addicts, to the recent resurgence of interest in anxiety and tranquilizers in the wake of 9/11.

Most historians wonder when the histories they tell truly begin. I start with a brief overview of the history and interpretation of anxiety, from the Catholic humanist Thomas More's first use of the term in 1525 through the Freudian turn during the twentieth century. On the eve of Miltown's release, psychoanalysis dominated the psychiatric establishment even as millions of Americans eschewed talk therapy and took addictive and dangerous barbiturates to battle frayed nerves and insomnia. As we shall see, the salience of neurosis in American thought and culture, the popularity of pharmacological nerve busters, and a cold war political establishment that ceaselessly reminded its citizens of the need for collective calm and individual achievement set the stage for the arrival of the nation's first prescription tranquilizer. The astonishing sequence of events that followed changed lives, made headlines, created commercial empires, and launched a pharmaceutical culture that, more than fifty years after it began, continues to celebrate the virtues of a quick and convenient calm.

(1)

Anxiety Before the Tranquilizer Revolution

When William Henry enlisted with the 68th Pennsylvania Volunteers in August 1862, doctors judged him to be in "good health." The records don't mention anything about his gallantry, patriotism, or youthful invincibility, but those qualities likely played a role, since Henry joined the Union army at a time when, by most accounts, the Confederacy was winning. At first the private did hard duty. But on the eve of the battle at Fredericksburg in December 1862, William Henry began suffering from various intestinal problems, notably diarrhea. If he had jitters, they were justified. In a decisive Confederate victory, the Union army suffered over 12,000 casualties. The carnage in the Virginia hills was so horrific that Confederate General Robert E. Lee reportedly said, with compassion, "It is well that war is so terrible—[lest] we would grow too fond of it." William Henry survived, but at a price. Army physician Jacob Mendez Da Costa chronicled the young man's miseries. After Fredericksburg, William Henry "was seized with lancinating pains in the cardiac region so intense that he was obliged to throw himself down upon the ground, and with palpitation. The symptoms frequently returned while on the march, were attended with dimness of vision and giddiness, and obliged him often to fall out of his company and ride in the ambulance."[1]

1

As Da Costa quickly discovered, William Henry's symptoms were not unique. At Turner's Lane Hospital in Philadelphia, which became famous for wartime neurological research, Da Costa encountered over three hundred otherwise healthy young soldiers with similar complaints: heart palpitations, dizziness, sweaty palms, insomnia, pain in the chest, digestive disorders, and a shortness of breath such "that he could not keep up with his comrades." Like most doctors of his time, Da Costa believed that illness was as unique as each patient's constitution. But he felt compelled to generalize as the number of similarly afflicted soldiers grew. Detecting no signs of organic disease, Da Costa ascribed their symptoms to an overactive heart, calling the ailment "irritable heart syndrome." Likely the heart had "become irritable, from its overactivation and frequent excitement and that disordered innervation keeps it so," he explained in an 1871 article later credited as being the first medical account of panic disorder. Da Costa treated the syndrome with the drugs at hand: digitalis, aconite, belladonna, opium, strychnine, and acetate of lead, among others.[2]

Da Costa believed that William Henry's symptoms were caused by an underlying coronary disorder and did not refer to his mind or psyche. Furthermore, he made no mention of the horrors of combat: the stench of the battlefield, the sight of shattered limbs, the shrill cries and whimpers that faded into silence.[3]

Nowadays, anxiety disorders, including panic disorder, are the province of psychiatric medicine. Classified as an illness, they are often treated with antianxiety medications or through therapy provided by mental health professionals. Neuroscientists have identified the brain structures and neurotransmitters implicated in anxiety, and visualization technologies, notably PET scans, offer kaleidoscopic snapshots of the anxious brain. The American Psychiatric Association (APA), presently the most influential organization of psychiatrists in the world with more than 36,000 members, recognizes several major types of anxiety disorders, detailed in the APA's *Diagnostic and Statistical Manual of Mental Disorders* (DSM). In addition to panic disorder, the most commonly recognized forms are obsessive-compulsive disorder, posttraumatic stress disorder, social phobia (also called social anxiety disorder), specific phobias, and generalized anxiety disorder.[4]

Nevertheless, vexing questions remain regarding the character and purpose of anxiety. Clinicians and researchers often disagree, for instance, over how to distinguish healthy from pathological anxiety, what defines appropriate treatment, and the prevalence of anxiety disorders. Most experts concur that *some* anxiety is desirable. Nervousness before a test or job interview may sharpen intellectual acuity and improve performance. Anxiety is also a natural response to real or perceived danger. A chance meeting with a grizzly bear or a stranger in a dark alley typically triggers the sympathetic nervous system in what is known as a fight-or-flight response: a state of hyperarousal appropriate to life-threatening situations. Usually, however, the threat is less immediate. Just as political leaders have channeled their concerns and frustrations into revolutions and reforms, so painters, performing artists, novelists, and poets have often linked anxiety and inspiration. Scientists also contest the origins of pathological anxiety. Even those who regard anxiety as a biochemical disorder of the brain generally acknowledge that genetics, biology, developmental, and behavioral factors interact in anxiety disorders in complex ways.[5]

Early Anxiety and Institutional Reality

Although it now falls under the purview of psychological medicine, anxiety has been experienced and interpreted differently for most of human history. The word "anxiety" is derived from the Latin *angere,* meaning to choke or throttle. Connoting a "troubled state of mind," the term first appeared in the writings of the sixteenth-century statesman and Catholic humanist Sir Thomas More. "There dyed he without grudge, without anxietie," penned More about Jesus of Nazareth in *Quattuor Novissima* (*The Last Four Things*) in 1522. Thirteen years later, More was sentenced to death by Henry VIII's newly Anglicanized court, and by all accounts he died without grudge and at peace with God.[6]

More's "anxietie" had nothing to do with psychiatric afflictions per se. Physicians had written about and treated insanity since at least the time of the famous Roman physician Galen (A.D. 129–200), but few had made it their life's work. Generally speaking, families looked after their own, although persons considered dangerously deranged could be confined to poorhouses or asylums. In More's time, a handful of asylums in Europe housed the insane as well as the homeless, some criminals, and the terminally ill. London's St. Mary of Bethlehem Hospital was built in 1247. It would become known to future generations as the notorious Bedlam and would be immortalized by William Hogarth's evocative sketches. It first admitted nine mentally ill patients in 1404. Prevailing patterns of institutionalization mirrored a broadly shared view that madness was a form of social transgression akin to vagabondage, prostitution, and thievery. In the absence of formal policies or a literature that dealt with insanity in medical terms, there remained a tacit understanding that these people were simply too dangerous or disruptive to be ignored. In hierarchical societies highly attuned to matters of convention and class, insanity, like all forms of deviance, fomented fear. Hence the alarmist tone of a 1751 petition to the colonial Pennsylvania Assembly which insisted that "Lunatiks . . . going at large are a Terror to their Neighbors."[7]

The horrors of asylum life in the premodern era have been well documented. The therapeutic vocation we associate with the modern psychiatric hospital traces its origins to segregated institutions for those with serious mental infirmities—psychosis, dementia, idiocy—established around the turn of the nineteenth century. The asylum movement found its strongest support among physicians in England, France, Germany, Italy, and the United States. Proponents championed the radically optimistic idea that suitable facilities could restore the mad to reason; therapeutic progress and institutional reform went hand in hand. In Williamsburg, Virginia, the Public Hospital for Persons of Insane and Disordered Minds, the first public institution dedicated to treating the mentally ill in British North America, opened in 1773. One of its few admission criteria was that patients had to be judged curable. At its inception, the Williamsburg hospital consciously distanced itself from its custodial and punitive predecessors, a symbol of the therapeutic and ameliorative optimism of a new institutional age.[8]

Despite the best of intentions, conditions inside were less than ideal and well shy of the English psychiatrist John Conolly's vision of places

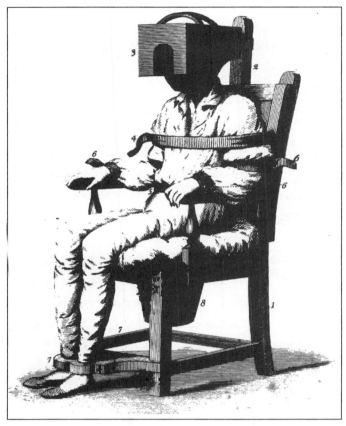

Rush's Tranquilizing Chair. Dr. Benjamin Rush designed this chair in 1811 to calm agitated psychiatric patients by restricting their sensory input and to provide a humane alternative to the "evils of the strait waistcoat." The widespread employment of restraint devices in asylums helped create a receptive audience for psychiatric medications, whose invisible workings made them seem more gentle and benign. Reproduced courtesy of the National Library of Medicine.

"where humanity, if anywhere on earth, shall reign supreme." Benjamin Rush's "tranquilizing chair" illustrates the limits of contemporary therapeutics. Rush, a signer of the Declaration of Independence, was renowned as a medical visionary. After practicing as a physician, he became a professor of medicine at the University of Pennsylvania. His clinical responsibilities included the psychiatric ward of the Pennsylvania Hospital, where his tranquilizing chair was used to pacify disruptive patients. Straps restrained the patient's chest, arms, and legs, and a wooden block around the head eliminated sensory input. Yet as psychiatrist Nancy Andreasen has observed, Rush's invention may be regarded "as the best that one of the most enlightened minds in a relatively enlightened era could come up with." Rush, it is worth noting, also wrote an early textbook based on his experiences, *Medical Inquiries and Observations upon the Diseases of the Mind* (1812).[9]

The early history of the psychiatric profession was intimately tied up with the new asylums. Until the twentieth century the "treatment of the diseases of the mind," as psychiatry was first defined, was synonymous with asylums or hospitals (such as Paris's Salpêtrière, where some of psychiatry's luminaries, including Philip Pinel, Jean-Martin Charcot, and Sigmund Freud worked or trained). One became an "alienist" (as psychiatric practitioners were then called) via a range of paths: general medicine, pathology, and particularly neurology. But it was the lunatic asylum that gave psychiatry an early, if inchoate, identity and a dubious legacy from which twentieth-century psychiatrists consciously distanced themselves, part of a wholesale effort to establish their therapeutic credibility and social legitimacy.[10]

Clearly, viewing anxiety as a form of lunacy made no sense. Lunatics were deranged outcasts who required institutionalization. Until mainstream psychiatry moved beyond institutions into private practice, before it laid claim to everyday problems in addition to dramatic mental diseases, anxiety remained off limits.[11]

Until relatively recently, anxiety and its offshoots—nervousness, tension, fear, and worry—were understood as a manifestation of a troubled spirit, a defective will, a lack of courage, or an unhealthy constitution. In the classical age, for instance, people might have invoked humoralist notions to explain their nervous temperament. This theory, which traced its origins to the Hippocratic authors of ancient Greece, remained influential until the mid-nineteenth century. It assumed that health, illness, temperament, appearance, and taste reflected the combined effects of the body's four humors—phlegm, blood, choler (yellow bile), and black bile (melancholy). Illnesses were caused by a surplus or deficit of one or more of them. Hence melancholia was thought to be due to an excess of black bile. Acrimonious or hot-tempered individuals were prey to excessive yellow bile. Healers used various means to adjust the humors: a corrective diet, exercise, tinctures, emetics, laxatives, cupping, and bloodletting. One appeal of humoral theory was that it explained pretty much everything, including idiosyncrasies that both patients and practitioners saw fit to leave alone.[12]

A nervous constitution might also be interpreted as a peculiarity of character or a social affect. Eighteenth-century journals often referenced phobias, but their tone alternated between thoughtfulness and outright derision: one might make allowances for fear of thunder (brontophobia), but a fear of cats (ailurophobia) was just plain silly. A 1786 article on the "different species of phobia" opens a window onto the cultural biases of the age. "Fear of dirt" was characterized as a nuisance "peculiar to certain ladies of . . . low Dutch extraction [who] make everybody miserable around them with their excessive cleanliness." It was their husbands Benjamin Rush presumably had in mind when he joked of the many male "home phobics" who "prefer tavern to domestic society." Affluent ladies had their own eccentricities. "A spider—a flea—or a musqueto [sic], alighting upon a lady's neck, has often produced an hysterical fit." God-fearing women's proclivity to seek divine protection from flying insects inspired the following medical ditty:

> *Say, O! my muse—say whence such boldness springs,—*
> *Such daring courage—in such tim'rous things?*
> *Start from a feather—from an insect fly—*
> *A match for nothing—but, the Deity!*[13]

Generally speaking, phobias were not medical illnesses but idiosyncrasies at once irrational (were parlor flies truly menacing?) and comforting, for they corresponded to and reinforced conventional behavioral norms. Stereotypes about the fragility of refined women made it normal for a lady to erupt in fits at the sight of a spider. A man doing the same? Much less so. To say that interpretations of phobias varied as a function of time and place is not to disparage or deny contemporary fears. Rather, culture was, and remains, the lens through which phobias and other fears were refracted.[14]

Neurasthenia

By the late nineteenth century, frazzled nerves drove countless Americans to seek relief at spas and from patent medicines and "nerve doctors": office-based neurologists, gynecologists, and those claiming expertise in hydrotherapy, physiotherapy, electricity, and massage. (Largely excluded were psychiatrists, who treated serious mental disorders and typically worked in asylums and hospitals, or in university posts.) The impetus was an outbreak of neurasthenia, an illness allegedly reaching epidemic proportions in the United States around the same time Da Costa was documenting soldiers' irritable hearts.[15]

Neurasthenia literally means tired nerves. To late nineteenth- and early twentieth-century doctors, however, neurasthenia was a catchall diagnosis for a range of nonpsychotic emotional problems that included worry, headache, fatigue, indigestion, muscle pain, inability to concentrate, and more. The American neurologist George Miller Beard, himself a neurasthenic, popularized the term and paved the way for the diagnostic frenzy that followed. Born in Connecticut in 1839, Beard was a minister's son and Yale graduate. His iconic status stemmed less from his intellectual acuity than his imposing publication record. Beard died of pneumonia at age forty-four, but not before convincing a wide audience that neurasthenia posed a threat to the civilized world. Thanks to Beard and other medical colleagues who supported the movement, including famed neurologist S. Weir Mitchell, by 1900 neurasthenia had become a household word. Reflecting the absence of standardized diagnosis in this era, neurasthenia was also referred to as nervous prostration, nervous fatigue, and nervous exhaustion.[16]

Like many contemporaries, Beard believed that each person is born with a finite amount of nervous energy, a vital force that facilitates health, vigor, and rational thinking. Its depletion can cause agitation. As such, Beard noted, "Nervousness is really nervelessness." Although neurasthenia lacked a clear pathogenesis (which compounded its mystery in an era when doctors and scientists were earning widespread praise for identifying the specific pathogens that caused infections such as tuberculosis), neurasthenia was regarded as an unfortunate but inevitable by-product of rapid social progress. The hectic pace of modern life, particularly evident in America's industrializing cities, had sapped the nervous vigor of a wide segment of the population. Americans' proneness to the disorder (another famous sufferer, William James, nicknamed it "Americanitis") made perfect sense to patriots such as Beard but conveniently overlooked the popularity of the diagnosis in other countries, notably England, imperial Germany, and Russia. In Beard's mind, the United States was simply more advanced than other nations. Nor was Beard surprised that wealthy, refined citizens seemed more prone. The affluent and the educated (people such as William James, Jane Addams, Theodore Roosevelt, Charlotte Perkins Gilman, and Charles Beard) occupied social stations that made them more likely than common laborers to confront the pace and accoutrements of modernity. The trappings of material and intellectual progress—steam power, the periodical press, the telegraph, advances in science and female education—had touched the country's most august and ambitious citizens. University education freed women from, or at least deferred, the domestic routines of marriage and motherhood. The fast pace of life advanced the nation but depleted the energies of its most determined denizens. In medical and cultural terms, neurasthenia in the late nineteenth and early twentieth centuries was regarded (much as anxiety would be in the 1950s) as the price Americans paid for their stunning success.[17]

Neurasthenics faced a dizzying array of treatment options. Newspapers, periodicals, dry goods stores, apothecaries, and itinerant peddlers marketed a cornucopia of potions and pills to calm bad nerves. Indeed, although the first prescription tranquilizer became available in the United States only in 1955, the nineteenth-century patent medicine market encouraged Americans' fascination with nerve nostrums. One contemporary ascribed the rising number of "opiate eaters" in 1895 to the increased nervous strain caused by

> our mechanical inventions, the spread of our commerce . . . our ambition
> for political honors; and grasping for petty offices for gain; our mad race
> for speedy wealth, which entails feverish excitements . . . a growth so
> rapid, and in some ways so abnormal, that in many directions the mental
> strain has been too much for the physical system to bear; till finally the

overworked body and the overtaxed brain must . . . find rest in the re-
peated use of opium or morphine.

Popular over-the-counter remedies included the cannabis-containing
"neurosine," purported to relieve neurasthenia, migraine, and neuroses, and
the ever popular "hop bitters," a tonic ideal for "a man of business, weak-
ened by the strain of your duties." The Rexall drug company marketed an
"Americanitis Elixir," a play on James's moniker for the seemingly ubiquitous American illness. Tonics such as Dr. Miles's Nervine, "the scientific
remedy for nervous disorders," and Wheller's Nerve Vitalizers were big
sellers before World War I. Most nostrums were laced with opiates or alcohol, a fact hidden from consumers until 1906, when the Food and Drug
Administration (FDA) required manufacturers to label ingredients.[18]
Ailing neurasthenics could also turn to their neighborhood druggists
for help. The 1899 *Merck Manual,* a compendium of preparations published by the pharmaceutical firm Merck and written for chemists, physicians, and pharmacists, catalogued nineteen neurasthenia remedies, all
"reported to be in good use with practitioners at the present time." These
included phosphorous, prescribed to Charlotte Perkins Gilman, and also
recommended to treat impotence, insomnia, and related nervous afflictions. For nervousness the *Manual* suggested opium, chamomile, and electricity. Drugs of choice for insomnia included belladonna, digitalis, and
opium: "a most powerful hypnotic." Interestingly, Da Costa had used all
three soporifics to calm soldiers' irritable hearts.[19]
Proprietors and retailers also promoted electrotherapy gadgets for home
use. Electric devices promised consumers cutting-edge technology without
the inconvenience or expense of a doctor's visit. Americans could purchase
belts, suspenders, and handheld massagers from their neighborhood pharmacy or order them from independent retailers or the Sears, Roebuck and
Montgomery Ward catalogs. An advertisement for Bryan's electric belts,
published in 1881 in the *Saturday Evening Post,* assured readers that it
would cure all nervous debilities "when every other means has failed."
Prospective buyers were encouraged to send statements outlining their
problems so that the company's "medical electrician" could advise them.[20]

Wealthier neurasthenics could recharge their batteries at exclusive nerve clinics and retreats. By 1900, multipurpose spas abounded in Europe, and in the United States those targeting neurasthenics were ubiquitous. The Jackson Sanatorium in western New York State was elegant and tastefully furnished. In addition to gourmet cuisine and high-class service, it offered state-of-the-art care to its harried guests: hydrotherapeutics, massage, and electricity administered by skilled attendants. Jackson was one of many nerve spas that offered the celebrated rest cure, the brainchild of neurologist S. Weir Mitchell. During the Civil War Mitchell had tended soldiers' gunshot wounds and nervous troubles at Turner's Lane Hospital, and he counted Da Costa a close colleague and good friend. After the war, Mitchell built on his success treating neurasthenic soldiers with a combination of rest, seclusion, high-fat diet, massage, and electrotherapy (which he believed infused electrical energy directly into the nervous system) creating a lucrative, office-based career dedicated to the treatment of civilian neurasthenia. After Beard died in 1883, Mitchell became the country's leading nerve specialist with a patient roster that included Gilman, Sarah Butler Wister (daughter of English actress and abolitionist Fanny Kemble), and Amelia Gere Mason, author, publisher, and society matron. Like Beard, Mitchell characterized neurasthenia as a disorder of capitalist modernity best remedied by scheduled vacations, caloric enrichment, and in extreme cases the rest cure: six to eight weeks of isolated bed rest punctuated by sponge baths, massage (to counter muscle atrophy), readings on lackluster topics, and a high-fat diet that included milk and raw eggs. In demand on the lecture circuit, Mitchell popularized his methods in talks, articles, and books such as *Wear and Tear* and *Fat and Blood*. Reflecting American's fixation with neurasthenia, the first of these sold out in just ten days.[21]

Though Mitchell initially gained experience from battle-scarred men, women were his primary office patients and most likely to be prescribed his hallmark rest cure. Their fragile constitutions were deemed particularly susceptible to wear and tear, and only a complete withdrawal from all forms of activity would return their health. Entrepreneurs sold ailing women variants of Mitchell's legendary treatment. The Newton rest cure offered a "limited number of ladies temporarily disabled through nervous diseases" a quiet,

medically supervised regimen in a private house in West Newton, Massachusetts. Men, in contrast, were subjected to rigorous back-to-nature regimens
that resuscitated their enervated bodies. A meat-based diet and physical labor
were the best antidote to debility caused by too much sedentary brain work.[22]

Two famous patients illustrate the gendered nature of care. After diag-
nosing writer and social critic Charlotte Perkins Gilman with postpartum
neurasthenia, America's top nerve doc confined her to bed. Mitchell ad-
monished Gilman to "have but two hours' intellectual life" a day and "never
to touch pen, brush, or pencil again." Gilman initially complied and subsequently "came so near the borderline of utter mental ruin that I could see
over." She finally "cast the noted specialist's advice to the winds and went to
work again . . . ultimately recovering some measure of power." She recounted her alienating and intellectually numbing experiences in her autobiography and the acclaimed short story "The Yellow Wallpaper" (1892), in
which the heroine bravely rejects the cure that worsens her disease. In stark
contrast to Gilman's medical misadventures, when Theodore Roosevelt's
doctor diagnosed him with asthmatic neurasthenia, he sent the future Republican president to a western dude ranch, a rough-and-tumble escapade in
the Dakota Badlands. The frontier respite was not only physically restorative
but an experience the naturalist found positively life transforming.[23]

The absence of psychiatry and psychiatrists in the early stages of the
neurasthenia craze may seem odd. One could make the case that neurasthenia was a form of mental illness; indeed, although the frequency with which
it was diagnosed began to decline in the 1930s, it was later classified as such
by the APA and the World Health Organization. But of the many specialties attached to nervous medicine, neurology was most prominent. This reflected both late-century patterns of professionalization and the negative
aura that continued to hang over psychiatry and its association with the incarcerated mad, in contrast to the affluent Americans who sought
Mitchell's care or recuperated at exclusive spas. While the professional divisions between neurology and psychiatry were porous in practice, in the
public mind, neurology appeared the more dynamic and scientifically advanced discipline. By the late nineteenth century, academic neurology had
coalesced around specialized societies, journals, and elite professorships; for

example, by 1870 most medical schools in New York City had established dedicated neurology chairs. Over time, various technological advances placed neurology squarely in the emerging world of laboratory medicine. Neurologists developed and applied a series of diagnostic technologies (the ophthalmoscope, the tendon hammer, neuropathology). Together with careful clinical observation and postmortem studies, they made high-profile discoveries in areas such as cerebral localization, motor deficits, and epilepsy. Eventually the pathological correlates of various neurological disorders—including paralysis, multiple sclerosis, and dementia—were elucidated. At the turn of the twentieth century, neurosurgery pushed the therapeutic boundaries of the neurosciences a critical step forward.[24]

American psychiatry, by contrast, languished. By the late nineteenth century, it seemed hopelessly backward. As historian Edward Shorter has observed, decades of research in neuroanatomy and neuropathology had yielded little of practical import to clinical psychiatry other than a clear picture of neurosyphilis. Unlike neurology, psychiatry had not developed a lucrative office-based practice, nor did it offer ailing patients a wellspring of effective treatments. The discipline remained rooted in the hospital and even more so in the asylum, which upheld its custodial tradition until the 1950s, when the advent of major tranquilizers permitted the discharge of large numbers of institutionalized patients. Medical school curriculums provided training in psychiatry that ranged from inadequate to absent, and prominent neurologists such as Mitchell apparently thought nothing of taking potshots at the discipline's shortcomings. "Where are your annual reports of scientific study, of the psychology and pathology of your patients?" he chided in an 1894 address delivered before the American Medico-Psychological Association, no less. "We commonly get as your contribution to science, odd little statements, reports of a case or two, a few useless pages of isolated post-mortem records, and these are sandwiched among incomprehensible statistics and farm balance-sheets." If psychiatrists felt chastised by Mitchell's rebuke, they got little validation from ordinary Americans. The stigma of having recourse to a "mad doctor" was at once dramatic and not wholly unjustified. Passage through a psychiatric asylum was a bleak experience. At Worcester Asylum in Massachusetts, five physicians oversaw the treatment of 1,200 patients in 1895. As

dedicated or gifted as an asylum's superintendent and staff might be, over-
crowding, relative neglect, and long-term (even lifelong) custodial care were
an inescapable reality for many of the institutionalized ill. Understandably,
people outside asylum walls rarely clamored to get in.[25]

In patients' minds, this was the all-important divide. Neurasthenics
may have welcomed the attention of nerve specialists and spa treatments,
but they did not want their ailments to be confused with psychiatric ones.
Indeed, one asylum psychiatrist cautioned that "nervous patients in particular find it undesirable to be in a psychiatric ward, even in separate units
or in special houses." The very presence of the mentally ill, many of whose
maladies were incurable, was oppressive. Mixed in with the mad, neurasthenics "start to be filled with dread, thus delaying their own recovery." As
we shall see, Americans in the 1950s would make a similar distinction between nervous tension—something for which one took a pill prescribed by
a family practitioner—and a mental illness requiring a psychiatrist's care.[26]

In an era when psychiatry was marginal to the realm of everyday problems, many nerve doctors set up business in private practice, treating the
relatively minor disturbances of the overly anxious and well-to-do. The
partnership between practitioner and patient was at once medical and
commercial. Psychiatrists didn't lose their jobs in hospitals or asylums
when they failed to cure the insane; indeed, driving the disparaging quips
about the discipline's failings was the assumption that they couldn't. The
economic livelihoods of nerve doctors, on the other hand, depended on
their capacity to make patients feel better. Dissatisfied, affluent patients
could go elsewhere—and did. This dynamic, which tied the treatment of
everyday problems to office-based practice that delivered patients personalized care, would play a decisive role in the paradigm shift in American
psychiatry and pharmacology in the decades ahead.[27]

Freud and the Neurotic Turn

Sigmund Freud began his office practice as a nerve doctor keenly aware of
the importance of keeping his clientele satisfied. Born in 1865 to a family
of merchants in Moravia (what is today the Czech Republic), Freud grew

up in Vienna, where he earned his medical degree in 1885. His original interests were neurobiology and neuropathology. In a letter written in May
1885 to his fiancée, Martha Bernays, he pronounced neuroscience his
great passion. "Precious darling," he wrote, "I am at the moment tempted
by the desire to solve the riddle of the structure of the brain. . . . I think
brain anatomy is the only legitimate rival you have or will ever have." After
a brief tutelage in Paris under the famed French neurologist Jean-Martin
Charcot, Freud returned to Vienna. There he set up a private practice in
1886 as a *Nervenarzt,* a nerve doctor. The morning edition of his favorite
Vienna paper, *Neue Freie Presse,* announced in its local news section that
"Herr Dr. Sigmund Freud, Docent for Nervous Diseases at the University
has returned from his study trip . . . and has consulting hours at [District]
1, Rathhausstrasse No. 7." Over time, Freud's Viennese patients supplied
the case histories on which he based his influential theories.[28]

Freud's clientele was typical of private practice neurology and nervous
medicine in Europe and the United States at the time: affluent and female.
His early years were undistinguished and gave no inkling of the international fame he would eventually enjoy. Like other nerve doctors, Freud experimented with electrotherapy. "If one wanted to make a living from the
treatment of patients with nervous ailments," he explained, "one obviously
had to do something." When this proved unsatisfactory, he tried hypnosis,
which Charcot had made famous in his treatment of female hysterics and
Freud later abandoned. Financially strapped, Freud scrimped on cabs
when making house calls and at one point considered working at a water
cure clinic to pay the bills.[29]

Freud of course is famous for his theories on the workings of the mind,
elaborated in a series of texts between the 1890s and his death in 1939. Initially intrigued by brain chemistry, Freud increasingly turned his attention to
the psyche, an elusive entity that encompassed the innate, often invisible
workings of the human mind. Some mental illnesses, he insisted, had no somatic correlate. They were entirely psychological. Freud focused his attention
on neuroses, the everyday worries and character foibles that troubled his otherwise normal patients. As he told a university audience in 1909, "Neurotics
fall ill of the same complexes with which we sound people struggle." Others,

like Charcot and Pierre Janet, had already described the clinical features of neurosis and ascribed it to intrapsychic process. Freud, however, ended up being far more famous. He turned neurosis into a household word and established psychoanalysis as a mainstream therapeutic approach. In the process, he persuaded physicians, including a growing number of influential American psychiatrists, to heed the inner turmoil of the worried well.[30]

Hoping to disaggregate the unwieldy number of disorders collectively called neurasthenia, in 1894 Freud divided neurasthenia into two distinct illnesses. "Actual neurasthenia" was associated with symptoms of somatic origin. A syndrome Freud called "anxiety neurosis" was psychogenetic—not the result of a physical problem.[31] In Freud's estimation, many, if not most, neurasthenics were neurotic. Rest cures, diets, electric gadgets, and other somatic therapies would not help them. Theirs was a disorder rooted in the workings of the mind.

Freud's theories were at once highly original and the product of their time. While in Paris, he was exposed to new ideas about the unconscious and the self. Charcot's private counsel to Freud—*c'est toujours la chose génitale*—partly explains his lifelong fascination with the sexual etiology of neurosis. If manifested in a variety of ways (compulsions, phobias, excessive emotions), most cases of neurosis, he insisted, could be traced to infantile sexuality. Freud's initial interest in neurasthenia and the physics of energy conservation also shaped his views. Like Beard's nervous system, the Freudian mind possessed a finite amount of energy. One of its most important and demanding functions was to balance a complex series of psychic forces or impulses. Unraveling the mind's mysteries required an understanding of the psychodynamic forces at work.[32]

Thus, even as German somatists searched for objective, microscopic correlates of psychiatric illness, Freud eschewed biology in favor of psychology. In his view, years of psychic conflict explained the neurotic's irritability, episodic unease, or even a woman patient's pessimistic tendency to think of influenza/pneumonia "whenever her husband . . . has a coughing spell." As children, most neurotic women experienced sexual desires and fantasies that they unconsciously repressed. There was nothing abnormal or shameful about children having sexual impulses; Freud believed all children did.

Whether these fantasies developed into neurosis depended on the "reactions toward these experiences, and whether these impressions responded with repression or not." Repression helped avoid immediate harm, protecting adults from the negative consequences of actualizing inappropriate desires. But it also set in motion a psychic tug-of-war between libido and repression. Neurosis signaled the uneasy "compromise between both psychic streams."[33]

Successful analysis depended on the recovery of the patient's repressed desires. This kind of psychic excavation took time. Had probing the unconscious been as simple, say, as taking a blood test, psychoanalysis likely would have been a professional dead end. In fact, psychoanalysis involved regular (ideally daily) conversations over months, even years. For this reason, it is sometimes called "the talking cure." The analyst's task is to build patients' trust, relax their inhibitions, and systematically explore the unconscious. Two important techniques closely associated with Freud are the interpretation of dreams ("the royal road to the unconscious") and free association. In 1899 he published his monumental *Interpretation of Dreams*, detailing the mechanics of free association in a series of essays on the psychoanalytic method. After comfortably installing the patient on the analyst's sofa, he wrote, the therapist was to remind them "to say out loud everything that runs through their head in this connection, even if they believe it to be unimportant or irrelevant, or that it is nonsense. With special emphasis, however, they are called upon not to exclude any thought or recollection from the account on the grounds that this information could be shameful or embarrassing."[34]

This caveat was critically important. One need only read a few of his case histories to appreciate Freud's investment in his patients' sexual lives. In clinical encounters, he relentlessly prodded them. No detail was peripheral. Freud's graphic discussions—which ran the gamut from incest taboos to oral fixation—challenged contemporary sexual strictures. While purity advocates, religious crusaders, and certain physicians tried to keep sex off limits, Freud stunned the world by insisting that patients' well-being depended on discussing it openly and unmasking it.

We need not find Freud's theories appealing or persuasive to appreciate why they were so influential for so long. The office-based management of neurosis provided psychiatrists with a way out of the asylum.[35] Freud also provided a grand, therapeutically constructive theory of causality to a discipline that traditionally had more questions than answers. His ideas were intellectually radical and to many, brilliant and shocking. Patients received time and attention in a safe, secular space from which—unlike the asylum—they were free to leave. Psychoanalysts listened to their patients and took their private experiences and stories seriously. One reason psychoanalysis endured was patients' conviction that they got something useful out of the encounter. If in the present age of biological psychiatry, we are comfortable dismissing the sum total of Freud's theories as an embarrassing detour on the march toward neuroscientific truths, it is possibly because some of his ideas, like the unconscious or the repression of desire, no longer seem controversial. We have set aside his more outlandish claims and assimilated bits and pieces of the rest. In the words we use to discuss human behavior and interpersonal relationships, in the causality we assign childhood events, Freudianism has seeped into the very sinew of American consciousness.

One of Freud's lasting legacies was to legitimize neurosis, both culturally and medically. In the early years of the psychoanalytic revolution, doctors of the mind were already dividing most psychiatric illnesses into one of two categories: psychosis and neurosis. Psychosis referred to certain particularly baffling illnesses, such as schizophrenia (also called *dementia praecox*) and manic-depressive disorder. Psychotics were out of touch with reality, a detachment generally accompanied by delusions and hallucinations. Neurotics, in contrast, remained rooted in "reality" but were subject to varying degrees of turmoil. The demarcation between psychosis and neurosis was rigidly cast; in some ways, it would become the most important distinction in early twentieth-century psychiatry. In *The Common Neuroses* (1923) T. A. Ross wrote, "The neurotic lives in the real world; . . . [his] are the same difficulties which all of us have. The difficulties of the psychotic arise from the fact that he is living in quite another world, in one that is not subject to the ordinary physical laws." In a 1935 self-help book on nervous breakdowns, the editors of *Fortune* magazine used biblical humor to convey these insights. "A man who thought he was Jesus was brought together with another psychotic Jesus," the psychiatric parable read. The psychotic Jesus "soon convinced him that, two Jesuses being an absurdity, he must be the prophet Elijah." Although not all readers may have been edified by the story, *Fortune*'s light-hearted narrative illustrates how commonplace psychiatric concepts had become.[36]

In its first *Diagnostic and Statistical Manual,* published decades later in 1952, the APA concretized the scientific validity of this binary classification. The handbook made neurosis a fundamental organizational category for mental illness, defining psychoneurotic complaints chiefly in opposition to psychosis:

> The chief characteristic of these disorders is "anxiety" which may be directly felt and expressed or which may be unconsciously and automatically controlled by the utilization of various psychological defense mechanisms. . . . In contrast to those with psychoses, patients with psychoneurotic disorders do not exhibit gross distortion or falsification of external reality (delusions, hallucinations, illusions) and they do not present gross disorganization of the personality.[37]

It is ironic that Freud had his greatest impact in the United States, where psychoanalytic teachings (based on the work of Freud and his many disciples) became fashionable in the 1920s and 1930s and became a staple of psychiatric medical training from the 1940s to the 1970s. Freud's only visit to the United States, in 1909, lasted all of two weeks. In fact, American enchantment with Freud had little to do with the man per se. Most American medical institutions were not as tradition-bound or as sophisticated as their European counterparts, and psychiatrists were eager to use Freudian insights to establish a "school" of their own. Leading European psychoanalysts who emigrated to the United States provided a critical mass necessary for its success. The psychoanalytically constructed concept of neurosis eventually spread like wildfire in certain communities. The concentration of psychoanalysts in New York and Los Angeles spawned neighborhood nicknames such as "Libido Lane" and "Nightmare Alley." In 1935, *Fortune* estimated the number of neurotics in the United States to be in the "hundreds of thousands—probably millions." Twenty years later, *Newsweek* put the count at a whopping 7 million, about one in every seventeen Americans.[38]

By midcentury, the problem with psychoanalysis in the United States wasn't so much its perceived legitimacy, despite its many detractors. Nor was the prevalence of neurosis at issue, an experience that one book declared as widespread as the common cold. Rather, the real issue that faced those struggling with debilitating worries, insomnia, and phobias was the cost and limited availability of professional treatment. Even in the heyday of psychoanalysis, there were only a few thousand psychiatrists (one report estimated a total of 4,000 in private practice) to help millions of neurotics. Psychoanalysis was costly and time-consuming, especially given that five visits a week for a year or even longer was the general rule. In the early 1930s, low-income clinics in Berlin, Vienna, and London admitted those who seriously needed analysis but could not pay for treatment. There was no equivalent in the United States; across the board, American psychoanalysts charged between $10 and $50 an hour in the 1930s. Together with certain ingrained biases against the profession, time and money kept most anxious patients out of analysts' offices. The talking cure was either culturally foreign or priced beyond reach, a privilege of the affluent rather than the birthright of all.[39]

Pharmacological Nostrums

The gap between therapeutic needs on the one hand and financial constraints and cultural aversions on the other was filled by a robust market in over-the-counter remedies. Antianxiety concoctions have had a long history. As writer and critic Aldous Huxley once observed, chemicals have been used "from time immemorial for changing the quality of consciousness . . . making possible some degree of self-transcendence and a temporary release from tension." British politician and philanthropist William Wilberforce was first given opium, a soporific narcotic known in the nineteenth century as either a "pick-me-up" or as a "calmer of nerves," to settle his nerves before giving important speeches in the Commons. William Gladstone likewise took laudanum (opium dissolved in alcohol) in his coffee for the same purpose. Military commanders have long used chemical remedies to vanquish fears among the rank and file. By whatever name doctors called it—irritable heart syndrome, soldier's heart, panic, or a rational reaction to the fight-or-flight impulse—combat anxiety was a serious problem. The fate of battles and empires turned on it. As recently as World War II, the penalty for desertion in Britain was death. In addition to threats of capital punishment, British commanders during World War I judged that occasional allowances of rum made it easier for soldiers to venture "over the top" and into enemy fire. After World War II, one prominent British physician observed that bromides and other sedatives had worked wonders coaxing men into battle after strategists realized that "immediate and heavy 'front line' sedation was generally more effective in the prevention of chronic neuroses, and so-called 'malingering' reactions, than all the threats of shooting for cowardice."[40]

In the United States, everyday worriers had long taken matters into their own hands. Americans' long-standing tendency to turn to over-the-counter chemical nostrums was duly noted by contemporaries. So vast was America's patent medicine market that one of the era's most respected medical minds, Sir William Osler, wondered if "the desire to take medicine is perhaps the greatest feature [that] distinguishes man from animals." Whether Osler's rumination was true or not, the brisk commerce in pharmaceutical tonics to quell anxiety established an important therapeutic foundation on which manufacturers of prescription-only tranquilizers would subsequently build.[41]

By the time Beard had popularized the term "neurasthenia," alcohol, opiates, chloral hydrate (a sedative-hypnotic introduced in 1869), and potassium bromide were common remedies for relief. Nostrums for neurasthenia introduced a plethora of new remedies and chemical combinations to the patent medication market. Those containing the sedative bromide were used so widely that by the early twentieth century the word "bromide" had come to be used figuratively to denote a dull and tiresome person, as popularized in Gelett Burgess's 1906 book, *Are You a Bromide?*[42]

In the early twentieth century, barbiturates provided a powerful new addition to the arsenals of the anxious. They come from a family of compounds of which barbituric acid, synthesized in 1864, is the parent. The first barbiturate, barbital, was marketed in the United States in 1903 as a hypnotic (a sleep-inducing agent) under the trade name Veronal. Less toxic than bromides and free of their bitter aftertaste, barbiturates caught on quickly and largely replaced bromides in asylum psychiatry, the burgeoning field of outpatient neuropsychiatry, and the expanding over-the-counter market. Veronal calmed the agitated and lulled insomniacs into a deep sleep. Laws regulating the sale of barbiturates, which varied by city and state, were inadequately enforced. New York City enacted a prescription-only municipal code in 1922, but elsewhere in the state, pharmacists could freely dispense them until 1939. Some states had no restrictions before 1951, when Congress created the category of prescription-only drugs to stem the rampant use of dangerous or addictive medicines outside of medical supervision.[43]

Even in places with prescription refill restrictions, pharmacists often refilled prescriptions on patient demand. In one case, a pharmacist dispensed six Veronal capsules ninety-six times without the physician's knowledge, on several occasions providing the patient with thirty capsules per visit instead of the prescribed six. This regulatory vacuum encouraged rampant self-medication. Americans who learned about Veronal from family and friends demanded their own supply. In New York City, a young schoolteacher plagued by insomnia asked a physician for a soporific, specifically "the new synthetic drug Veronal." The doctor had never heard of it, but he wrote the prescription as requested, dutifully asking the man to spell the drug's name. Unfortunately the incident ended tragically when the medical neophyte authorized a lethal amount. The schoolteacher fell asleep and never awoke. In a jeremiad decrying "quick-cure nostrums," the *New York Times* reminded readers that the sedative was not "to be used at the request of laymen or to be prescribed offhand."[44]

The admonition had little impact on Americans' taste for antianxiety remedies. Barbiturates quickly gained a foothold in the sedative-hypnotic market, which expanded on the coattails of Freudian ideas about neurosis. Barbiturates were a quick, reliable, and easy way to transcend anxiety, a poor man's alternative to psychoanalysis. The 1930 *Merck's Index* recommended Veronal for the treatment of "extreme nervousness, neurasthenia, hypochondria, melancholia [and] conditions of anxiety." Barbiturates also began to be used for surgical anesthesia, obstetrics, alcohol withdrawal, ulcers, hyperthyroidism and, because of their anticonvulsant properties, epilepsy. Until the arrival of tranquilizers, however, they were primarily used to treat anxiety-related conditions. Indeed, one senior psychiatrist recalled that before the advent of minor tranquilizers, "the prevailing anxiolytic was elixir Phenobarbital," a reference to Bayer's long-acting barbiturate, introduced in 1912.[45]

Pharmaceutical companies happily kept American worriers well stocked with barbiturate options. Because the barbiturate molecule was easily modified, company chemists were able to create hundreds of new derivatives, each with a slightly different therapeutic effect. By 1947, firms had produced some 1,500 variants, thirty of which were sold under their trade name on the American market. In addition to barbital and phenobarbital, popular barbiturates included the shorter-acting Amytal (amobarbital), Nembutal (pentobarbital), and Seconal (secobarbital), whose use was immortalized by Jacqueline Susann in her bestselling novel, *Valley of the Dolls.* Hundreds of compounds also combined barbiturates with other drugs. Barbiturates came in so many different shapes, colors, and forms (pills, capsules, and elixirs) that users assigned them affectionate nicknames: yellow jackets, blue angels, pink ladies, and reds. On the street, they were known collectively as goofballs.[46]

Production and sales of barbiturates mushroomed during World War II, rising from 531,000 pounds in 1941 to 900,000 pounds, the equivalent of over 1.5 million doses, in 1947. Some of the increase reflected expanded military use. Army physicians employed barbiturates to sedate the wounded and comfort the dying, relieve combat fatigue, thwart shock, and, in keeping with new ideas about treating battle anxiety, help soldiers confront traumatic memories. When narcotics were scarce, barbiturates were given liberally to potentiate the analgesic effects of supplies that remained.[47]

Increased use of barbiturates also spread into civilian life. Rampant nervous and mental disorders among military recruits, active-duty soldiers, and veterans both medicalized and normalized neurosis. Psychiatrists successfully treated war neurosis in field camps and postcombat rehabilitation centers, elevating the stature of the profession and giving talk therapy a big boost. Psychiatrists' ability to return soldiers to a healthy psychological state reminded Americans everywhere that even normal men—farmers, machine workers, truck drivers, schoolteachers—had a breaking point. Neurosis was a normal reaction to environmental stress. Indeed, one of war psychiatry's great take-home messages was that battle trauma differs little from trauma affecting the rest of the population. Although wartime psychiatry played up the virtues of psychoanalysis, it also cleared a path for broader acceptance of barbiturates as a civilian anxiolytic by giving the pharmaceutical treatment of neurosis pride of place. A report issued by the *New York Academy of Medicine*, while highly critical of the "indiscriminate and ill-advised" use of barbiturates, acknowledged that it was ethically unacceptable to withhold a prescription from anxious patients who needed it. "The wide prevalence of psychiatric complaints among the population must add up to a large volume of legiti-mate therapeutic need," conceded the Committee on Public Health.[48]

Notwithstanding barbiturates' legitimacy, many came to fear their abuse. Two issues framed medical and political debates. One was safety. Barbitu-rates have a low and highly variable therapeutic window. Overdoses were common and often deadly. Worse, the threshold is individually variable; a dose that is therapeutic for one person could kill another. Barbiturates are also addictive. Sudden cessation after prolonged use may trigger a panoply of excruciating symptoms: perspiration, elevated blood pressure and pulse, tremors, aggression, anxiety, convulsions, and rarely death. In 1951 the di-rector of the Federal Narcotics Hospital at Lexington, Kentucky, insisted that withdrawing from barbiturates was more unpleasant and medically complex than was the case with narcotics. As with many other habit-form-ing medications, users require increasingly higher—and potentially toxic—doses to sustain a therapeutic benefit. In an unregulated or poorly regulated barbiturate economy, such as existed in the United States prior to 1951, self-medication resulted in countless poisonings and accidental deaths.[49]

In one case, a thirty-year-old mother got a prescription to take one bar-biturate before retiring. When the first capsule failed, she took another. Still awake an hour later, she took three more. She regained consciousness in a hospital, the victim of barbiturate poisoning. In another instance, a man took pills for insomnia induced by "business worries." Over time, he developed tolerance. One pill no longer sufficed. He took a few more but nothing happened. Desperate for a good night's sleep, he eventually took a total of ten. "The bottle wasn't marked poison," he explained later. "I thought it would be all right." Luckily for him, he survived.[50]

Thousands of others were not so lucky. In New York State, deaths from barbiturate poisoning increased nearly fivefold between 1937 and 1946; in 1950, national barbiturate-related deaths numbered at least 1,000. Alarmed health officials implicated user ignorance. Like the man who overdosed because the bottle wasn't marked as poisonous, most patients weren't aware of the dangers. Self-medication, pharmaceutical hubris, naïveté about addiction, and the barbiturates' inherent toxicity made for a deadly combination. "The matron who regards a pink pill as much of a bedtime necessity as brushing her teeth, the tense business man who gulps a white capsule to ease his nerves before an important conference, the college student who swallows a yellow 'goof ball' to breeze through an examination, and the actor who takes a 'blue angel' to bolster his self-confidence are aware that excessive use of barbiturates is 'not good for the system,' but are ignorant of the extent of the hazard," railed the *New York Times,* in an article that declared barbiturates "more of a menace to society than heroin or morphine."[51]

If legitimate use engendered alarm, their recreational uses were even more disturbing. In the late 1930s, reports suggested that barbiturate misuse among teenagers had caused a steady rise in traffic accidents. By the mid-1940s, social commentators increasingly portrayed barbiturates as dangerous street drugs, popular among juvenile delinquents, petty criminals, thrill-seeking partygoers, and trouble-making GIs. Tranquility in this case could be a liability, insisted a senior psychiatrist who treated adolescents at Bellevue Hospital. It effectively lowered people's inhibitions and incited acts they would not otherwise dare to perform. Hence "the very quality that makes physicians prescribe barbiturates for anxious, nervous patients is one of the things that make dangerous their uncontrolled use. The pills bring a feeling of well-being, a relaxation of fears and inhibitions. This is good in many illnesses, but a bad thing for potential trouble-makers who are held back only by their inhibitions of fear of committing anti-social acts." One report warned of a nationwide "cult of youths who take sleeping pills with beer to get a 'high' feeling." The cocktail earned its street name, the Wild Geronimo.[52]

Ties to the illicit drug trade, especially black market narcotics, further tarnished barbiturates. In 1947 the chief of the Eastern Division of the Federal Narcotics Bureau declared that "90 percent of persons involved in the violation of narcotic laws used barbiturates also." Narcotics addicts used them to boost the effects of morphine, cocaine, or heroin. When their narcotic supplies dwindled, they also took them to offset withdrawal symptoms. The assistant commissioner of health in New York City estimated that most addicts "carry a bottle of the pills for use as a tide-over if they should find themselves cut off from their supply."[53]

Availability and affordability drove the barbiturate panic. Goofballs were ubiquitous and cheap. Even in states that regulated their sale, pharmacists who viewed restrictions as an unwelcome curtailment of professional prerogatives regularly flouted the law. Druggists' violations incited well-publicized stings to ferret out dishonest merchants. These raids made for good news copy but had little impact on the barbiturate market. The commerce became subdued but not contained.[54]

Desperate users could also score a stash from bootleggers who did a brisk trade at saloons, truck stops, hotels, and other public venues. Whether sold by pharmacists or more marginalized vendors, barbiturates made for a cheap fix, especially compared to other drugs. Admittedly, when Veronal was introduced in 1903, it was too expensive for many public asylums, which continued to rely on cheaper standbys to calm garrulous inmates. Increased production and competition caused a rapid and dramatic price drop, putting barbiturates within the reach of even the less affluent. By the 1940s, barbiturates cost about fifteen cents per capsule and by 1950, about a dollar a dozen.[55]

Given that Pandora's box had effectively been opened, what was to be done? The barbiturate crisis put physicians, law enforcers, and countless anxious Americans in a bind. Psychoanalysis had normalized neurosis as a medical disorder and set the stage for the psychopharmacological revolution that followed. While the prevailing therapeutic dogma favored the talking cure, millions of nervous Americans had turned instead to pharmaceuticals for relief. In choosing to do so, they created a robust, unevenly regulated commerce in antianxiety drugs. Unfortunately, a taste for tranquility had exacerbated a host of medical and social problems. On the eve of Miltown, the troublesome question of how to deal with American neurosis remained unresolved.

(2)

The Making of Miltown

Miltown, the first of the so-called minor tranquilizers, was discovered in 1950 and approved for sale by the FDA in 1955. It quickly became a national phenomenon. By 1956, an astounding one in twenty Americans had tried it. No drug in the United States had ever been in such demand.[1]

Given the drug's blockbuster status, its historical obscurity is curious. For most of us, tranquilizers mean Valium or Xanax. Miltown is the tranquilizer we tend to forget. Yet the little white pill left an indelible imprint on modern medicine and psychopharmacology. Its arrival, one psychiatrist later observed, changed everything: Miltown "*was* the revolution." The drug's popularity and efficacy challenged Freudian ideas about the etiology and treatment of neurosis. It bolstered the claims of a new biological psychiatry that attributed mental disorders to imbalances in the brain, and it rendered anxiety, in the words of psychiatrist and historian Tom Ban, "accessible to scientific scrutiny." Miltown gave the nation's worried well a useful pharmaceutical treatment. It helped normalize the use of psychiatric drugs for outpatient disorders and shifted the practice of front-line psychiatric diagnosis from the psychiatrist to the family doctor.[2]

In addition, the drug's appeal fomented a fundamental and lasting change in how Americans viewed and used prescription medicines: it was okay to see doctors for drugs to make them feel better about the vagaries of life, not just to treat diseases. Miltown's success inaugurated an era of lifestyle drugs familiar to Americans today. Pharmaceutical executives awestruck by Miltown's unexpected popularity made a gamble. If people were willing to line up to buy drugs for anxiety, they might buy pills for other problems too: depression, difficulties concentrating, a weak libido. Prozac. Ritalin. Viagra. Each owes something to the Miltown moment, when anxious Americans reached for their pocketbooks and bought into the elusive promise of better living through a pill.

More than a medical phenomenon, the little white pill shaped an era. For millions of Americans, Miltown was a new and seemingly harmless drug to be experienced, experimented with, and enjoyed. Miltown inspired new beverages and jewelry. It was discussed and joked about in magazines, on radio, on Broadway, and on television. Salvador Dali paid artistic tribute to Miltown's capacity to rid the mind of troubling distractions and free it for genius; Aldous Huxley proclaimed that Miltown would inaugurate an era of great fun. So far-reaching was its cultural import, so seamless was its integration into America's social and linguistic fabric, that by the late 1950s Miltown needed no explicit explanation. The word had become shorthand for a cultural phenomenon people intuitively understood.

The Man Behind Miltown

After the fact, the stunning profitability of tranquilizers seemed inevitable and, to some, the fruitful realization of a premeditated plan. Yet evidence from the 1950s shows that the birth of the tranquilizer industry was marked by corporate intransigence, scientific contingency, and widespread societal and patient enthusiasm. In fact Miltown was discovered accidentally by a researcher who struggled for years to convince his bosses to make the drug available.

That researcher was Dr. Frank Milan Berger. Gracious and introspective, Berger was more comfortable with the solitude of a book or research lab than with the grandstanding so often required of pharmaceutical executives at medical meetings. One journalist described him in 1945 as having the build of a rugby halfback, the penetrating look of the scientist, and

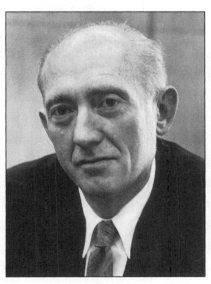

Frank Berger, 1913–2008. Although his most profitable discovery was Miltown, he downplayed its importance throughout his career and refused to allow detail men at Carter-Wallace to promote it. Medical science, he insisted, should not be confused with salesmanship. Copyright © 2000; undated picture. Reproduced courtesy of the Collegium Internationale Neuro-Psychopharmacologicum.

the slight stoop of a scholar. In quiet moments, he turned to classical literature and philosophy, particularly the writings of seventeenth-century rationalist Baruch Spinoza. A left-leaning humanist whose principles were hedged by a pragmatism culled from decades of struggle, Berger never abandoned his belief in humanity's capacity to eradicate suffering. Though his professional success was tied to drug development, he rarely took medications (just the occasional pill for insomnia) and worried that Americans took too many of them. In conversations, he consistently downplayed Miltown's importance and discussed what he considered his greater scientific achievement: research to develop compounds to increase the body's resistance to infection and disease. Berger's commitment to socialized medicine and his aversion to drug promotion made him an unlikely candidate to spearhead a psycho-pharmaceutical revolution. Yet history is replete with unexpected twists. The interconnected histories of Frank Berger and Miltown are among them.[3]

Berger was born in 1913 in Pilsen, the capital of West Bohemia in the Austro-Hungarian Empire. His father, who sold textiles to factories, was German; his mother was Czech. As a child, Berger struggled with the hostility toward a native German speaker in a province that became, in October 1918, part of the new republic of Czechoslovakia. He attended Czech schools where "they taught that the worst enemies of the Czechs were the Germans." The chilly reception he received from schoolmates and neighbors was exacerbated by his moderate deafness. "People erroneously believed," he recounted later, "that my inability to respond to [their] comments . . . was due to a lack of knowledge of Czech." In fact, Berger spoke the language proficiently and was a true Czech patriot. His boyhood hero was the republic's founder and first president, Thomas Masaryk, an erudite man whose trek from the countryside to the center of Czech culture and whose advocacy for persecuted minorities inspired the young Berger, who himself felt frequently misunderstood. When Masaryk died in 1937, Berger felt the pall of a new political order and correctly predicted that "the Republic would not be able to maintain its independence for very long."[4]

By 1937 Berger had already made a name for himself as an acclaimed scientist, moving, like Masaryk before him, from the social margins to the hub of Czech intellectual life. Berger's father had hoped his son would enter the textile trade, but Berger consciously distanced himself from a vocation he regarded as too tied to the crude mechanics of buying and selling. He flourished in his high school Latin classes in Pilsen, relishing what he called the how-to books of his youth: Homer's tales and Ovid's *Art of Love*. After graduation, he decided to pursue a medical degree at the German University in Prague. He saw medicine as an all-encompassing intellectual undertaking that would help him unlock the "great mysteries of life such as birth and death, suffering, sex, and love." Berger approached medicine as part of a broader impulse to discern how the universe itself worked, not simply as a specialized vocation.[5]

In medical school, Berger combined coursework and independent research. Fascinated by his experimental physiology class, he obtained his professor's permission to carry out a study at the university's Institute of Physiology on estrogens in the treatment of gonorrhea, a therapy widely used in Europe prior to the development of sulfa drugs and antibiotics. Berger's findings, which suggested that the topical application of hormones might be as effective as injections, were published in the prestigious medical journal, *Klinische Wochenschrift*, and captured international attention. Berger went on to do research in bacteriology and immunology at the

Institute of Hygiene. His discovery of new techniques for identifying sal-
monellas—important in tracing the sources of diarrheal disease—earned
him a Czechoslovak National Prize for Scientific Research in 1938, only a
few months after he received his medical degree in December 1937. Thus,
at the age of twenty-five, Berger was already recognized as a gifted and
promising scientific luminary. Encouraged by his success and attracted by
the lure of laboratory investigation, Berger decided to devote himself full-
time to a career in research.[6]

The best-laid plans are often derailed by politics and love. Such was the
case here. A few years earlier, in 1935, Berger had met Bozena Jahodova,
a nurse in the Department of Internal Medicine in Prague. They fell in
love, and Bozena agreed to move in with Berger in 1936. In March 1938
Hitler annexed Austria. In September, the German dictator demanded the
absorption of the Sudetenland, the German-speaking portion of Czechoslovakia. Hoping to prevent war and to appease Hitler, Great Britain,
France, and Italy signed the Munich Agreement and surrendered the
Sudetenland. Czechoslovakia, excluded from the talks, became a truncated
state. While Czechoslovakia mourned, British Prime Minister Neville
Chamberlain optimistically proclaimed that the geopolitical shuffling
would bring "peace in our time." Chamberlain, of course, was wrong.
Berger learned that Germany would occupy all of Czechoslovakia and
knew that the new regime would be hostile to a man with a Jewish heritage and socialist sympathies. He married Bozena immediately and, on
March 15, the newlyweds boarded an overnight train to Holland, where a
Quaker organization provided papers to get the couple to London. Berger
joined a diaspora of scientists fleeing Hitler's Europe, an exodus of talent
including Albert Einstein, Leo Szilárd, and Niels Bohr. All of them would
profoundly shape scientific research in the decades to come.[7]

The first weeks in London were difficult. Barred from exporting
money, the Bergers arrived in England poor and alone. After learning she
was pregnant, Bozena found refuge in the Jewish shelter in the East End.
Quarters were crowded, however, and there was no room for Berger. He
ate at the Salvation Army soup kitchen and slept on park benches. En-
forcing the wartime midnight curfew, the police rounded him up daily and

escorted him to Brixton prison. He passed his nights in a room with hundreds of other homeless men.

Berger finally found work as a physician at a camp for refugees from occupied countries, mainly Germany, Austria, Poland, Romania, and Italy. Here, he learned English. Yet tragedy struck when Bozena suffered an agonizing and nearly fatal delivery that claimed the life of their infant son. Decades later, Berger admitted that he never recovered from the anguish of that loss. In search of more stable living arrangements, Berger accepted a job as an assistant bacteriologist in the Public Health Laboratory in Wakefield, south of Leeds. Bozena was hired as his assistant, and the two worked side by side. Immersed in research on antibiotic preservation, Berger would, through circumstance and luck, identify a compound whose tranquilizing properties laid the chemical groundwork for Miltown.[8]

On the Heels of Penicillin

Like most medical researchers, Berger was familiar with Scottish scientist Alexander Fleming's earlier work on penicillin. Returning from a short vacation to his germ lab at London's St. Mary's Hospital in 1928, Fleming was astonished to find a dark green felt-like mold (a "contaminating colony") inhibiting bacterial growth in one of his staphylococcal cultures. The mold was *Penicillium notatum;* on Fleming's dish, it was suspended in a liquid substance that physically buffered it from the staph bacteria. In moist environments, the mold can grow on a variety of moist surfaces, from bread to shoe leather to strawberry jam. What vexed scientists, Berger among them, was how to isolate and stabilize the antibacterial agent from the mold and broth it produced. Legend has it that there was a colony developing in a laboratory below Fleming's and a single wayward spore drifted through an open window into Fleming's lab, settled in a Petri dish, and began its destructive work. Had there been no vacation, open window, or unwashed dish, or had Fleming not hesitated before discarding the Petri dish with the altered staphylococcal culture, the course of medicine would have been radically different. Instead, Fleming published a report on his observations in the *British Journal of Experimental Pathol-*

ogy, calling the bacteria-destroying broth penicillin. Doubtful that it could stay active long enough in the human body to fight infections, and unable to isolate the antibacterial agent in the juice exuded by the mold, he stopped studying it in the early 1930s.[9]

Two bacteriologists, Australian Howard Walter Florey and Ernst Boris Chain, a German refugee biochemist, pushed Fleming's observations to the next level. At the pathology department of Oxford University, Florey and Chain used a novel freeze-drying technology to isolate a biologically active powder from the original broth. Further research showed that penicillin cured not only mice but humans with common bacterial infections too. The scientists' results were published in the British medical journal *Lancet* in August 1941.[10]

Florey and Chain's findings were path-breaking news for a world again at war. Twenty years earlier, World War I had created a new set of medical priorities. For the first time, mortality rates from wounds outstripped those from infectious diseases such as typhus, typhoid, smallpox, and malaria. Trench warfare and its signature weapons—machine guns, artillery, gases (debilitating tear gas but also the more lethal mustard gas and phosgene), and infantry weapons such as the rifle, bayonet, shotgun, and grenades—wreaked carnage on the battlefield. Military doctors scrambled to stem the rising tide of infection-related fatalities and amputations, for even minor injuries could lead to serious complications. Yet there was only so much they could do, for humans' capacity to maim and kill vastly exceeded their ability to heal. Between 1914 and 1918, one of an estimated seven or eight wounded soldiers died of infection.[11]

The advent of sulfa drugs in the 1930s, which stopped germs from multiplying but did not eliminate them outright, helped injured soldiers at the start of World War II. But the sulfa drugs were ineffective against some bacterial infections, and their side effects, which could include confusion and severe nausea, were potentially debilitating. Penicillin, on the other hand, was effective in combating man's fiercest bacterial foes, but it could not be manufactured and preserved in quantities large enough for civilian or military populations. A single patient might require 100,000 units of penicillin a day to treat a serious infection, a dose that required 100 liters of culture. The mold was grown in big, bulky containers that required large amounts of incubator space. Penicillin was extracted from the fluid the mold produced. Because penicillin was inherently unstable, it was not uncommon for half a culture to be destroyed by contaminants—acid, alkaline, even airborne germs—before it could be harvested. A frustrated pharmaceutical executive complained that "the mold is as temperamental as an opera singer, the yields are low, the isolation is difficult, the extraction is murder, [and] the purification invites disaster." The demand for penicillin was so great that patients lucky enough to get it were often asked to save their urine so that the antibiotic could be isolated and reused.[12]

In 1944, Frank Berger became one of hundreds of scientists in Britain and the United States striving to break the bottleneck in penicillin production. Settled in his Wakefield lab, Berger obtained subcultures of the mold, which he described as looking like a "crusty Camembert cheese," directly from Sir Alexander Fleming. Putting his microbiology training to work, he identified new and improved extraction and purification techniques. Berger grew the mold in an ice chest, filtered off the coffee-colored liquid containing penicillin, and treated it chemically to isolate, purify, and stabilize the venerated antibiotic. The method was simple and inexpensive, yet it managed to preserve for about two months an astounding 85 to 95 percent of the potency of the harvested penicillin. Berger's penicillin was tested on local hospital patients: two children suffering from pneumonia, a young housewife with meningitis, and an elderly man with a gaping abdominal wound caused by a bomb. Miraculously, all of them recovered.[13]

Refusing to profit from his discovery, Berger released his findings to the wider medical community "so that no commercial exploitation may deprive any human being" from benefiting from his work. His research led to publications in the widely read journals *Nature* and the *British Medical Journal,* and landed him a prestigious post with a London manufacturing firm, British Drug Houses. There Berger continued his penicillin research, screening chemical compounds that might protect this magical but rare amalgam from the bacteria that destroyed it.[14]

By 1945, monumental breakthroughs in penicillin production had been achieved. U.S. pharmaceutical firms, in partnership with the government's

Committee on Medical Research (CMR), launched a major initiative to find a way to manufacture penicillin. Vast sums of federal money (more than $2 billion on penicillin alone) and countless hours were invested in the quest to mass-produce this lifesaving drug. CMR scientists and executives in the Big Three pharmaceutical houses—Merck, Pfizer, and Squibb—initially focused on artificially synthesizing penicillin but could not figure out how to do it. Instead, it was deep-tank fermentation, a prewar technology that involved growing penicillin cultures in giant vats, that saved the day. Pfizer mastered the method first, but by 1943, twenty-five other drug companies were manufacturing enough antibiotic to meet demand. By the end of the war, commercial production—which rose from 400 million units per month in the first half of 1943 to a staggering 650 billion units by August 1945—had saved thousands of soldiers' lives. In civilian medicine, antibiotics offered doctors and patients their first real cure for syphilis, gonorrhea, and bacterial pneumonia, as well as for other infectious diseases that had plagued humankind for thousands of years.[15]

While Berger's penicillin research had helped pave the way for these important developments, it also proved fruitful in an unexpected way. One compound Berger had tested as a penicillin preservative was mephenesin, a chemically modified version of a disinfectant on the European market. Berger injected it into mice to evaluate its toxicity for human use. The mice became relaxed and their muscles went limp yet they remained conscious: "their eyes were open and they appeared to follow what was happening around them." Berger was intrigued by this result. Had he unwittingly discovered a relaxant less sedating than barbiturates? To his astonishment, he had. The side effects he observed with the mice—muscle relaxation and temporary paralysis but also full consciousness—were replicated in subsequent studies.[16]

This exciting discovery had profound implications for neurology, surgery, and anesthesia. Berger described the drug's tranquilizing properties in an article in a British pharmacology journal in 1946: "Administration of small quantities of these substances to mice, rats or guinea pigs caused tranquilization, muscular relaxation, and a sleep-like condition from which the animals could be roused." Although other substances, including alcohol, were recognized as tranquilizing agents, Berger's article represented the first time in the annals of modern medicine that a drug's capacity to tranquilize had been singled out as an attribute worth testing and discussing in a pharmacology journal.[17]

Indeed, mephenesin is one of many accidental innovations—penicillin and Viagra (an offshoot of the search for angina medications) are other examples—that have shaped pharmacology. As a distinct class of drugs, tranquilizers began as an unexpected side effect of a compound developed not to soothe frayed nerves but to kill penicillin-destroying bacteria. As Berger said, "Discoveries in medicine are often made in indirect, roundabout ways. Back in 1945, I did not have any plans to discover either a muscle relaxant or a tranquilizer." In the end, he came up with both. What would eventually become the bestselling drug in medical history began as a curious footnote to a far more pressing problem: increasing the antibiotic supply. By 1947, Berger's mouse relaxer was being used on humans. Retailed in the United States by E. R. Squibb under the trade name Tolserol and in the United Kingdom by British Drug Houses as Myanesin, the drug was administered intravenously in surgical wards to induce preoperative relaxation. By March 1948, more than 10,000 patients in the United Kingdom had reaped the benefits of Berger's calming drug. The medication also found a faithful following among patients afflicted with multiple sclerosis, cerebral palsy, Parkinson's disease, strokes, and back injuries. In such cases, a person's muscles contract continuously or uncontrollably, causing pain, tightness, and stiffness, sometimes severe enough to impede movement or speech. Mephenesin attenuated spasms and other debilitating symptoms. In 1949, only a year after its American debut, Tolserol had become one of Squibb's most prescribed drugs. It's still used as a muscle relaxant today.[18]

The drug had its drawbacks, however. It was rapidly absorbed after injection, and its effects lasted only a few hours. In oral form it was far less potent. It was thus typically administered intravenously, but this technique posed its own problems. Solvents used to transform the drug into an injectable solution could cause adverse effects, from local inflammation to severe venous thrombosis. Berger vowed to create a medicine that would be as effective as mephenesin, last longer, and remain as potent in pill form.[19]

In 1949, however, this was one man's dream. The availability of mephenesin failed to generate broader commercial interest in the development of a tranquilizer for everyday use. There was no race to develop Miltown that would parallel the frenzied and high-stakes rush to develop the benzodiazepine tranquilizers Librium and Valium. In fact, the president of Carter Products, which would eventually manufacture Miltown, psychiatry's first mass-market blockbuster, was initially unconvinced that a tranquilizer would sell at all.

What Works for Monkeys . . .

In 1947, as mephenesin was receiving widespread medical attention in the United Kingdom and the United States, Frank and Bozena Berger moved to the United States. Berger's parents and many of his friends and relatives had died in Nazi death camps, and the couple decided to make a new life for themselves in America. Taking stock of his professional triumphs and personal tragedies, the thirty-four-year-old pondered the next phase of life. He and Bozena were passionate about starting a family. But what of his career? Did he want to teach at a university (he imagined a professorship with an endowed chair in pharmacology), practice as a physician, or develop new drugs for a pharmaceutical firm? He wasn't sure. After a brief stint as a research professor in the Pediatrics Department at the University of Rochester Medical School, Berger tossed his hat into the pharmaceutical arena. In June 1949, he accepted an offer from Wallace Laboratories, a branch of Carter Products of New Brunswick, New Jersey, to become its president and director of medical research.[20]

Today, America's pharmaceutical industry is a financial powerhouse. With annual sales exceeding $200 billion, the prescription drug business is the most profitable in the nation. In the 1940s and 1950s, however, its financial future, from the perspective of industry analysts and executives, seemed bleak. Excitement about the new wonder drugs—penicillin, cortisone, and antihistamines—had increased prescription medication sales from $1.57 million in 1939 to $1.1 billion in 1952. Yet it was drugstores, not pharmaceutical manufacturers, that benefited first. Whereas tobacco, toys, and soda fountains had been their previous commercial staples, prescription drugs and cosmetics were the new cash cows. In 1947, prescriptions represented a mere 16 percent of drugstore sales; by 1958 they accounted for 25 percent. Most retail pharmacists, trained in the science of pharmacology, welcomed the change. It made sense to them that university-educated druggists dispensed medicines rather than toys and milkshakes. "I don't think [soda] fountains are necessary anymore," one relieved California pharmacist professed. "They're dirty and smell bad. And besides, druggists don't know the first thing about running fountains."[21]

While pharmacists embraced this new commercial terrain, drug manufacturers suffered. Particularly hard hit was the ethical drug market, comprised of companies that made prescription medicines only. (The proprietary drug market, in contrast, sold over-the-counter medicines directly to the public.) Companies that had rushed into the initially lucrative antibiotic market at the end of the war suffered from the slump caused by overproduction and a precipitous drop in penicillin prices, from $3,955 a pound in 1945 to a meager $282 in 1950. This, coupled with the gradual revival of the European drug trade (whose stymied operations during the war had spawned the expansion of the American market) checked the industry's fortunes and dampened its wartime optimism. To reduce costs, some firms temporarily shut down production facilities. Even industry leaders were hard hit. In 1952, eight of the twelve largest American pharmaceutical firms, among them Merck, Parke Davis, Pfizer, Searle, and Sharpe & Dohme, reported a *decrease* in profits. As one industry analyst observed, "The rise in earnings [is] extremely small in comparison with the added dollars of business done."[22]

Executives looked for a way out of the financial quagmire. With consumer confidence in medical research high, prescription sales brisk, and household incomes rising, the answer seemed clear. Companies needed to create a wider range of patentable drugs whose manufacture could be monopolized and whose retail price could be kept high under patent protection. In 1953, one pharmaceutical president presciently predicted that the viability of the trade would require companies to devote "an increasing portion of their time to [the] investigation, production and sale of non-antibiotic drug specialties, products packaged under a company's trade name, and intended for the treatment of specific ills." He identified the development of innovative drugs for the prevention of cardiovascular disorders, degenerative diseases of aging, and mental disorders as the most promising path to commercial salvation.[23]

This strategy, embraced by a large number of pharmaceutical companies in the 1950s, was not without risk. In the short term, businesses would have to invest more in research and development. In addition, there was no guarantee that their investments would pay off. The image of men in white lab coats busily churning out batches of newly invented pharmaceuticals was a projected fantasy rather than a historical fact. With the exception of phenothiazine antihistamines, hatched by pharmacologists at Rhône-Poulenc's laboratories in France, most drugs had been discovered by chance. The supposition that scientists sequestered in laboratories could develop a cornucopia of profitable drugs in a timely fashion took more than generous funding; it required a leap of faith that drug development could be rationally planned. It was a gamble, but the profits could be huge.[24]

This uncertainty bedeviled American pharmaceutical executives when Frank Berger joined their ranks. Competition was stiff. Profits were down. The industry's fate was tied to unproven laboratory research. The stable profits the industry would come to enjoy in the 1960s were still a pipe dream. And no one could have predicted the astronomical earnings that would begin in the 1980s and persist until this day.[25]

Carter Products was one of hundreds of drug companies trying to shore up its earnings during difficult times. The firm was founded by Dr. Samuel J. Carter, a graduate of the University of Edinburgh who served in the Medical Corps during the Civil War and decided to remain in the United States to practice pharmacy in Erie, Pennsylvania. The company's best-known product was a laxative, Carter's Little Liver Pills. Carter compounded the pills in the 1870s for patients who felt "under-par and listless." The pills, which he euphemistically claimed would increase the flow of intestinal bile, were a success, and patients began to ask for Dr. Carter's Pills by name. Carter formed the Carter Medicine Company in 1880 to develop a national market for his local one-pill wonder. The strategy worked. The old saying, "He has more money than Carter has pills" reflected the company's success in creating a mass market and cultivating brand recognition. In subsequent years, Carter's Little Liver Pills, shrewdly merchandised under the peppy slogan, "Wake up Your Liver Bile!" remained a fixture on the American patent medicine market. Other patent drugs came and went, but Carter's Little Liver Pills endured.[26]

Incorporated in the 1930s as Carter Products, the company remained a small outfit with twenty employees and annual sales of $550,000. During this decade it expanded its product line, adding Arrid deodorant and Nair depilatory. These products upped sales, but by the time Berger was hired in 1949, Carter was still a minor entity in the pharmaceutical economy with annual sales of about $7 million. Carter was looking for products that would enable Wallace Laboratories, a spin-off subsidiary established in 1938 to develop prescription-only medication, to break into the coveted prescription market. Manufacturers of ethical drugs faced uncertain times, but they commanded the greatest respect in the medical world. In the early twentieth century, the dangers of patent medicines and the recklessness of some manufacturers had unleashed a barrage of prosecutions, further stigmatizing a trade whose cultural authority had long been tenuous. Such actions discredited companies like Carter while simultaneously cementing the legitimacy of firms that sold drugs exclusively to doctors and hospitals, the recognized ambassadors of respectable medical commerce.[27]

Carter's reputation had been further tarnished by a protracted legal dispute with the Federal Trade Commission (FTC). Underlying the conflict were Carter's claims about the therapeutic indications for its Little Liver Pills. In addition to being a laxative, the pills were said to be effective for biliousness, liver trouble, headaches, bad complexion, and that "worn out feeling." In 1943, the FTC filed charges against Carter for false and misleading advertising. At issue was not only Carter's advertising claims, but also its status as a reputable pharmaceutical firm. The company engaged in seventeen years of legal wrangling and spent over $1 million trying to clear its name. When Carter lost the case in 1959, it also lost a larger public relations campaign to seal consumer confidence and goodwill. Against this backdrop, Carter's bid for the prescription drug market was as much about distancing itself from its dubious roots as about making money.[28]

Henry Hoyt, the president of Carter Products who recruited Berger in 1949, was a short, middle-aged man who had purchased an interest in the company in 1929 when he became its managing director. He knew a lot about making laxatives and money, and though he knew very little about producing prescription drugs, he was eager to give it a try. When Berger joined the company, Wallace Laboratories had little to show for a decade of operation. It manufactured mainly dermatological creams and gels with a combined annual sales of about $87,000. Its laboratory comprised a few disheveled rooms in the company's main factory in North New Brunswick, in which a couple of chemists performed quality checks on Little Liver Pills. There was no pharmacological laboratory to support drug development or animal house to test new agents. It was, in Berger's eyes, an unimpressive outfit, "a small, financially unsuccessful subsidiary." Hoyt began to search for a scientist who could turn Wallace into a first-class research facility, making it more than the "dormant province of his small kingdom." In Frank Berger he found a medical researcher with impeccable credentials and a track record for drug development, a man with ambition, talent, energy, and youth. Berger, he believed, was just the sort of scientist to enhance the reputation and sales of both Carter and Wallace.[29]

What Berger got from Hoyt was a financial offer he couldn't refuse. In 1949, Berger remained a liberal idealist who extolled the virtues of socialized medicine. He chafed at the idea of being a physician forced to charge fees for services he believed "were the birthright of every sick person." He continued to believe that the medical researcher's primary responsibility was to assuage suffering. His work on estrogens, penicillin, and mephenesin had convinced him that such optimism was well founded. But recent events had instilled a newfound pragmatism. He had lost his immediate family, he had lost his first child, and when the communists came to power in the former Czech Republic, he had lost his claim to his family's property too. He had arrived in the United States and accepted a post as assistant professor of pediatrics at the University of Rochester. But with few resources he had amassed increasing debt. Bozena was pregnant again, joyous news that was also a source of worry. There was no nest egg Berger could tap to provide long-term care; he had to borrow money from his uncle merely to buy a refrigerator. What if he should get injured? What if he should die? "I felt that I had to take steps to give Bozena some security," he recalled.[30]

He applied for life insurance but was rejected because his blood pressure was too high. Berger surveyed his alternatives. He had ruled out clinical practice because he was "too sensitive a person to be a practicing physician. I was too deeply affected by the suffering of my patients." He had given up on academia; university professors, he avowed, didn't make enough money. His salary of $5,400 at the university was insufficient to pay off debts and support a family. In addition, his deafness made teaching difficult. Ardent about applied research, he relished the freedom and flexibility to work unfettered by the pressures of endless grant writing—something incompatible with university life.[31]

Allying himself with the pharmaceutical industry seemed the best way to meet his professional goals and take care of his family. Berger was sufficiently well-known and respected to receive offers from a number of firms. He chose Carter because Hoyt promised Berger a yearly salary of $12,000, more than double what the University of Rochester paid. But it was the generous royalty clause that sealed the deal. Hoyt offered Berger royalties of 1 percent of sales up to $7 million for every marketable product he developed. An incentive scheme of this magnitude was unprecedented. Although it seemed remarkably generous at the time, in the long run it would restrict Berger's share of the superlatively profitable tranquilizer pie. But Berger couldn't predict the future, nor could he resist the deal on the table. He and Bozena moved from New York to New Jersey in the summer of 1949.[32]

As the new president and medical director of Wallace Laboratories, Berger immediately got to work transforming the small workspace into a modern facility, hiring pharmacologists, buying equipment, setting up an animal research laboratory, and drafting a strategic plan. His burning ambition did not waver; he remained committed to the development of an orally active and longer-lasting version of mephenesin. He and Hoyt had

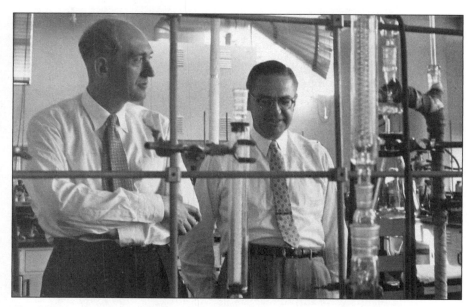

Frank Berger and Henry Hoyt. Berger and Hoyt during a lighter moment in Berger's laboratory at Wallace. Reproduced courtesy of the Berger Family.

discussed this prospect during Berger's recruitment interview, and Hoyt had tentatively approved Berger's plan. With Bernie Ludwig, the brilliant Columbia University–trained organic chemist hired to head Wallace's new laboratory, Berger tested compounds he believed might outperform mephenesin. The two men synthesized some five hundred of them. A dozen seemed particularly promising and were tested on animals. The dozen was narrowed down to four. One caught Berger's fancy—meprobamate, synthesized in May 1950. They submitted a patent application for it that July.[33]

In addition to relaxing the muscles of mice, meprobamate soothed irritated Rhesus and Java monkeys. Berger remembered how surprised he and Ludwig were by the drug's calming effects on the notoriously volatile primates. "We had about twenty Rhesus and Java monkeys on hand," he recalled. "They're vicious, and you've got to wear thick gloves and a face guard when you handle them." After being injected with meprobamate, they became "very nice monkeys—friendly and alert. Where they wouldn't previously eat in the presence of human beings, they now gently took grapes from your bare hand. It was quite impressive." Berger and Ludwig decided they had found their sought-after drug. Meprobamate's muscle relaxant properties lasted longer than those of mephenesin, and it relaxed patients more safely than barbiturates.

As Berger and Ludwig toiled in their lab, two important events changed the fate of the tranquilizer story. The first was medical reports on the therapeutic benefits of mephenesin for patients with psychiatric disorders. A small-scale study published in 1949 in the *Journal of the American Medical Association* (*JAMA*), the most prestigious and widely read medical journal in the country, was soon followed by other positive reports. In 1950, physicians at the University of Oregon published in the *American Journal of the Medical Sciences* the results of a study using Tolserol on 124 adult patients seen in private practice for a range of "anxiety tension states." The results were impressive. Whether administered as a tablet or an elixir, Tolserol eased a majority of them into a state "commonly seen in individuals who are pleasantly and comfortably at ease." The authors praised the drug's value as a supplement to psychoanalytic therapy. By inducing relaxation in patients, it enabled psychiatrists to employ "re-educative or psychotherapeutic measures" more effectively.[34]

A 1951 report on institutionalized patients presented more dramatic testimonials of mephenesin's psychiatric benefits. In one case, a patient prone to angry outbursts when questioned by his psychiatrist was given mephenesin. He "became noticeably calmer, ceased threatening the therapist and answered questions which previously produced rage in a calm, objective manner." In another, a "suspected homosexual" was given intravenous mephensin. He had a long history of being reticent when interviewed and emotionally withdrawn. Within thirty minutes of the drug's administration his speech became calm, he answered questions directly, and he "freely admitted overt homosexuality."[35]

These and other articles portrayed the drug as a valuable supplement to psychotherapy, suggesting that the therapeutic profile of mephenesin could be expanded to help psychiatric patients. In addition, by underlining the fundamental compatibility of drug therapy and psychotherapy, they established a new way of talking about anxiolytics that cast them as agents complementary to, rather than at odds with, psychoanalysis. In the view of these researchers, no drug could match talk therapy. All the same, by acknowledging the drug's ability to induce a state of mental relaxation, they raised the possibility of a tranquilizing pill for clinical use.[36]

The other monumental event with a direct bearing on the future of Miltown was the 1951 Humphrey-Durham amendments to the 1938 Food, Drugs, and Cosmetic Act. This important law responded to widespread concerns that Americans were consuming potentially dangerous drugs, particularly unchecked quantities of barbiturates, without medical supervision. In the early 1900s, federal prescription labeling status had applied only to narcotics. By law, a pharmacist could dispense narcotics only with a written prescription from a doctor or a dentist. By the late 1930s, the FDA had publicly acknowledged that other drugs also required a minimal degree of medical monitoring. By 1941, the agency had identified over twenty medications that fell into this group, including barbiturates and sulfa drugs. But because the FDA did not want to appear to be encroaching on the turf of manufacturers or pharmacists, it issued guidelines prohibiting only their "indiscriminate" sale. It left it to pharmaceutical manufacturers to decide what other drugs should be restricted to prescription-only status. As historian John Swann has argued, this industry-friendly compromise was no way to instill order in the pharmaceutical trade. States and municipalities had their own drug regulations that, like FDA guidelines, were frequently ignored and unevenly enforced.[37]

The Durham-Humphrey amendments strove to protect the public from the health hazards of self-medication. The new rules changed how medicines could be marketed, distributed, and refilled at the national level. It became the FDA's job to decide which drugs were safe enough to be sold over-the-counter and which required the added safeguard of medical supervision. Drugs that fell into the restricted category had to be labeled: "Caution: Federal law prohibits dispensing except on prescription." Consumers who had previously acquired potentially dangerous drugs directly from pharmacists could now get them only with a physician's script. The amendments also curbed laissez-faire refill practices, forcing druggists to secure a physician's authorization before issuing a refill. Durham-Humphrey sought to protect the public health by establishing doctors as the expert gatekeepers to drugs. It also positioned reputable and, increasingly, large-scale pharmaceutical companies as the primary suppliers of prescription medicines.[38]

Manufacturers of proprietary medicines howled in protest. The Durham-Humphrey amendments diminished their prerogatives and undercut the authority of retail druggists. Outraged by what it saw as the expansion of FDA authority at its expense, the proprietary industry assailed the new law as a handmaiden of socialized medicine. (Interestingly, pharmaceutical firms today invoke the same inflammatory rhetoric to criticize the expansion of FDA regulations.) At the annual meeting of the Proprietary Association in New York in 1951, a spokesman called the measure a dangerous threat to the freedom of medical care, and warned that the Durham-Humphrey amendments trammeled the traditional right of self-medication and patient choice.[39]

The new measures distressed companies such as Carter that depended on over-the-counter drug revenue. Lawyers at Carter were still haggling with the FTC over how Little Liver Pills could be advertised. Now Carter executives had to worry about whether their flagship product (or any new product, for that matter) would be restricted by the FDA to prescription status. The amendments meant that the new compounds Berger and Ludwig were synthesizing at Wallace would be available only by prescription. Courting doctors' support was new territory for Carter, and Hoyt and his colleagues were worried. While contemporary critics of the pharmaceutical industry often regard physicians as accomplices in a pharmaceutical cabal—willing pushers of the latest drugs—Hoyt and his cronies considered them fiercely independent agents whose loyalty would have to be carefully wooed and won.[40]

By the end of 1951, Berger was ready to begin testing meprobamate on humans and to conduct toxicity tests on animals. But he needed a larger supply of the powder than Wallace's facilities could furnish. Like most drug firms at the time, Carter and Wallace were not vertically integrated— they lacked the capacity to transform raw materials into finished products on a large scale. Berger needed a manufacturing ally, a chemical firm able and willing to produce a few hundred pounds of an experimental compound. But as he cast about for an industrial partner, Berger found that reputable chemical companies didn't take Carter seriously. When he approached Union Carbide and DuPont, both turned him down. Neither had enough faith in Carter to risk the venture. A lesser known outfit, Berkeley Chemicals, finally agreed. Bob Milano, its president, became fast friends with Berger. Milano's willingness to help would later be handsomely rewarded with a contract to produce meprobamate powder.[41]

Small-scale trials of meprobamate began on patients suffering from neurosis, psychosis, epilepsy, and muscle spasms. The results confirmed what Berger's monkey trials had previously demonstrated: meprobamate diminished patients' anxiety. Berger was thrilled and rushed to share the good news with Hoyt. To his dismay, the businessman balked and put the Miltown project on hold.

Hoyt's reaction may seem surprising given the subsequent profitability of minor tranquilizers. But in the context of the pharmaceutical economy and psychiatry practice of the early 1950s, it possessed a certain logic. There was no preexisting market for prescription-only tranquilizers and no one could predict how they would perform. The use of mephenesin had been largely hospital-based, whereas meprobamate was intended for non-institutional patients too.

Augmenting company concerns, commercial prospects for a prescription antianxiety agent seemed bleak. Psychiatry departments throughout North America were still enamored with Freudian theories of neurosis, which taught doctors to regard anxiety as the product of unresolved conflict bubbling from the unconscious mind. Indeed, as one contemporary observed, psychoanalysis was about as "controversial as the American flag." Biological psychiatry was not yet in vogue. Personal history rather than brain chemistry remained the therapeutic focus.[42]

Hoyt's reservations were compounded by the company's internal research on the likely market for an antianxiety agent. Wallace Laboratories had commissioned the Harris Poll to survey two hundred doctors to gauge interest in a prescription anxiolytic. Doctors were asked if they would be willing to prescribe a drug for everyday anxiety. The vast majority said no. Hoyt wondered whether a pharmaceutical market for anxiety even existed.

And if not, how could Carter, of all companies, create one? Unwilling to assume the risk, he refused to sanction Berger's bid to perform the next steps to secure FDA approval.

Although frustrated, Berger persevered. He regarded excessive anxiety as an impediment to clear thought and reason, the hallmarks of enlightenment and progress. In Berger's mind, there was nothing fundamentally noble or beneficial about being nervous. Rather, anxiety prevented individuals from having honest and clear discussions. The virtue of meprobamate, he told me, was that after taking it "you are more settled down [and] have a little more peace of mind to consider the world." In addition, Berger believed that tranquilizers eliminated unnecessary anguish in the stricken and uplifted humanity as a whole. In his writings, Berger liked to quote Spinoza: "Human bondage consists in the impotence of man to govern or restrain [their] effects . . . for a man who is under their control is not his own master. A free man is one who lives according to the dictates of reason alone."[43]

Berger believed that doctors and patients would share his vision of anxiety and be interested in a pill to combat it. He pressed on. With Bob Milano's help, Berger acquired enough tablets to send to practicing psychiatrists in the field. In January 1953, a batch went to Dr. Joseph C. Borrus, a New Jersey psychiatrist who had agreed to test it on patients suffering from a range of psychiatric disorders (although the largest number were affected by anxiety). A second batch was sent to Dr. Lowell S. Selling, a psychiatrist in Orlando, Florida, to be used on patients being treated for outpatient anxiety. Far removed from the corridors of Carter or Wallace and unknown to Henry Hoyt, the two physicians began their trials.

Borrus treated 104 patients, 45 females and 59 males, over a twelve-month period. Meprobamate was found to have no therapeutic benefit on patients with a "psychopathic personality" or schizophrenia, but it helped 78 percent of those with anxiety symptoms. They were less tense and irritable. They slept better. They returned to work. They were socially productive. And the drug seemed safe. Blood tests and urine analysis showed no signs of toxicity, even after long-term use. Patients withdrew from the drug with ease.[44]

Selling was equally sanguine about the results of his trial, conducted over a fifteen-month period during 1953 and 1954. So too were his patients. "When I first came in here, I couldn't even listen to the radio," one patient told Selling. "I couldn't stand to have company, and . . . in April I thought I was going crazy." A few months after taking meprobamate, her life had improved. "I want you to know I now go to football games, shows, and even watch TV. My husband can't get over how relaxed I am." The woman's experiences were not atypical. More than 90 percent of Selling's tense patients improved or recovered after taking a 400 mg tablet after each meal and at bedtime. Selling endorsed the drug's effectiveness not only in controlling tension and anxiety, but also "fear, headaches, mild depression, insomnia, and neurodermatitis."[45]

Compared to today's large-scale, randomized clinical trials, which often involve several thousand people, the protocols used to test meprobamate were different. Enrolled patients numbered in the hundreds, not thousands, and no control group was used. Borrus told his patients: "I am going to give you this medicine to see if it will help you." Yet the designs of the meprobamate trials were consistent with other clinical trials in this era, and nothing about them alarmed researchers or regulators. Doctors and FDA officials evaluated what qualified as good science in the context of their times. In 1955 Selling and Borrus's studies were considered so resolutely sound and path-breaking that *JAMA* decided to publish them as sequential articles on April 30, 1955. The articles spawned medical interest in and scientific enthusiasm for meprobamate, what Selling referred to as a "new tranquilizing drug."[46]

Even before the *JAMA* studies appeared, Berger used their results to leverage Hoyt's permission to file a new drug application with the FDA to authorize meprobamate's sale. Hoyt's response was tepid, but he gave Berger his okay. Berger submitted the application to the FDA in December 1954. While Berger's confidence in the drug had grown, Hoyt struggled with looming practical questions. How could small-scale Carter mass-manufacture a drug? What should it be called? How should it be classified? And how could the company overcome the kind of physician resistance indicated by the Harris Poll? Luckily, Berger had some answers. The manufacture of meprobamate powder would continue to be outsourced to freestanding chemical firms, including Milano's Berkeley Laboratories. This would leave to Carter the more manageable task of tableting and bottling.[47]

Finding the right trademark, the brand by which meprobamate would be sold, was trickier. The advertising industry had already created a naming tradition for new pharmaceutical products. Ad men favored names with a classical ring to them, words that connected a new drug to a venerable past. The class of drugs known as ataractics took their name from *ataraxia*, the Greek word meaning freedom from mental disturbance. The marketing mission was to give doctors and patients the security associated with the aura of antiquity, conferring on new products what historian Eric Hobsbawm has called an "invented tradition."[48]

Berger drafted a list of possibilities. He liked "Mepheton" and was disappointed to discover that it had already been claimed by A. H. Robbins, another pharmaceutical firm. He had equally bad luck with other suggestions: "Meprodriol," "Mepromate," and "Meprodil" sounded too similar to drugs already on the market. Berger was stumped. He could come up with nothing better. Not being a man enamored by "the niceties of pharmaceutical nomenclature," neither could Hoyt.[49]

The solution sprang from Wallace Laboratory's peculiar custom of coding experimental compounds not by their chemical names but by the names of nearby New Jersey towns. One drug in the experimental stage was called Princeton, another was Newark. Meprobamate had been dubbed Milltown after a bucolic village lined with picturesque cottages about three miles from Wallace's New Brunswick laboratory and about thirty miles outside of New York City. Before the drug made Milltown famous, a guide book prophetically described it as "tranquil little Milltown." It would make for a terrific study in contrasts: a drug to combat the frenzied pace of modern life would be linguistically linked to a quiet, tree-shaded town founded in 1664. In the 1950s, the hamlet was still so peaceful that its 3,800 inhabitants required only a six-man police force and a two-cell police station to keep order. Hoyt knew that places could not be trademarked, so he unceremoniously struck a letter *l*. And so it was that with a stroke of the pen, Berger's new baby was christened Miltown.[50]

Having settled on a trademark, Berger wrestled with ways to change medical minds. In a move befitting the cinematic temperament of 1950s America, he and Carter colleagues Thomas E. Lynes and Charles D. Hendley made a film. Might a short documentary convince people? It had worked for political propaganda. Why not for drugs? The low-budget motion picture entitled *The Effect of Meprobamate (Miltown) on Animal Behavior* was shot in Berger's lab. Rhesus monkeys were featured in three distinct chemical states: naturally vicious, unconscious on barbiturates, and calm but awake on meprobamate.[51]

The film was first screened at the April 1955 meeting of the Federation of American Societies for Experimental Biology in San Francisco. It generated widespread excitement and caught the attention of executives at Wyeth Laboratories. Wyeth was an established firm, one of several subsidiaries and the primary ethical division of the conglomerate American Home Products Corporation. Founded in 1860, Wyeth manufactured an extensive line of medical products and sported a phalanx of 800 pharmaceutical sales representatives to promote them. Wyeth's men talked to Berger and Hoyt about purchasing a license to market meprobamate under a different name: in effect, the same drug (whose manufacture Wallace would control) would be sold under two competing trademarks. Wyeth's representatives reviewed the drug's pharmacological, toxicological, and clinical data. They were impressed. Berger told them that FDA approval was expected in May.[52]

Wyeth then made Carter a lucrative offer. It agreed to purchase meprobamate powder for $10 per pound, about twice what Carter paid for it. It offered Carter a supplemental 5 percent royalty fee for the right to sell meprobamate under the trade name Equanil. It was a generous offer, and Hoyt knew it. He agreed to a licensing arrangement that would allow Wyeth to sell meprobamate as Equanil in the fall. Hoyt realized Miltown would benefit from Wyeth's retailing push as much as it would from the royalty arrangements, which delivered Carter profits each time a prescription for Equanil was filled. From Hoyt's perspective, there were no losers in this agreement. He was relieved. Wyeth's bid offered Carter a financial safety net. If Miltown failed, Wyeth's financial contributions would offset the cost of bringing the drug to market. Carter had nothing to lose.[53]

The final issue was how to classify the drug. Once again, chance intervened. Berger was having dinner with Nathan Kline and Paul Janssen, two rising stars in the field of psychopharmacology. Kline was an ambitious psychiatrist with degrees in psychology and philosophy who had recently become the research director of Rockland State Hospital in Orangeburg, New York (featured in the acclaimed 1948 film *The Snake Pit*). Janssen was a pharmacologist who had established a small, research-oriented drug firm in 1953. In a Manhattan restaurant, Berger talked enthusiastically about the upcoming launch of meprobamate and his difficulties sorting out its classification. He was toying with the idea of calling it a sedative, a traditional label with a solid sales record. Kline talked him out of it. "You are out of your mind," Janssen remembered Kline saying. "The world doesn't need new sedatives. What the world really needs is a tranquilizer. The world needs tranquility. Why don't you call this a tranquilizer? You will sell ten times more." Persuaded, Berger called his new creation a tranquilizer.[54]

Wallace's Miltown became available in May 1955, a full five years after Berger and Ludwig had concocted it. Wyeth released Equanil a few months later. The march to Miltown had been long, and on the eve of its release, no one was certain what the future might bring.

(3)

The Fashionable Pill

Miltown debuted on Monday, May 9, 1955, with little fanfare. It was the day after Mother's Day, and the newspapers were filled with discussions of the previous day's church sermons, imploring the faithful to honor their mothers. Across the country, medical reporters paid little heed to the release of a tranquilizer intended for everyday nerves. Instead, they focused on the federal government's May 7 decision to suspend the polio inoculation campaign. Fifty cases of paralytic polio had been confirmed among the 5 million children who had received the new vaccine since January 1955. Most of those infected had received injections made by a single laboratory, and the government wanted to inspect the safety of the remaining inventory before the campaign resumed. Parents were frantic. Were their inoculated children going to get polio too? School boards were fielding angry calls, and state health departments weren't sure what to do. Dr. Leonard A. Scheele, the U.S. surgeon general, was struggling to reassure parents that although the government's decision had been prudent, the health of the nation's schoolchildren was not at risk.[1]

If the polio panic was the perfect setup for a worry-busting pill, no one seemed to notice. In its first few months on the market, Miltown was roundly ignored. Sales of the tranquilizers, which cost about ten cents each, totaled just $7,500 in its first month, and June sales were equally unimpressive.[2]

Then unexpectedly, things picked up. By August, sales of Miltown had climbed to $85,000; by September, $218,000. The momentum continued. By Christmas, total sales for 1955 exceeded $2 million. Carter Products began the new year with a surprising and welcome challenge: how to fill a million dollars' worth of back orders for the new drug. Carter executives were pleased but puzzled. What curious psychology had reversed Miltown's fortunes so precipitously? No one understood what sparked this burst of interest, but Miltown mania had begun.[3]

Henry Hoyt, Frank Berger, and the pharmaceutical and psychiatry establishments never could have predicted the impact Miltown would have in a single community. Sometimes the projections of Madison Avenue marketing experts are foiled by the unforeseen behavior of consumers, and the hoopla surrounding a new product can take on a life of its own. In the winter of 1955 and spring of 1956 Miltown mania was powered by events and fashions that converged in forceful and sometimes volatile ways. But nothing was as unexpected or as newsworthy as Hollywood's fascination with the little white peace pill.

Hooray for Miltown!

Drugs were nothing new in the arts and entertainment industry. Indeed, today's fascination with celebrity pill popping reflects a long history of use and abuse. Studios have often supplied cast and crew with drugs to help them meet demanding production schedules and long film shoots. Silent screen heartthrob Wallace Reid, whom *Motion Picture* magazine called "the screen's most perfect lover," succumbed to morphine addiction in 1919 after a doctor prescribed the powerful and habit-forming narcotic for injuries incurred from an accident on location in Oregon. Morphine alleviated Reid's pain and enabled him to keep up with the studio's frantic pace, but it likely hastened his premature death at age thirty-one in 1923. Some speculate that MGM launched Judy Garland's lifelong struggle with substance abuse when it supplied amphetamines to the teenage actress to help her slim down and give her extra "oomph" to endure the punishing filming of the *Wizard of Oz*. Garland used barbiturates (to which she became famously addicted) to offset the insomnia caused by amphetamines until she suffered a fatal overdose in 1969. David O. Selznick's legendary twenty-two-hour *Gone with the Wind* shoots were said to be fueled by a steady diet of the stimulant Benzedrine. Omar Sharif allegedly popped speed to get extra energy for the filming of *Lawrence of Arabia*. Worried about Sharif's drug habit, cast mate Jack Hawkins pulled him aside. "Dear boy," he counseled Sharif, "the secret is to relax; you need energy, but relaxed energy."[4]

Miltown promised relaxed energy to an industry comprised of overwrought women and men struggling with nervous pressure, exhaustion, grueling schedules, and the fear that a single bad performance could cost them their careers. Playwrights and journalists racing against deadlines, stage and television performers under the scrutiny of the spotlight, dancers auditioning for career-making parts: it is no wonder that Miltown took this harried celebrity culture, already familiar with drugs on demand, by storm.

In addition, many Angelenos considered Miltown hip and fun. Never simply a drug to help Hollywood denizens deaden stress, Miltown carried a star power all its own. In a community where taking pills was part of the social scene, in a town where people tracked trends and fads, the pills enjoyed a double identity as fashion and medicine. Movie stars and television personalities gushed about Miltown, gossip reporters wrote treatises on it, and at celebrity galas, illicit Miltown was passed around as casually as canapés. Doctors prescribed it frequently—some would say permissively. If one's own physician refused, there were other ways to secure a supply. Miltown was a bit like the latest lipstick sensation or a newly discovered restaurant. It was novel and exciting. It was something to try.

Los Angeles was the drug's first big market, "Miltown-by-the-sea," according to one contemporary. In time, Miltown mania would infuse the New York entertainment industry too, but initially Miltown was, in the words of one Broadway journalist, "strictly a Hollywood success story." Hollywood's most famous pharmacy at the time was Schwab's on Sunset Boulevard, where Harold Arlen composed "Over the Rainbow" and Marlene Dietrich was spotted buying face powder. The "Drugstore of the Stars" sold a whopping 250,000 meprobamate pills and turned away more

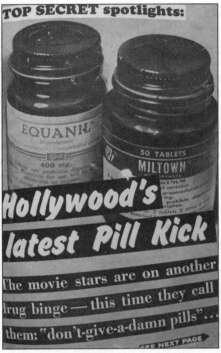

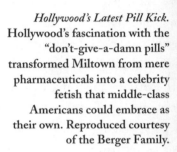

Hollywood's Latest Pill Kick. Hollywood's fascination with the "don't-give-a-damn pills" transformed Miltown from mere pharmaceuticals into a celebrity fetish that middle-class Americans could embrace as their own. Reproduced courtesy of the Berger Family.

scripts than it could fill in four months during the winter of 1955–1956. Leon Schwab, the store's owner, wouldn't disclose the names of his famous Miltown clients but admitted that they included "the biggest names in movies and television," including one songwriter who called them his "uranium tablets" and a TV comedian who left a standing order for all the tablets he could get.[5]

The consumer frenzy stumped distributors' best efforts to keep area pharmacies stocked. "When you have 600 drugstores and only 400 bottles of Miltown, how can you ration them?" wondered one frustrated buyer. A new shipment was something to celebrate, and pharmacies were quick to communicate the good news to doctors and passersby. A *Los Angeles Times* ad in December 1955 proclaimed, "Attention physicians: just arrived by air, another shipment of MILTOWN. Your prescriptions can now be filled." Some stores posted giant banners that communicated the drug's availability. "Yes, we have Miltown!" announced the red placard on the window of a Hollywood drugstore at the corner of Sunset and Gower.[6]

While Hollywood's Miltown obsession was sometimes ridiculed by critics of celebrity fads, many in the entertainment business considered it a reasonable response to industry demands. Tranquilizers, concluded one nightclub comedian in 1957, are "the most revolutionary thing in show business. . . . Tension is the killer in this business and this is the answer." Kendis Rochlen, a columnist for the Los Angeles *Mirror-News*, agreed. "If there's anything this movie business needs, it's a little tranquility," she explained. "Once you're big enough to be 'somebody' in filmtown you've just got to be knee-deep in tension and mental and emotional stress. The anxiety of trying to make it to the top is replaced by the anxiety of wondering if you're going to stay there. So, big names and little alike have been loading their trusty pillboxes with this little wonder tablet."[7]

A movie mogul explained to a journalist what compelled him to take the drug. "Most everyone who is anyone in Hollywood is excitable, jumpy, nervous, tense—ready to jump out of his skin." It only stood to follow that "Hollywood has been one of the best markets for the emotional aspirins," a nickname that captured a view of tranquilizers as casual and carefree. He had started taking Miltown as soon as he heard about it, he admitted, and had felt less overwhelmed ever since.[8]

On crowded movie sets and in writers' quiet studies, in smoky nightclubs and in the solitude of studio cutting rooms, some of America's most talented and creative minds took Miltown. Lucille Ball's assistant kept a supply on the set, once offering Ball a Miltown in her coffee to calm the star after a stormy argument with husband Desi Arnaz. Lauren Bacall remembers being prescribed Miltown for insomnia after the death of husband Humphrey Bogart. While working on rehearsals of his taut drama *The Night of the Iguana*, which opened on Broadway in December 1961, Tennessee Williams added Miltown to the list of substances to which he was addicted. He told *Theatre Arts* magazine that only "Miltowns, liquor, [and] swimming" could tame his driving restlessness and creative tension. "Last night after the cutting session, I took two Miltowns," he admitted. The drugs helped him fall sleep and wake up refreshed enough for his three-hour writing stint, a morning ritual he had cherished for more than thirty-five years.[9]

In his frank disclosure of Miltown use, Williams was consistent with many other celebrities and literati who discussed their relationships with pills. In an era when the use of prescription drugs had not yet been stigmatized, many devotees in the arts and entertainment world readily shared their experiences with the press. These confessions, overwhelmingly positive in tone, depicted the drug as simultaneously glamorous, necessary, and routine. A nightclub singer told *Uncensored!* magazine that Miltown was the greatest thing that ever happened to her. Before going on stage, she "used to get the shakes and felt extremely nervous at times." Taking Miltown before each show made her confident. Gone, too, was her insomnia from being keyed up by the evening's performance. Before bed, she would take two more and sleep "like a baby." Film and stage actress Tallulah Bankhead joked that the amount she ingested probably obligated her "to pay taxes in New Jersey," the now well-known birthplace of Miltown. Norman Mailer also admitted to consuming massive quantities in addition to plenty of other pharmaceutical concoctions while revising *The Deer Park,* his 1955 novel about power, corruption, and sex in Hollywood. Others raved about their Miltown substitutes. When a reporter asked Jayne Mansfield if she took tranquilizers, the blonde bombshell playfully retorted, "Miltown, schmiltown. Who needs Miltown when I've got Mickey (the muscle man) Hargitay?" a reference to the Mr. Universe boyfriend she would soon marry. Whether they boasted of Miltown use or denied it, celebrities made the drugs the talk of the town.[10]

Tranquilizers were easy to get because doctors prescribed them liberally and pharmacists often refilled prescriptions without authorization. Rumors abounded that some California pharmacists sold them over the counter. In addition, a vibrant bootleg market surfaced to meet the extraordinary demand that legitimate purveyors were unable to satisfy. Miltown's many markets, both legal and illicit, gave the drug a wide circulation. In Los Angeles it was easy to procure tranquilizers from friends, relatives, hosts, and business associates. One Hollywood reporter identified only one prescription holder out of the fifty tranquilizer users he interviewed in 1956. A top modeling agency kept a stash at the receptionist's desk for "cover girls who [felt] nervous or fatigued after a hard day before the cameras." At the headquarters of a daily newspaper, Miltown was available on demand from the head copy boy.[11]

Miltown was frequently handed out at parties and premieres, a kind of pharmaceutical appetizer for jittery celebrities. Frances Kaye, a publicity agent, described a movie party she attended at a Palm Springs resort. A live orchestra entertained the thousand-odd guests while a fountain spouted champagne against the backdrop of a desert sky. As partiers circulated, a doctor made rounds like a waiter, dispensing drugs to guests from a bulging sack. On offer were amphetamines and barbiturates, standard Hollywood party fare, but guests wanted Miltown. The little white pills "were passed around like peanuts," Kaye remembered. What she observed about party pill popping was not unique. "They all used to go for 'up pills' or 'down pills,'" one Hollywood regular noted. "But now it's the 'don't-give-a-darn-pills.'"[12]

The Hollywood entertainment culture transformed a pharmaceutical concoction into a celebrity fetish, a coveted commodity of the fad-prone glamour set. Female entertainers toted theirs in chic pillboxes designed especially for tranquilizers, which became, according to one contemporary, as ubiquitous at Hollywood parties as the climatically unnecessary mink coat. In 1956, Tiffany jewelers reported brisk sales of "ruby and diamond-studded pill coffers for those who wished to glorify their new-found happiness." Cartier sold a bracelet charm shaped like a pill with enough room for two peace pills for $20 and a $148 gold box with sapphires and rubies that held six. One cosmetic firm marketed Tranquilease, a cream said to iron out the unsightly facial features of tension and emotional upset. Miltown even inspired a barrage of new alcoholic temptations, in which the pill was the defining ingredient. The Miltown Cocktail was a Bloody Mary (vodka and tomato juice) spiked with a single pill, and the Guided Missile, popular among the late-night crowd on the Sunset Strip, consisted of a double shot of vodka and two Miltowns. More popular still was the Miltini, a dry martini in which a Miltown replaced the customary olive.[13]

Reflecting how deeply embedded Miltown had become in the language and identity of Angelenos, manufacturers appropriated the image of the frazzled Hollywood tranquilizer user to market nonpharmaceutical goods.

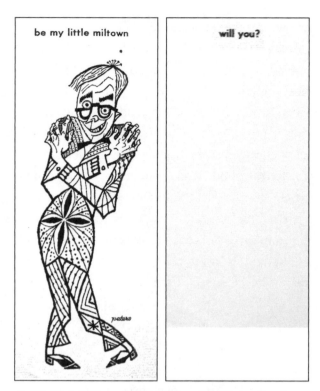

Be My Little Miltown. Although its cultural appeal and
medical popularity would largely be forgotten by a
subsequent generation of Americans, Miltown enjoyed an
almost iconic status in the 1950s. The little white pill
inspired television skits, cocktails, and even greeting cards,
such as this enterprising 1957 Valentine's Day card, which
coupled romantic bliss with drugged tranquility.
Reproduced courtesy of the Berger Family.

Baskin-Robbins even used the Miltown name to sell ice cream in cartoon
ads featuring a bespectacled director overwrought to the point of shaking.
Clutching his telltale megaphone, the nervous director would approach a
Baskin-Robbins vendor and demand, "Give me a gallon of Miltown Ice
Cream!" The vendor's reply was always the same: "Sorry, Mister, no Miltown but our Hazelnut Toffee Ice Cream [or any one of the company's
thirty-one flavors] is mighty relaxin.'"[14]

Miltown's promise of the peaceful life was also used to sell railroad trips
and cars. The Union Pacific Railroad promoted its Domeliner passenger

cars as nerve tonics. "Tense and on edge lately? Desk drawer stocked with Miltown?" If so, a trip on the Domeliner's peaceful, quiet Pullman accommodations was just the thing. Promoting its sleek new car designs, the Holiday Motors Company of Los Angeles psychologized that tension from driving the wrong car was implicated in the stress that caused thousands of Californians to take Miltown. "Why not curb [the problem] at its source?" the company asked. Ads invited the road weary to visit Holiday's showroom, where the year's newest models—Ford Zodiacs, Consults, Zephyrs, and the Renault Dauphine—"will allow anybody taking 'happy pills' to toss them out the window for good." Stop "buying those tickets to Miltown," the company beseeched, "and drive home one of Holiday's new Peace of Mind Autos."[15]

Miltown and the National Media

As local advertisers sought to cash in on Miltown's allure, writers introduced Miltown to a broader audience. The 1957 film *Feliz Año* tells of an overworked concert violinist who ignores his doctor's advice to take Miltown and a vacation. Instead, the burned-out performer has an adulterous fling, a detour that estranges him from his saintly wife, who dies before our hero realizes his mistake. The film's subtext suggests that the violinist should have heeded his doctor's advice and just taken his pills. In the musical *Portofino*, romantic lead Helen Gallagher belts out, "When I think of him kissing me, I don't know whether to fall down, sit down, or Miltown."[16]

Even writer and political satirist Aldous Huxley gave the drug a glowing review. His futuristic and dystopian 1932 novel, *Brave New World*, envisaged a society in which citizens enjoyed comfort and security. Science had extinguished human error, but also its spirit. Political control was achieved through civilian pacification with a drug called Soma, possibly suggesting that the always didactic Huxley would have been intellectually predisposed to be a stern critic of meprobamate. But in fact Huxley became an early advocate of the drug. Huxley gave a headline-grabbing plenary lecture on the history of tension at a symposium in New York City in

1956. He characterized the discovery of meprobamate as "more important, more genuinely revolutionary, than the recent discoveries in the field of nuclear physics." Nuclear physicists might give humans "cheaper power and its corollary of gadgets" but pharmacologists had the power to grant something greater: "loving kindness, peace, and joy." By 1956 the skeptical materialism of Huxley's earlier years had yielded to a fascination with mysticism and chemical mind-bending. The advent of Miltown was a vast improvement over the "dangerous and degrading poisons" that mankind had turned to since ancient times, from the poppy heads found in the kitchen middens of Swiss lake dwellers to opium and alcohol, in search of "self-transcendence and relief from tension." Asked if he was worried that Miltown might tranquilize the world into political and spiritual oblivion, Huxley was dismissive. Fiction was fiction. "My prediction was made for strictly literary purposes," he explained about Soma, "and not as a reasoned forecast for future history. All that one can predict," he enthused, "is that many of our traditional notions about ethics and religion, many of our current views about the nature of the mind, will have to be reconsidered and reevaluated in the context of the pharmacological revolution. It will be extremely disturbing; but it will be enormously fun."[17]

Huxley would continue to endorse the revolutionary possibilities of consciousness-changing drugs, including meprobamate, until his death in 1963. Health problems curtailed his ability to deliver lectures, but Huxley continued to publish, including several essays in mainstream journals such as *Esquire* on the political and spiritual benefits of pharmaceutical transcendence. "More than a thousand million doses of meprobamate were swallowed, last year, by the American public," he enthused in one piece. "And the numbers of those who regularly turn to the tranquilizing drugs for that relief from psychological distress, without which there can be no pleasure, is likely to increase with every passing month." This was cause for optimism, as was future pharmaceutical innovation. "Within the next few years we may expect to see the development of a physiologically costless stimulant and a physiologically costless transfigurer of perceived reality . . . capable of transforming time into eternity, of making the soul say yes to the world instead of no, of imparting to the most dismal or commonplace scene unsuspected and unimaginable qualities of beauty—even of making the average TV program seem absolutely wonderful."[18]

Miltown left its mark on television programs too. Television actors likely used them more than anyone else in the entertainment industry. Today most television broadcasts are prerecorded, subjected to multiple re-takes, and painstakingly edited to deliver a flawless finished product. But in the mid-1950s, a majority of shows and commercials were broadcast live. This placed tremendous pressure on performers, whose every move and word could be scrutinized by millions. Television commentator Virginia Graham empathized with colleagues who took tranks. "Take the young lady who practices at least six hours a week for a one-minute live commercial," she explained. "For one minute, three times a week, [this actress] has to be utter perfection. What if a curl should fall out of place while she is in the midst of this all-important tense minute?" Before Miltown, Graham's acquaintance had knitted her way through her jitters, right up until she went on air. Now the actress took Miltown and left her knitting needles at home. Small wonder, as Graham observed about Miltown use, that many television entertainers "live on the things." [19]

Like others in the entertainment business, comedians openly discussed their Miltown habit, even on live television. This was the golden age of American television, and the demographic reach of such testimonials was potentially huge. By the end of the 1950s, nine of every ten households owned a television and audiences could number in the tens of millions. In 1954, for example, the popular *I Love Lucy* show counted 50 million regular viewers among 163 million Americans.[20]

Of the dozens of television personalities who discussed Miltown's appeal, no one was more vocal than Milton Berle. The high-energy host of NBC's *Milton Berle Show* was television's first superstar. Watched by millions, Berle's variety show commanded such a loyal following that restaurants, theaters, and other establishments often closed when it aired on Tuesday nights between 8:00 and 9:00 P.M. There were Uncle Miltie comic books, chewing gum, T-shirts, and wind-up toys. On the air, Berle raved about how good Miltown made him feel and how often he took it. Loaded on the goodwill pills, he began to call himself "Uncle Miltown."

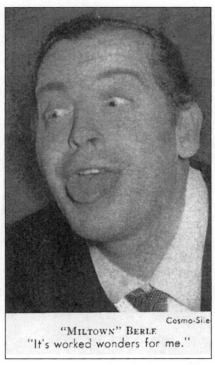

"Miltown Berle." Television superstar Milton Berle, whose weekly evening variety show was watched by millions, raved about how good Miltown made him feel and how often he took it. His frequent on-screen testimonials and jokes about the goodwill pills earned him the nickname of "Uncle Miltown." *Time*, February 27, 1956.

"MILTOWN" BERLE
"It's worked wonders for me."

Cosmo-Site

On one occasion, he gloated to viewers that "it's worked wonders for me. In fact, I'm thinking of changing my name to Miltown Berle." On another, he reassured viewers that they were addicted only if they were taking more than their doctors. "Heard about the 'new vitamin pill?'" he quipped on a later episode. It's "half oyster juice and half Miltown. [It] gets you romantic but puts you to sleep before you get in trouble."[21]

Berle's numerous testimonials and jokes prompted his wife, Ruth, to make a series of public statements about her husband's drug use. Worried that Berle was working too hard, she encouraged him to scale back his television appearances for the 1956–1957 season. For herself, she wanted "more Milton and less Miltown." Discussing the tranquilizer, she explained that "most of the comedians in television are taking it now. This is such a grueling business that most of them couldn't stand the pace without it." Alarmed by the possibility that Berle's frequent and casual references to the drug were encouraging indiscriminate use, she made an unusual disclosure. She and Milton "had a long discussion about it," she admitted in 1957, "and we decided Milton shouldn't boost something that was helping him but could possibly have a different effect on someone else." Whatever the impact her cautionary remarks had on viewers, they did little to silence Berle. A review of the show's scripts reveals that Miltown jokes endured well into the 1960s.[22]

Taking their cue from Berle, writers made Miltown a staple of television humor. According to one contemporary, comics jested about Miltown in 1956 almost as much as they did about Elvis Presley. These jokes may not seem particularly funny today, but they were common at the time. Comedian Red Skelton, host of the long-running *Red Skelton Show*, joked about what one Miltown in his pillbox said to another. "I feel so terrible I think I'll take a Perry Como," a reference to the Italian American crooner whose soothing, velvety ballads were the butt of many jokes. "Miltown is now coming out in four strengths," teased NBC's Bob Hope. "Quiet, very quiet, rest in peace, and Perry Como." On another occasion, Hope asked his audience if they had heard about Miltown. He went on: "The doctors call Miltown the 'I don't-care-pill.' The government hands them out with your income-tax blanks."[23]

Miltown jokes could engage both the superficial and the serious. Humor and jest can create a safe cultural space for people to discuss difficult topics. During the cold war, a drug to offset anxiety became an ideal pretext for politically freighted jokes. A Hope skit that aired in the spring of 1956 captured the flavor of the political ribbing:

HOPE: Whether you like them or not, Khrushy and Bulgy are two of the smartest Russians alive. [Laughter.] The fact that they're alive still proves it. Now they want to come to the United States and sell us peace. Is this a switch? They must be spiking their vodka with Miltown. [Laughter.][24]

At its annual roast in 1957, the Gridiron Club in Washington, D.C., concerned itself with controversies surrounding Eisenhower's 1956 southern victories and civil rights initiatives by lampooning southern Democrats. The Democrats were depicted as taking "jolly pills" prescribed in

"Dr. Lyndon B. Johnson's Jolly Pill Pharmacy in Miltown, U.S.A." to forget their north-south troubles. Sometimes the gags were more solemn. The day after the Russians launched Sputnik, the first earth satellite, one journalist wrote that "President Eisenhower gave the Soviet satellite the Miltown treatment at his weekly press conference." Eisenhower was being accused, albeit in jest, of being too placid in his handling of what many saw as a calamitous assault on American military supremacy.[25]

Media Improprieties

Eventually media coverage of Miltown, particularly recurrent television endorsements from celebrities, caught the attention of the FDA. Was Wallace covertly paying celebrities to endorse their drug? Were television testimonials kindling a bootleg market? By the late 1950s, FDA agents had documented a counterfeit tranquilizer business sustained by a network of small drug manufacturers and peddlers that included New Jersey, New York, Florida, Louisiana, and Texas. In New York City in 1956, for instance, a tablet of meprobamate could be had for nine cents with a prescription and upward of forty-two cents without. The illicit trade was so vast that the FDA's Division of Regulatory Management hired private investigators to document counterfeit sales. One woman wrote the FDA, demanding that it flex its regulatory might to stamp out the counterfeit commerce she had observed in her hometown of Daytona Beach. She alleged that large quantities were peddled at "cut-rate prices" by an individual "who [was] neither a licensed physician nor pharmacist." In Manhattan, police nabbed a pusher offering "hot Miltown" on the street.[26]

The FDA decided to investigate a possible link between celebrity endorsements and inappropriate tranquilizer use. In March 1956, FDA headquarters contacted its Los Angeles division. It observed that at the Emmy and Academy Award shows in 1955, Miltown was explicitly praised by Bob Cummings, Jimmy Durante, and Jerry Lewis. "The references of these screen and TV stars to the drug, and the rumor that the product can be bought over the counter in California, makes us inquire as to whether or not you have any knowledge of such type of sale in your

District area." A decoy agent in a covert investigation to secure Miltown without a prescription came up empty-handed. The pharmacist he approached at a Sunset Boulevard drugstore offered to phone the agent's physician on his behalf, but "assured me that I would need a prescription" before an order could be filled.[27]

The FDA dropped its investigation. Investigators sought but found no hint of advertising impropriety. Celebrities, it seemed, were simply smitten with their Miltown. At the next year's Academy Awards presentation, emcee Jerry Lewis happily revived his Miltown repertoire, promising nominees who failed to take home an Oscar that buttered Miltowns would be available in the lobby to help them deal with disappointment.[28]

Back on Madison Avenue, a spellbound advertising community monitored the media circus in awe. The Ted Bates Agency, Carter's advertising firm, had landed itself a winner. "Namewise, you'd think Miltown would never have had a chance in this business," marveled one advertising rival. "It just didn't have that ethical ring to it." But "what identity it turned out to have!" The agency was giddy over its product's success. "It was a dream campaign," gushed one Bates man. But the agency claimed only partial credit. The publicity was "partly [our] slugging away in there, partly just letting the thing roll on its own—you couldn't have stopped it," an associate recalled. At Carter, Henry Hoyt couldn't believe his good fortune. "I was frankly amazed at all the exposure we were getting," he recalled. The celebrity plug? "We never anticipated such a development. Those television actors—hell, we hadn't even sent them free Miltown or anything."[29]

While his boss basked in the Hollywood hype, Frank Berger was uneasy. The attention, he feared, would tarnish the company's reputation as a proprietor of ethical medicines and test the goodwill of physicians, who were not trained to prescribe prime-time fads. In Berger's mind, the media had responded "excessively and improperly," parlaying a serious matter—anxiety—into a "stupid joke."[30]

The conflicting views indexed a tension between the two men that would have profound implications for how Carter and other pharmaceutical firms courted medical support for new psychopharmaceuticals in the years that followed. In the mid-1950s, the future of biological psychiatry was as unclear as the commercial viability of an ethical psychotropic market. Would psychiatrists beholden to psychoanalytical concepts accept prescription pills as a useful adjunct to therapy? Would other doctors groomed to see anxiety as a cause or symptom of illnesses welcome tranquilizers into their expanding pharmaceutical arsenal? Neither Hoyt nor Berger was certain. Clearly the success of such a market hinged on doctors' willingness to prescribe drugs. Although not everyone agreed on the best strategy for securing doctors' prescription allegiance, companies and their advertising arms pioneered new forms of psychiatric salesmanship designed to build a loyal and dependable prescription base among a wide constituency of physicians. But deft medical marketing was only one part of the commercial creation of psychopharmacology. Even as advertising firms worked tirelessly to finesse the perfect message to sell psychiatric medicines, economic and political exigencies unexpectedly nudged even the most recalcitrant doctors down a pharmaceutical path.

(4)

Psychiatry in the
Medicine Cabinet

W hile Hollywood publicized Miltown to the general public, the tranquilizer revolution could not have happened without the cooperation of doctors who signed patients' scripts. Pharmaceutical companies aggressively courted doctors' new and vaunted economic power as gatekeepers to new psychiatric medications. Yet it would be a mistake to dismiss physicians as mere accomplices of the pharmaceutical industry or pawns of patient pressure. The therapeutic paradigm that propelled Miltown and other tranquilizers to a pivotal place in modern medicine was engineered by many forces. Indeed, as the age of biological psychiatry began to unfold, political and social circumstances shaped how doctors interpreted and prescribed Miltown.

From Detail Men to Doctors' Scripts

In the late spring of 1955, when Wallace was planning the market debut of Miltown, Berger and Hoyt found themselves locked in a serious advertising dispute. The 1950s had seen the rapid rise of the pharmaceutical salesman, or detail man, and Hoyt was among the many pharmaceutical executives clamoring to hire an army of them. The ranks of detailers (as they were also called) had swelled as the prescription drug industry grew. Patent medicine peddlers had been a familiar presence in American communities since the eighteenth century, and by the early twentieth, traveling medicine shows, picture postcards, ads in newspapers and magazines, and even radio sponsorships were used to promote proprietary drugs, such as cough syrups, hair tonics, and laxatives. The advertisement of ethical (prescription-only) drugs followed different rules. In an effort to place physicians above the fray and to distinguish the legitimacy of prescribed medications from the nostrums of quacks, the advertising of prescription drugs to the lay public was discouraged. Pharmaceutical outfits specializing in ethical medicines had few sales representatives, and product advertisements in medical journals favored the descriptive and the discreet. Before the Durham-Humphrey amendments were enacted in 1951, there was little incentive for active promotion. The vast majority of drugs consumed by Americans were over-the-counter remedies.[1]

The restructuring of the industry into prescription and over-the-counter markets, as well as the advent of promising and pricey ethical drugs, spurred companies to restrategize. After 1950, consumer spending on prescription drugs overtook proprietary sales; between 1929 and 1969, the portion of the drug market cornered by prescription medicines grew from 32 to 83 percent. In this new and competitive commercial landscape, where doctors controlled patient access to prescription drugs and patents gave companies a limited time—about twenty years—to profit from their products, securing physicians' brand loyalty was essential.[2]

The mushrooming pharmaceutical sales force reflected these new marketing imperatives. In the late 1920s there were 2,000 detail men (and pharmaceutical sales representatives were almost exclusively males) in the United States. By 1959, their numbers exceeded 15,000. These emissaries "detailed" doctors on the chemical properties and therapeutic advantages of their wares. Their objective was to persuade doctors to prescribe their employer's products. The pharmaceutical powerhouse Wyeth considered its detail men the most important link in its promotion and distribution system. Each had been groomed to perfection. A Wyeth detail man was typically a college graduate; biology, chemistry, and pharmacology majors were prized because their training equipped them with the scientific vernacular necessary to communicate to physicians. After joining the firm, a Wyeth man underwent an intensive eighteen-month training program. Upon graduation, he began making his rounds, spending about 75 percent of his time visiting doctors. Whether he worked for Wyeth or another pharmaceutical outfit, the detail man upheld an industry-wide code of style and deportment. Conservatively dressed, respectable in appearance, the detailer's demeanor bore all the trappings of medical objectivity and commercial neutrality. Only his mission—to cultivate product partisanship—betrayed the scientific facade.[3]

In this new era of pharmaceutical salesmanship, drug companies spared few expenses and opportunities to push their wares. Indeed, this marketing approach continues to guide drug promotion today. Journalist and mental health advocate Mike Gorman remembered the largesse showcased at psychiatry conventions in the 1950s. Doctors and other participants would be wooed by expensive cocktail parties and elegant dinners while being shadowed by ubiquitous sales representatives. Gorman recalled that it was difficult to walk five feet without encountering a detail man. It was equally unfathomable to pay one's own tab in a restaurant or a bar. Corporate lavishness was, in Gorman's eyes, akin to Roman splendor.[4]

It was precisely this commercial grandstanding that Frank Berger opposed. Immersed in the cutthroat world of pharmaceutical development, he retained his ideal that medicine ought to be a science unvarnished by materialist excess. He wanted Miltown to succeed—his royalties depended on it—but he found detailing distasteful and crass. He thought doctors should learn about drugs through independent trials published in journals free of industry ties. Neither medical meetings nor articles should have "an invested interest in the drug that is being discussed," he insisted. However good the sales pitch, it would never be science.[5]

Berger vowed to buck the detailing trend and in the spring of 1955, he met with representatives of the Ted Bates Agency, which handled the company's accounts. The advertising agency had no previous experience with prescription drugs and Berger, with the authority that came from being medical director and president of Wallace Laboratories, laid down the rules. There would be no detail men employed under his watch. Promotion would be restricted to journal advertising and mailings to physicians. Advertising was to be factual and educational.[6]

Until the day Berger retired in 1973, the company retained no detail men. This policy respected Berger's wishes but made the company an anomaly in the increasingly aggressive world of pharmaceutical marketing. As a result, Wallace Laboratories was largely unknown to doctors. Nor did its parent organization, Carter, still best known as a laxative manufacturer, have a track record that inspired physicians' confidence.[7]

As sales of Miltown floundered in the weeks after it went on the market, a worried Henry Hoyt sprang into action. At the end of June, he verbally accepted Wyeth's offer to sell meprobamate as Equanil. Strategizing about Equanil's imminent release, Hoyt gave Miltown a timely promotional push, instructing the Ted Bates Agency to initiate an aggressive print and mailing campaign. In the absence of detail men, the agency relied on the U.S. postal service to spread word of the new tranquilizer. In their morning mail, physicians across the country began receiving offprints of clinical studies and company reference manuals touting the wonders of Miltown. Equally important, Hoyt urged the agency to gather anecdotes of tranquilizer triumphs that, together with scientific studies, could be used to tip the lay press. FDA regulations forbade direct-to-consumer advertising, but nothing proscribed planting stories about the new drug to magazines and newspapers, a strategy that helped achieve the same results. "We supplied dope on Miltown for pieces in *Time, Newsweek,* the *Saturday Evening Post,* and so many I could hardly name them," a Bates man recalled. As Hoyt knew from his Little Liver Pill experience, patients were often the greatest enthusiasts of drugs.[8]

But Berger's perspicacity about doctors' loyalties and prescribing behavior proved prescient. The street popularity of Miltown and Carter's commercial background gave doctors pause. In 1956 physicians began to back Wyeth's Equanil, the "other meprobamate." Wyeth sold 100 million Equanil tablets—enough for 2 million prescriptions—in January alone. Within months, Wyeth had eclipsed Wallace's share of the meprobamate market. Try as it might, Wallace never caught up. By 1960 Equanil outsold

Miltown three to one. Both would later be dwarfed in the 1960s by the phenomenal success of the benzodiazepine tranquilizers Librium and Valium.[9]

Wyeth's ability to harness the prescribing power of the doctors owed something to the company's carefully guarded reputation as a dignified outfit that would not stoop to cavort with the lay press. But Equanil's success also gathered momentum from Wyeth's energetic and slick campaign to win the loyalty of physicians, exactly the sort of drug promotion Berger had vetoed for Miltown. While ordinary Americans heard about Miltown from Uncle Miltie, doctors learned of Equanil, chemically identical to Miltown but lacking its crass popular baggage, from hundreds of suited men distributing samples, paraphernalia, and pamphlets. In the words of one advertising executive, Equanil was the tranquilizer no one joked about.[10] To doctors, that distinction was golden. The company played up this difference to its advantage, using traditional and conservative images and language to strengthen the drug's identity as a dignified medicine. While Miltown was being hyped in tabloids, promotions for Equanil advertising turned to the words of William Shakespeare. One Wyeth brochure, an example of the company's adroit marketing maneuvers, displayed a world map entitled "Equanimity . . . the universal need," showing a pair of human eyes anxiously surveying the equatorial latitudes. The caption came from *Macbeth:*

Canst thou not . . .
Raze out the written troubles of the brain
And with some sweet oblivious antidote
Cleanse the stuff'd bosom of that perilous
Stuff
Which weights upon the heart?[11]

The answer was yes, with three tablets of Equanil a day.

Carter tried in vain to countermand Wyeth's coup. Twice it had bungled, misjudging the marketing psychology of doctors. It had stalled the launch of meprobamate by deferring to a survey of doctors' prescription preferences that subsequent sales had proven wrong. Now it had alienated doctors in bypassing physicians and promoting the drug indirectly to patients. Hoping to make up for past blunders and restore Miltown to market supremacy, Carter made a concerted effort to influence medical minds.

The Ted Bates Agency stepped up Miltown's mailing campaign, sending not only offprints and manuals but specially produced Miltown phonograph records—seven different albums by 1960. Doctors could play them in well-equipped waiting rooms or listen to them at home. One side featured soothing, usually classical, music; on the other was what Hoyt called a scientific discussion of Miltown. One LP combined a recording of violinist David Oistrakh playing Smetana melodies with an endorsement for Miltown use by pregnant women. Another, mailed during the stressful holiday season, offered "The Twelve Days of Christmas" and an infomercial for Wallace's new appetite suppressant, Appetrol. The compound combined dextro-amphetamine with meprobamate "to relieve the tension of dieting." Eventually promotional mailings included not only records and reprints, but also free drug samples, which reached more than 92,000 physicians, roughly half of all practicing doctors in the United States. The company estimated that its advertising cost $9.22 per physician, mostly general practitioners and psychiatrists.[12]

The agency likewise made the most of Aldous Huxley's timely and widely reported endorsement of meprobamate in his lecture at the New York Academy of Sciences. The proceedings of the symposium Huxley participated in were published in *Meprobamate and Other Agents Used in Mental Disturbances*. The Ted Bates Agency made 153,000 copies of the report and sent them to physicians, courtesy of Wallace Laboratories.[13]

Wallace also increased the number of ads it published in medical journals. To disarm critics worried that tranquilizers would try to muscle out psychoanalysis in the treatment of neurosis, the company advertised Miltown as a valuable adjunct to psychotherapy. Fearing that some doctors would regard drugging the brain as incompatible with the personal and subjective orientation of talk therapy, Carter positioned minor tranquilizers as just another tool in the analyst's arsenal, a chemical aid that would enable psychiatrists to relax their patients, peel back layers of repression

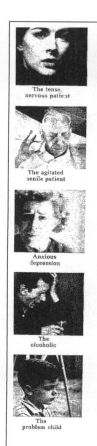

Belongs in Every Practice. Versatile, dependable, and easy to use, Miltown was touted for its "outstanding record of safety," a claim that would be challenged in the 1960s and 1970s. As did other tranquilizer firms, Carter-Wallace tried to create a broadly based demographic market that would encourage tranquilizer use from cradle to grave. *American Journal of Psychiatry*, July 1964.

and inhibition, and identify the crux of their problems sooner. An advertisement in the *American Journal of Psychiatry* showed a psychiatrist, pen in hand, consulting a young man whose face was seized with worry. Bold letters delivered the advertisement's main message: Miltown "improves rapport when anxiety blocks therapeutic progress in private practice." Miltown merely helped the psychoanalyst do his job better (the doctor in Miltown ads was always male). It reduced anxiety levels and helped the patient overcome "neurotic inhibitions," improving patient cooperation and facilitating productive sessions. Ads such as these reinforced the importance of neurosis as a medical disorder while acknowledging the centrality of the psychiatrist's therapeutic role.[14]

Journal ads were not exactly high art but, intriguingly, Carter's promotional tactics included that too. As luck would have it, Gala Dali, wife of the Spanish surrealist painter Salvador Dali, took Miltown. (Another famous "Miltown wife" was Jane Cheney Spock, whose husband Benjamin drew heavily on psychoanalytic theory in his bestselling and hugely influential *Baby and Child Care*.) Frank Berger recalled that Gala Dali approached him to suggest that the company commission her husband to depict through art the experience of being pharmaceutically liberated from anxiety. Hoyt consented, as did Dali. So began one of the oddest collaborations in the history of medical marketing. Berger remembers Dali as eccentric and theatrical: "he liked to be photographed in urinals . . . and had flies in [tailor-made] glass frames so that there was constant movement around him." Fittingly, in 1958, Dali produced one of the most unusual exhibits ever to grace the halls of the annual meeting of the American Medical Association.[15]

The *Crisalida*, Dali's Miltown masterpiece, consisted of a two-and-a-half ton tunnel shaped like a cocoon, braced by undulating silk walls that mimicked the appearance and texture of skin. Doctors who dared enter the head passed through its pulsating, ribbed body and exited via the tail. Elongated murals showed the stages of transformation from anxiety, depicted as a gnarled figure full of holes, to tranquil peace, portrayed as a figure whose head was crowned with flowers. On the figure's staff was a butterfly, the symbol of transformation and, according to Dali, the "nirvana of the human soul." In addition to the installation, Dali painted images of the pharmaceutical metamorphosis that were reproduced in a commemorative Miltown pamphlet doctors could take home.[16]

Dali suggested that tranquility was a precondition of genius and, he exclaimed, "I am the only artist today who has this." In an immodest and misleading assessment of the rationale for his commission, he told the press that Wallace had approached him "because in Dali pictures there is found the most extraordinary tranquility." He added, "I alone was capable of designing the Crisalida. Picasso? Almost, but he is too much of a modern man. . . . I am the only one who combines all—philosophy, psychology, science, and love." Although one observer referred to the exhibit as

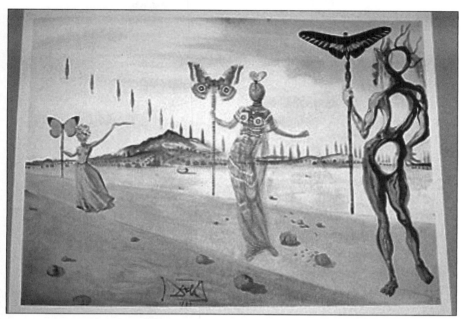

Dali's Crisalida/Crisalida at the Convention. In an intriguing chapter in the history of pharmaceutical marketing, Carter-Wallace commissioned Salvador Dali to commemorate the experience of being liberated of anxiety with Miltown. Dali's *Crisalida*, which premiered at the 1958 meeting of the American Medical Association, included a sixty-foot, pulsating, walk-through cocoon, said to depict man's metamorphosis from "the evils of nightmares" to "divine and paradisiac dreams" and a souvenir pamphlet featuring original artwork. *Business Week*, June 28, 1958. Program image, pictured above, copyright © 2008 Salvador Dali, Gala-Salvador Dali Foundation/Artists Rights Society (ARS), New York.

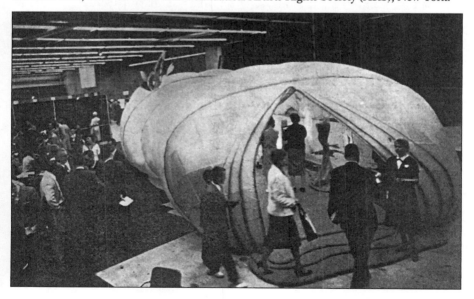

about as aesthetically appealing as a piece of army equipment, Dali insisted that it captured how Miltown enabled mortals to pass "through the evils of nightmares to divine and paradisiacal dreams."[17]

What doctors thought about the *Crisalida* and Wallace's other bids for their support is unknown. What *is* clear is that a critical mass of physicians came to regularly prescribe the drug. Only fourteen months after it had been made available, meprobamate was the country's fastest-selling prescription medication. And although Equanil outsold Miltown, Wyeth's licensing agreement delivered Carter hefty profits. By the end of the decade, Wyeth's annual payments defrayed the cost of manufacturing the pills for both companies and still cleared Carter $1 million in profit. With Miltown and Equanil sales booming, it is no wonder that Carter Products and American Home Products were declared the two most profitable companies in the nation.[18]

Tranquilizers and the Rise of Psychopharmacology

Clearly doctors were influenced by the promotional campaigns of pharmaceutical companies and patient demands, but they were also guided by the conviction that new psychiatric medicines were doing some good. One year before meprobamate's release, McGill University psychiatrist Heinz Edgar Lehmann had transfixed the psychiatric world with reports of the first clinical trial of the drug chlorpromazine. Lehmann was clinical director of Verdun Protestant Hospital, a psychiatric institution in Montreal, later renamed Douglas Hospital. The rise of psychoanalysis hadn't made much of an impact on patients institutionalized at psychiatric hospitals such as Verdun. Such "incurables" filled the wards of asylums throughout Canada and the United States. Most institutions were publicly funded, overcrowded, and understaffed. At Verdun, Lehmann was one of only a handful of physicians assigned to treat some 1,600 confined patients; his personal patient load exceeded 600. Beginning in the late 1940s, the mental asylum, derogatorily referred to as the "snake pit" (the title of the stirring 1948 film starring Olivia de Havilland that showcased the horrors of psychiatric institutions) became a lightning rod for public criticism as journalists, filmmakers, and health lobbyists exposed the mistreatment and neglect of psychiatric patients. At the same time, politicians denounced the millions of dollars taxpayers spent keeping these institutions afloat. Compounding these criticisms was the fact that many medical treatments of the time failed to cure patients. A significant number were discharged only after undergoing lobotomy, a surgery performed on over 5,000 patients in 1949 in the United States alone.[19]

Lehmann was a physician's son whose interest in psychiatry was kindled by his own experience with depression in early adolescence. During these difficult years, a tutor steered him toward the work of Sigmund Freud. Many psychiatry books later, Lehmann was hooked. After graduating with an M.D. from the University of Berlin, Lehmann immigrated to Montreal, where in 1937 he was hired as a junior psychiatrist at Verdun.[20]

While working at the hospital and teaching psychiatry at McGill University in the early 1950s, Lehmann stumbled across an article left by a sales representative from the French pharmaceutical firm Rhône-Poulenc. The study reported on a newly synthesized drug being used on psychotic patients in France, a sedative called chlorpromazine. Unlike many of his North American colleagues, Lehmann was fluent in French (his wife Annette was French Canadian), and he read the article during a Sunday evening bath; he ordered a supply from the company the following day. With the help of a colleague, he launched a clinical trial in 1953 on seventy patients suffering from schizophrenia, severe depression, mania, psychomotor excitement, and organic dementia. The results were remarkable. In a matter of weeks, patients who had previously entertained no hope of recovery or discharge found themselves symptom-free. "We knew we had something very unique," Lehmann remembered. "In fact, we had never had anything like it."[21]

Lehmann published the results of his study in 1954. Even before the article came out, word of his results had reached the United States. As a result, chlorpromazine, sold by Smith Kline & French Laboratories under the brand name Thorazine, was quickly adopted in mental health institutions such as Pilgrim State Hospital in New York, the nation's largest. Tales of miraculous remissions and unexpected discharges spread like wildfire. No one doubted the drug's significance. As Lehmann put it, the coming of chlorpromazine represented nothing less than "the most dramatic breakthrough in psychopharmacotherapy since the advent of anesthesia more than a century before."[22]

Thorazine inaugurated the massive deinstitutionalization of psychiatric patients, chiefly schizophrenics. In 1955, for the first time in twenty-five years, the annual intake of hospitalized mental patients declined. Thorazine's clinical efficacy, attributable to its action on neurotransmitters, served to buttress a theory that would become the bedrock of the new biological psychiatry: the notion that mental illnesses were caused by malfunctioning brain biology rather than patients' bad upbringing or flawed character. This was a startlingly new way to conceive of mental illness. Chlorpromazine's success provided scientists with a promising research agenda. If mental illness was caused by chemical deficiencies, then finding the right chemical cocktail could return the brain to a normal state and make sick people well. Helping schizophrenics would be only the beginning.[23]

A gradual shift in how psychiatrists understood the etiology of mental illness from a psychodynamic to a biochemical model helps explain the hyperbole of a new generation of biological psychiatrists who identified effective drugs as evidence of progress and cause for hope. Researchers, government agencies, and drug firms searched for pharmaceutical answers to baffling psychiatric problems. The widespread adoption and demonstrated value of drugs such as chlorpromazine and reserpine, known as the major tranquilizers in the United States (and more likely to be called antipsychotics or neuroleptics in Europe), lent credence to the claim that synthetic solutions might exist for other psychiatric disorders too.[24]

A spirit of pharmaceutical optimism thus underwrote medical responses to Miltown's release. As much as physicians objected to Miltown's tabloid-and-television popularization, few could deny its clinical efficacy. Doctors' evaluations of the benefits of psychopharmacology were also shaped by political and economic concerns. Whether disorders were severe enough to require periodic hospitalization or treatable on an outpatient basis, they were disrupting families, undermining workplace efficiency, and depleting the nation's financial reserves. Throughout the 1950s, psychiatrists, lawmakers, and lobbyists continued to discuss psychiatric illness as the nation's leading public health problem. Mike Gorman's explosive *Every Other Bed,* published in 1956, described mental illness as a billion dollar a year problem, given that "every other bed" in tax-supported hospitals was occupied by the mentally ill. In 1956, 10 million Americans were estimated to be psychologically unwell—about one of every seventeen people. By 1959, the figure had been revised upward to 17.5 million—one of every ten. Of these, only a fraction was thought to need hospitalization. The vast majority had disorders such as neurosis that could be treated on an outpatient basis. Indeed, some psychiatrists believed that neurosis affected as many as a third of all Americans, ordinary folks "not operating on all eight cylinders because of psychological sludge."[25]

Lobbyists looked to the pharmaceutical industry for cost-saving drugs and a way out of this psychiatric morass. This was the golden age of applied science, when the fruits of laboratory research seemed bountiful. The invention of a war-ending atomic bomb and the discovery of the insecticide DDT (which won the Nobel Prize in 1948) were powerful tributes to the success of institutional research in the United States. Pharmaceutical firms had recently produced a batch of new wonder drugs. Penicillin was capped by a succession of other stunning achievements: corticosteroids, broad-spectrum antibiotics, antidepressants, and the first pills to treat hypertension and diabetes. Children survived what a few years earlier might have been a deadly bout with bacterial pneumonia, and adults with rheumatoid arthritis were liberated from wheelchairs through cortisone. These well-publicized triumphs provided tangible evidence of the wonders wrought by pharmaceutical science.[26]

No problem seemed beyond science's reach. New drugs gave doctors an armamentarium of therapies to treat a wide array of disorders. In the eyes of many, these agents were nothing less than magic bullets: medicines that acted on specific illnesses while leaving patients otherwise intact. Illnesses once treated with potentially toxic remedies or regarded as medically insurmountable could now be controlled, even cured, by a pill. After World War II, the mass expansion of federally funded research by the National Institutes of Health and the National Science Foundation had encouraged

Americans to believe that they would personally benefit from the work being conducted in laboratories across the country. The arrival of a cornucopia of life-saving drugs further fueled this expectant optimism. Nor in the 1950s was there cause to doubt the safety of prescription medications. The Thalidomide tragedy and diethylstilbestrol (DES) disaster had yet to occur. (In the early 1970s synthetic estrogen, DES, prescribed since the 1940s to millions of American women, often to prevent miscarriage, was linked to a higher incidence of cancer in female offspring.) Against this backdrop, Americans looked to laboratory-driven science for answers to vexing medical problems. [27]

In a political environment captivated by the possibilities of pharmaceutical medicine, scientists demanded government support for psychopharmaceutical research. The National Mental Health Act of 1946 had called for a freestanding National Institute of Mental Health (NIMH), which became operational in 1949. In 1956 Congress funded the Psychopharmacology Service Center within the NIMH to support the development and testing of psychiatric drugs, largely in response to the persuasive testimony of psychopharmacologist Nathan Kline, renowned for his pioneering work on reserpine, and journalist and lobbyist Mike Gorman. Testifying before the Senate Appropriations Subcommittee on Labor, Health, Education, and Welfare in 1956, Gorman asked the government to support scientists who "conduct fundamental research leading to the development of new and more effective drugs in the field of mental illness." Gorman was optimistic about pharmaceutical research because, like many in this era, he believed it was helping the mentally ill. Researchers inspired by the chlorpromazine breakthrough were searching for psychiatry's other wonder drugs: medicines to "compensate for some particular defect in body chemistry, much as insulin shots used for treating diabetics compensate for a failure of the pancreas."[28]

Many clinical psychiatrists were equally sanguine. No symbol in the 1950s conveyed scientific might more forcefully than the atomic bomb, and it is telling that psychiatrists often invoked cold war metaphors of apocalyptic power to describe psychopharmaceutical development. Nathan Kline characterized the advent of psychopharmacology as comparable to a thermonuclear explosion that marked the end of one era and the beginning of another. Indeed, he said, the creation of psychiatric drugs may "be of markedly greater import in the history of mankind than the atom bomb since if these drugs provide the long-awaited key which will unlock the mysteries of the relationship of man's chemical constitution to his psychological behavior and provide effective means of correcting pathological needs there may no longer be any necessity for turning thermonuclear energy to destructive purposes."[29]

It was a lot to ask of research, to treat psychiatric illness and to establish world peace. But Kline's remarks captured the rising confidence in biochemistry as a tool to engineer both better brains and a better world. Cold warriors enthralled by pharmacology's powers imagined a society where drugs and other mind-altering technologies might be employed to safeguard state secrets, force spies to reveal them, or allow Americans to be productive on three hours' sleep. This kind of thinking, propelled by cold war paranoia, prompted horrible abuses, such as the CIA's clandestine mind control program, a series of sinister experiments that involved brainwashing, drugging, sleep deprivation, and blitzkrieg electroshocks. The CIA's covert activities were a far cry from therapy, but they reflected how cold war fears and the optimism of neurobiology could overlap, even merge. Also undergirding researchers' zeal was the daunting fear that if Americans didn't invent such agents first, then surely the Russians would. "I'd be surprised if the Russians aren't on to these drugs," Kline told the *Wall Street Journal* about preliminary tests of sleep-deprivation pills. "What would a few more hours of work a day mean to Russian industrial output?" Apparently, quite a lot. Psychopharmacology's ability to heal ordinary individuals was inextricably linked to its power to help the world's richest and most capitalistic country function at full capacity. Drugs that freed schizophrenics from institutions saved taxpayers millions. Drugs that boosted workplace efficiency were a powerful lubricant to the industrial machine. In the new era of psychopharmacology, political, economic, and medical imperatives converged.[30]

Doctors thus encountered Miltown in a milieu deeply invested in pharmaceutical panaceas. At a time when ethical drugs were enjoying

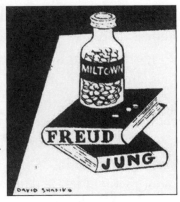

Miltown on Top. Given the popularity of psychoanalysis, executives at Carter-Wallace initially doubted that there would be medical interest in a pill for everyday anxiety. Instead, Miltown became a runaway bestseller, the first psychotropic blockbuster in U.S. history. "Drugs for the Mind," by David Shapiro from the July 21, 1956 issue of *The Nation.* Reprinted with permission from *The Nation.*

unprecedented cultural legitimacy and psychopharmacology was a beacon of hope, the debut of an antianxiety pill induced much enthusiasm. Medical researcher and clinical psychiatrist Frank Ayd, one of the founders of the American College of Neuro-Psychopharmacology, remembered the buzz surrounding Miltown at the American Psychiatric Association (APA) meeting in 1955. Chlorpromazine and reserpine were getting plenty of attention, but what really had psychiatrists atwitter was Miltown. Ayd recalled that few psychiatrists or science writers returned from the conference unaware of its existence.[31]

Doctors who prescribed meprobamate welcomed it to their expanding pharmaceutical options. No one disputed that meprobamate was a marked improvement over traditional sedatives such as bromides, chloral hydrate, and the discredited but still popular barbiturates. Carter's claim that "suicidal attempts with Miltown have been unsuccessful despite the ingestion of large amounts of the drug" would subsequently be challenged, but at the time doctors believed it. As Frank Ayd observed in 1960, physicians were keenly aware of the disadvantages and limitations of older compounds. When newer drugs became available and "it was obvious that they represented a distinct advance," doctors naturally started to prescribe them "for millions of people for whom there was previously no satisfactory medicinal agent."[32]

Others emphasized the superiority of tranquilizers to other anti-anxiety substances. "No drug is wholly without side effects," counseled *For-*

tune. "But by and large [tranquilizers] carry fewer physiological penalties than . . . alcohol, and they seem to be less habit-forming than cigarettes." Indeed, meprobamate won rave reviews from doctors seeking to shepherd alcoholics through the psychologically and physically painful stages of withdrawal. In studies at Yale and in Boston, the drug had controlled some of its most common and debilitating symptoms: anxiety, tremors, and depression.[33]

Doctors also had sound political reasons for prescribing Miltown. By helping individuals coexist with life's everyday challenges, the drug allowed America collectively to cope. "What is important to me as a practitioner who treats patients only outside of hospitals," Frank Ayd told a Senate subcommittee, "is the fact that the drugs have permitted many patients to remain at home and to work, despite the persistence of their basic disorder. To me, this is not a small accomplishment." Kline also trumpeted the virtues of a drug that could keep the engine of economic output humming. The use of meprobamate restores "full efficiency to business executives" and puts artists and writers "suffering from long periods of nonproductivity because of 'mental blocks'" back on track. Productivity, efficiency, social stability—these were watchwords of political strength as well as mental health.[34]

Not every doctor supported the use of tranquilizers. Psychiatrists and other physicians have never been a monolithic group, and their theories and therapies in the 1950s varied, much as they do today. In the age of Miltown, doctors discussed the pros and cons of tranquilizers and heatedly debated when the threshold separating normal and pathological anxiety had been breached. As psychologists Raymond B. Cattell and Ivan H. Scheier explained in a pioneering medical article in the late 1950s, for "researchers as well as laymen, this is the age of anxiety." Plenty of work had been undertaken by scientists, theorists, clinicians, and philosophers to pinpoint anxiety's causes and cures. But, Cattell and Scheier asked, "can we honestly claim that our understanding of anxiety has increased in proportion to the huge research effort expended or even increased perceptibility? We think not." For all of the pontificating on its meaning, measurement, and treatment, anxiety remained a field of "conceptual chaos."[35]

Discussions among the New York Academy of Medicine's Subcommittee on Tranquilizing Drugs, which first convened in the fall of 1956, the divisions gripping the psychiatric community. One doctor worried that high prescription rates in New York City, estimated to range from 5 to 10 percent of all prescriptions filled, pointed to indiscriminate use, while another insisted that other drugs, such as the stimulant Benzedrine, posed a greater social problem. Several psychiatrists on the committee wondered about meprobamate's adverse effects, including depression and habit formation; others insisted they had observed no such complications among patients. The subcommittee's final report, approved in December 1956, raised a series of unresolved questions mirroring the disparate views of committee members. "Anxiety and tension seem to abound in our modern culture and the current trend is to escape the unpleasantness of its impact," it proclaimed. "But when has life ever been exempt from stress? In the long run is it desirable that a population be ever free from tension? Should there be a pill for every mood or occasion?" These insightful comments presage current debates about the intrinsic value of using lifestyle drugs (tranquilizers but also drugs for sexual dysfunction, baldness, or acne) to treat what some construe as nonmedical problems. The subcommittee offered no definitive answers but called on empirical research, specifically the putatively objective science of epidemiology, to resolve the question of toxicity and therapeutic merit. "It should be clearly stated that the magnitude of prescriptions for tranquilizing drugs does not prove that they are a menace to public health," the report insisted. Until "science" weighed in, the drugs should be used judiciously and always under medical supervision. In 1957 the APA issued a statement declaring tranquilizers a "useful adjunct in the psychiatric treatment of certain patients in private practice and on an outpatient basis in clinics and hospitals." But it warned that casual and daily use of tranquilizers by the public to relieve everyday tension was medically unsound because insufficient time had elapsed to determine the drugs' side effects. The APA left it to individual doctors to decide what constituted medically appropriate use.[36]

Several analytically oriented physicians expressed more tendentious views. Oregon psychiatrist Henry Dixon insisted that learning how to coexist with anxiety was a necessary prequel to mental wellness. People who go too long in a state of tranquility, he cautioned, were unable to benefit from the trial and error that comes from learning. The long-term implications were troubling. "We then face the prospect of developing a falsely flaccid race of people which might not be too good for our future." Dr. Janet A. Kennedy, a New York psychoanalyst, agreed. She insisted that tension and working out problems by oneself was normal. It was the completely worry-free individual who was mentally ill. Kennedy rarely used tranquilizers in her practice. "Nor do I know many psychoanalysts who do."[37]

Some doctors and researchers in the 1950s went a step further, proclaiming anxiety as nothing less than the seedbed of human artistic and intellectual talent. "Van Gogh, Isaac Newton: most of the geniuses and great creators were not tranquil," enthused one contemporary. "They were nervous, ego-driven men pushed on by a relentless inner force and beset by anxieties." To mollify those demons might purge society of its most brilliant or creative members.[38]

Reflecting their ambivalence about neurosis as psychopathology, some psychiatrists drew contrasts between major and minor tranquilizers and the different illnesses they treated. Chlorpromazine and reserpine's benefits for the hospitalized mentally ill should not be confused with meprobamate's benefit as a tranquilizer for the masses. Although he would later modify his views, Heinz Lehmann was initially critical of meprobamate's widespread use. "You cannot cure an anxiety state with pills," he told a Senate subcommittee in 1960. Like others in the field, he believed pills diminished feelings of anxiety by stifling a patient's "spontaneity, his creativeness, his independence." Because anxiety was not comparable to psychosis, doctors should not assume that a pharmacological compound could treat it. With schizophrenia, "it is likely that some physical factor is involved and, therefore, a physical agent like a pill . . . would be logical as a weapon against it." Anxiety and tension states were different. They were caused by "psychological reasons, and to fight a psychological condition with a physical agent doesn't make sense." Yet even Lehmann recognized that meprobamate was better than barbiturates. He put one of his patients, a barbiturate user for ten years, on meprobamate. In Lehmann's mind, it represented a switch to a "lesser evil." He reported that the patient was doing well.[39]

Psychiatrists expressed their opinions in interviews, before Congress, on radio, and even on television. NBC's *The American Forum of the Air*, a live weekly radio and television production that discussed controversial issues, dedicated a broadcast to the subject of "Tranquilizer Drugs—Blessing or Danger?" in July 1956. Dr. Herman Denber, director of psychiatric research at the Manhattan State Hospital, criticized the widespread use of minor tranquilizers. Echoing Lehmann's demarcation between psychosis and neurosis, Denber urged viewers to differentiate between "patients in a psychiatric hospital who have had a psychiatric breakdown, and . . . the man in the street who is a little nervous because he has to make a speech or a man who has had a battle with his wife and they are about to break up, or a person who feels he doesn't like his job and therefore he is anxious, or a person who doesn't get along well with his boss." The former was medication worthy. The latter was not. Learning how to manage these social problems required time and a therapist's care, not vials of pills. Mike Gorman, another guest, decried the elitism of Denber's method. At an average of $25 an hour, psychoanalysis had become "inaccessible to 90 percent of the income groups in the country." It cost too much and took too long. Should people suffer psychologically for want of money? Surely not, Gorman raged. "We are born into a world where there is insecurity and where there is anxiety," he proclaimed in a sideswipe at psychoanalysis. "If we cannot afford the detailed, long analyses—which have their own side effects, incidentally, some of them quite disastrous, economically and otherwise—I think it is good for many people in the out-patient world [to] be calmed down and helped during this thing."[40]

Gorman's rebuttal touched on a critical component of the psychopharmaceutical revolution. However much psychiatrists—only about 20 percent of whom practiced office-based psychiatry when Miltown hit the shelves—disagreed about the merits of a little anxiety or the therapeutic value of tranquilizers, patients themselves were increasingly turning to their family doctors rather than psychiatrists for help. As psychiatrists debated the virtues of couch time versus pill time, the American public over-whelmingly endorsed the latter. It is an interesting paradox that Miltown's phenomenal success in spawning the development of biological psychiatry and the expanded use of psychiatric medications was carried out by nonpsychiatrists.[41]

Psychiatry Goes Mainstream

The marginalization of psychiatry in the mid-1950s owed much to the fact that it lacked the same social and scientific credibility as other medical disciplines. This stigmatization shaped the profession in ways that de-terred doctors from entering its ranks. In 1955 the average psychiatrist earned $18,000, significantly less than the $25,000 average salary of a surgeon. Family members and academic mentors discouraged medical stu-dents from selecting psychiatry as a specialty. Heinz Lehmann remem-bered his father's scorn over his decision to become a psychiatrist. Before the psychopharmaceutical turn, he recalled, psychiatry was viewed as "a rather derelict career. People only went there if they couldn't do anything else—or were alcoholic."[42]

Decades later, psychiatrist Stephen Stahl remembers his family's am-bivalence about the field. As a medical student in the 1970s, when psy-chiatry departments remained divided between analytic and biological schools, he "thought that psychiatrists were a little loony," often lacking the scientific and quantitative rigor of other clinicians. Stahl was leaning toward a career in neurology when he decided that the field of biological psychiatry had advanced sufficiently for him to become a "pharmacolo-gist of the brain." His parents, hoping that he'd become an obstetrician, took longer to forgive him; in their minds, psychiatry was still profes-sionally dubious.[43]

The field's identity crisis meant a shortage of psychiatrists and linger-ing doubts among patients who feared being stigmatized if they needed a shrink. Psychoanalysis was more firmly rooted in American psychiatry than anywhere else. In Germany the Nazis had purged it, and in the So-viet Union it was banned. But the grip of psychoanalysis on the nation's psychiatry profession was often at odds with the desires and needs of ordinary Americans, who frequently challenged its tenets, its methods, and the financial and time commitments it demanded. Many Americans were uneasy with the prospect of disclosing their dreams or fantasies on a therapist's couch. In addition, no one could demonstrate conclusively that psychoanalysis worked. One study compared rates of improvement between groups of anxious patients who received psychoanalysis and those kept on the waiting list who received none. The outcomes for the two groups were identical.[44]

For the budget conscious and the time strapped, for the hesitant and the skeptical, pills provided a seemingly more straightforward route to treat run-of-the-mill anxiety. Relatively cheap and easy to take, they bypassed the time and possible discomfort of therapy. They fit snuggly within the confines of a doctor-patient relationship: an ordinary person talking to a physician about a routine problem that a seemingly benign "emotional aspirin" or "peace pill," as Miltown was variously called, could fix. The fact that anxiety was being blamed as the cause of a myriad medical disorders, from ulcers to asthma, made its treatment the legitimate domain of nonpsychiatrists. Indeed, like Heinz Lehmann, patients stridently distinguished themselves from people afflicted with serious psychiatric illnesses. In most patients' minds, Miltown enhanced the functionality of successful people; it was, one contemporary averred, "just the thing" for "perfectly normal people who need temporary help." It was no surprise, then, that with the advent of Miltown, Americans consulted the doctors they were most likely to see for routine problems—family practitioners, internists, pediatricians, and obstetrician-gynecologists.[45]

The popularity of new psychiatric drugs promoted the rise of biological psychiatry and shored up psychiatry's scientific credentials. The biochemical revolution also fueled the diversification of psychiatric practice by transferring it from the specialist's office to the generalist's prescription pad. In the age of Miltown, frontline psychiatric diagnoses and treatment became the therapeutic province of physicians who had little advanced training in psychiatry. By 1960, nearly three-quarters of all doctors in the United States prescribed meprobamate. Of these, only a small minority were psychiatrists.[46] The medical management of anxiety had gone mainstream.

This was one of Miltown's lasting contributions to the psychopharmacology revolution. Miltown's success, fomented by the prescription practices of nonpsychiatrists, forged a new patient-doctor relationship in which Americans increasingly came to regard mental health—first anxiety, then depression, attention deficit disorder, bipolar disorder, and so on—as grounds for routine medical consultation and pharmacological intervention. More than just an effective tranquilizer, Miltown encouraged greater social acceptance of and dependence on lifestyle drugs. It stitched together patients, doctors, and pharmaceutical companies in a web of psychotropic drug consumption, setting the stage for the massive expansion of the country's psychopharmaceutical armory.

Behind the rising tide of scripts and profits lay not only physician acquiescence but also patient enthusiasm. The pill phenomenon launched in Hollywood quickly broadened its reach. Indeed, as important as inventors, manufacturers, and doctors were to the Miltown story, the greatest agents of change in the rise of a tranquilizer culture were indubitably patients themselves.

(5)

Arsenals of the Anxious

On August 29, 1949, the unthinkable happened. In a remote corner in Kazakhstan, the Soviet Union detonated its first atomic bomb. U.S. spy planes positioned off the coast of Siberia detected the atmospheric disturbance, and Geiger counters registered a surge of radioactivity that could only be explained by an atomic explosion. Since July 16, 1945, when the United States detonated its first thermonuclear device in the New Mexico desert, the government had been responsible for eight detonations. Then, without forewarning, the Russians shattered America's nuclear monopoly.[1]

President Harry Truman struggled to find the right moment to deliver the devastating news. At 11:00 A.M. on September 23, he updated his cabinet at its weekly meeting. Elsewhere in the White House, Charles Ross, Truman's secretary, detained correspondents an extra half-hour after a routine press meeting. He filed the apprehensive journalists into his office, closed the door, and posted a member of the Secret Service to stand guard. Clutching pens and paper, they waited. Ross waited too, delivering the news only after he was certain Truman had finished his cabinet briefing. Reporters' yells shattered the uneasy silence. "Russia has the atomic bomb!" one shouted. They dashed through the door to the telephones in the nearby press room.[2]

It was a milestone in the loss of nuclear innocence that opened a new chapter in what W. H. Auden had declared the "Age of Anxiety." The country's vulnerability to nuclear attack incited widespread worry, notwith-standing the soft-spoken quips from the chair of the Joint Chiefs of Staff that the "calmer the American people take this the better." Americans' distress was the foreboding attendant to having their fate held hostage by men in the White House and the Kremlin. There were gnawing doubts about America's leadership too. Nuclear scientists had miscalculated by at least three years the time the Russians needed to reach atomic parity. Even in April, *Business Week* had breezily announced, "Few atomic people are inclined to think the Russians have made much progress."[3]

The months that followed brought more bad news. In late 1949, China's communist leader Mao Zedong ousted Chiang Kai-shek, toppling the Nationalist government the United States had spent $3 billion propping up. The world's most populous country had gone red. John Foster Dulles, a leading Republican voice on international affairs, called Mao's victory "the worst defeat the United States has suffered in its history." Things got worse on June 27, 1950, when Truman announced that he had committed American troops to Korea.[4]

For a country that had defeated Hitler, won a war with Japan, and invented the atomic bomb, problems of this magnitude were not to be taken lightly. Americans prepared themselves to withstand a nuclear attack, if only because they believed they could. Call it patriotism, call it denial; some later called it foolish. But across the forty-eight states, men, women, and children got ready. They stocked family bomb shelters with canned soup, flashlights, portable radios, and first aid kits. They built warning sirens and established community evacuation plans. Schools taught children to "duck and cover" as if it would enable them to withstand the heat and debris of a nuclear strike. These readiness rituals reflected an equal measure of terror and faith. The apocalypse *could* be prepared for. And with the right tools and techniques, the nuclear devastation might be endured.

The flush of enthusiasm surrounding Miltown needs to be understood within this political ambit. When journalists in the United States announced the discovery of minor tranquilizers, they broke the news in a culture suffused with atomic anxiety and striving to find a means of attenuating and containing it.

The Frantic Fifties

What had begun as Hollywood's hottest drug sensation swept the nation. A Gallup Poll conducted in early 1957 found that among the 7 million Americans who had tried it, northeasterners had become as familiar with meprobamate as those on the West Coast. Soon the frenzy had spread inland to the Midwest and the South. A second study in mid-1957 funded by *Fortune* determined that the meprobamate market was about the same "in every part of the United States and in cities of every size." In 1957, the manager of Hollywood's famed Schwab's Drug Store conceded that his tranquilizer business was still booming but his clientele had changed. Since 1955, the store had sold less to celebrities and more to "just plain people." In a few years, tranquilizers had migrated from the mouths of movie stars to those of mere mortals.[5]

Glowing press coverage and positive scientific testimonials about Miltown invigorated consumer demand. Newspapers and magazines gushed about the new, effective, harmless, "ideal tranquilizer." Today's debates about the adverse impact of direct-to-consumer advertising (DTCA) on Americans' prescription practices may have caused us to overlook how information about drugs circulated more informally but no less powerfully in the past, forging a culture that bred familiarity with and interest in new medications. Americans in the 1950s discussed with neighbors, friends, and relatives what being on tranquilizers felt like, which doctors readily prescribed them, and which pharmacies were most likely to have them in stock. Americans could also learn about tranquilizers through a range of media, from literary magazines to tabloids to television shows, where references to Miltown were, as in the case of Milton Berle's show, written into scripts. Probably no drug in modern times, mused one contemporary, "has the glowing word-of-mouth reports that these little pills could have enjoyed."[6]

From the beginning, patients were among the drug's most ardent enthusiasts. Patient influence and demand should not be equated with unlimited agency, what some economists call "consumer sovereignty." Consumer choices have always been framed by technological, social, professional, and financial constraints. Yet characterizing the commercial success of

Miltown as a top-down process engineered by pharmaceutical executives and physicians mistakenly portrays patients as passive recipients of medical change. It also occludes patient-driven negotiations that have consistently imparted a dynamic character to medical practice. In order to "be on Miltown" patients had to make a medical appointment, see a doctor, find a pharmacy to fill their script, and swallow their pills. The historian Roy Porter has urged scholars to pay heed to patients' economic power. The paying consumer, he notes, "simply by possessing choice and the power of the purse [can] exercise considerable sway in the medical marketplace." This observation seems particularly apt in the case of Miltown, a drug that practically flew off pharmacists' shelves. "I had no idea at the outset of the potential size of the meprobamate market," an awed Henry Hoyt declared in 1957. "Let me tell you, when you're dealing with the general public, you're dealing with the great unknown."[7]

If activists and scholars later blamed doctors for pushing tranquilizers on patients, doctors' recollections suggest that power often flowed in the opposite direction. Confident that they would personally benefit from the pills and insistent that they were entitled to them, Americans actively sought prescriptions. As a London newspaper reported in 1956, Miltown mania was built on the backs of a society comprised of citizens conditioned to believe they had a right to take tranquilizers for the stresses of "civilized living." The frequency and forcefulness with which patients lobbied physicians was widely noted and often disparaged. "Physicians are constantly confronted by patients who, brandishing press clippings, demand prescriptions," observed one contemporary about the tranquilizer trade. Dr. Leonard Weil, president of the Dade County Academy of General Practice, acknowledged that physicians realized that if they didn't accommodate patients' demands for tranquilizers, others would. Doctors who might have second-guessed the wisdom of a prescription often relented, boxed in by the exigencies of the situation and an earnest desire to help patients requesting aid. In the end, doctors prescribed tranquilizers they might not have if they "had more time." Another family practitioner disclosed the despair he felt fruitlessly trying to convince patients that pills were *not* the answer. "Patients are far from passive recipients of these drugs," he insisted.

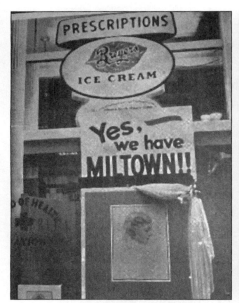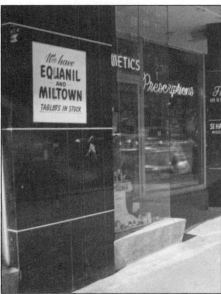

Yes, We Have Miltown!/New York City. In the mid-1950s, consumer enthusiasm for Miltown was so vast that demand frequently exceeded supply. In tranquilizer-happy Los Angeles (left) and New York City (right), merely having the drug in stock was cause for celebration and commercial promotion. Reproduced courtesy of the Berger Family.

Many arrive at doctors' offices "requesting, and even demanding medication to relieve their anxiety." When he suggested nonpharmaceutical remedies, they got angry, "as if [we] are holding back this wonderful panacea."[8]

Physician acquiescence created a stampede of script-toting patients whose hunger for made-to-order tranquility emptied drugstores of their inventory. In tranquilizer-happy Los Angeles—but also in Baltimore, Charlotte, Newark, and Louisville—patient demand frequently surpassed supply. Try as it might, Carter Laboratories couldn't manufacture meprobamate powder fast enough. "Our inventory," admitted a company official in May of 1956 "is zero. We're working overtime . . . but we can barely fill our orders."[9]

Pharmacists invented creative strategies to ride out the frenzy. Some rationed the coveted pills, filling only part of a given prescription; tranquilizers were like a scarce commodity, as milk and eggs had been in World War II. Others kept waiting lists or preferentially filled the prescriptions of certain customers. A few drugstores asked patients to wait in line before the store opened, rewarding only the most tenacious of the early birds with their desired allotment. No matter how hard pharmacists tried, customers frequently left drugstores empty-handed.[10]

The 1950s are often seen as a prelude to a more interesting, culturally dynamic time. Black-and-white photos, the main medium through which photographers captured the decade for posterity, suggest a static, stale world sometimes referred to as the age of conformity. In reality, of course, life was animated and colorful. Indeed, many Americans who lived in this era remember it as frenetically busy rather than static. Beneath the "nuclear numbness" that seemingly paralyzed the population, millions labored and millions more worried.

Albeit differently paced from the tumultuous late 1960s, it was nonetheless a world in constant motion. Newspapers and television sets briefed Americans on the daily struggle to quash communism and survive nuclear annihilation. If the destructive might unleashed by the atomic bomb could not be controlled, the resulting political exigencies could not be ignored. Feelings of fear and fortitude commingled as Americans struggled with life in the atomic age. By 1959, two-thirds of Americans saw the threat of nuclear war as the country's most pressing problem.[11]

The political and cultural rhetoric of the era oscillated between abject terror and robust confidence in America's ability to stave off enemy threats, domestic and foreign. The political pendulum swung from dejection to elation: the Soviet Union's atomic bomb was overshadowed by America's hydrogen bomb. Fears of nuclear disaster were offset by medical triumphs such as cortisone and the Salk vaccine. Joseph McCarthy's boorish behavior and doctored list of "known Communists" were checked by his televised downfall in 1954. The era had the feel of a barroom brawl: just when things appeared to be slipping into chaos, order was reaffirmed.

The government had learned a painful lesson about the importance of emotional management after the mass panic following the 1938 Halloween radio broadcast of H. G. Wells's *The War of the Worlds*. Life imitated art as thousands of terrified radio listeners in the United States and Canada fled into the evening darkness to protect themselves from Martian invaders who'd purportedly disembarked in New Jersey. In a single block in Newark, over twenty families abandoned their homes, their faces covered with wet handkerchiefs and towels, fleeing what they feared were gas raids. In Indianapolis, a distraught woman disrupted a church service shrieking, "New York destroyed; it's the end of the world. You might as well go home to die." In Pittsburgh, a man returned home during the broadcast to discover his wife clutching a bottle of poison in the bathroom. She yelled, "I'd rather die this way than like that." If people panicked in response to radio fiction, imagine the effects of a genuine attack.[12]

On the heels of the Soviet Union's nuclear test and the start of the Korean War, Congress and the Truman administration created the Federal Civil Defense Administration (FCDA) in January 1951. Its daunting mandate was to teach citizens to prepare for and survive a biological, chemical, or nuclear attack. Through its pedagogical projects the FCDA amplified the likelihood of a nuclear invasion even as it proffered routines to allay civilian insecurities. Few questioned the permissibility or the political value of terror; fear of communist Russia was a necessary mechanism for rallying support to the government's cold war policies. But mass panic and hysteria were a different matter. Buttressed by an exhaustive, multivolume report of Project East River, a government-sponsored study undertaken by a consortium of universities, the administration concluded that panic and hysteria, left unchecked, could weaken America's moral resolve. [13]

Civilian defense training thus endeavored to dampen atomic anxiety by teaching people how to manage their fears, offering a sense of mastery over the vicissitudes of fate. Education was America's "first line of defense," and the FCDA fought panic through a panoply of programs in schools, on radio, and on film. Schools distributed metal dog tags to children, intended to identify the dead and wounded after an attack (tattoos had been considered, but officials concluded that metal was more resilient than human flesh). Educators portrayed them as protective devices designed to keep children accounted for and safe. The FCDA sponsored air-raid drills in cities assumed to be Soviet targets, including Pittsburgh, New York City, and Mobile.[14] Students were instructed to drop to the ground, crawl under their desks, and assume the "atomic clutch," shielding their heads from heat and debris. The capstone of these drills was the 1951 cartoon film *Bert the Turtle*. Filmed in Public School 152 in Astoria, Queens, and watched by millions of Americans in schools and on television, the nine-minute "documentary" used the antics of a turtle named Bert to teach survival techniques. If Bert's composure under attack could save *him*, the message ran, surely anyone could survive. An atomic explosion, the film explained, would create a "bright flash, brighter than the sun, brighter than anything you have ever seen" and "things will be knocked down all over town." To cheery music the background chorus sang:

> *There was a turtle by the name of Bert*
> *And Bert the turtle was very alert*
> *When danger threatened him he never got hurt*
> *He knew just what to do . . .*
> *He ducked!*
> *And covered!*
> *Ducked!*
> *And covered!*[15]

The film's release was supplemented by a companion radio broadcast, a sixteen-page color booklet of Bert's thoughtful instructions, newspaper serialization, and a featured spot in the Alert America Convoy: three motorized caravans that toured the country for nine months in 1952 imploring Americans to do their best to prepare for the worst.[16]

Miltown thus arrived in a society preoccupied with anxiety and committed to its containment. The government's political discourse legitimized fear while urging patriotic citizens to take measures to stay calm. Fallout shelters and air-raid drills were daily reminders of what might happen, yet they were also an invitation to be more than passive bystanders. If anxiety was ubiquitous and impossible to eradicate, it could also be managed and controlled.

Indeed, the drug was often linked to atomic anxiety. A 1958 story in the *New Yorker* observed that tranquilizers could not have emerged at a better

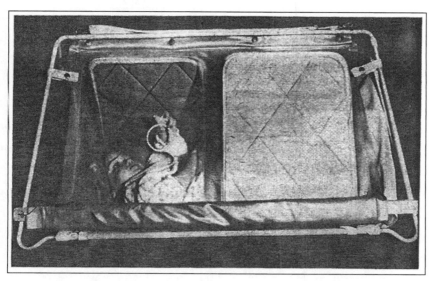

Baby Pup Tent. Like tranquilizers themselves, this baby shelter, created by the U.S. Army, was lauded as an invention that lionized America's ingenuity in the cold war race for scientific supremacy even as it promised to protect the country's most vulnerable population in the event of an atomic attack. *Newsweek,* January 9, 1956.

time: "An age in which nations threaten each other with guided missiles and hydrogen bombs is one that can use any calm it can get, and calm is what the American pharmaceutical industry now abundantly offers." *Newsweek* juxtaposed an article on the benefits of meprobamate for alcoholics with a paragraph trumpeting the Army Chemical Corps's latest invention, an infant nuclear shelter. The crib-size tent, outfitted with a ventilator that had been treated with chemicals to filter out poison gas, bacteria, and radioactive particles, promised to keep America's most vulnerable population safe and peaceful. As if to drive home the point, the magazine included a photograph of the high-tech shelter, a placid-looking baby happily toying with the air filter designed to save her. The visual and rhetorical coupling of tranquilizers and the shelter vividly suggested that in an age of international peril, home-grown technologies would allow Americans to endure.[17]

A government-sponsored civilian defense film was even more explicit, encouraging Americans to keep the new pills stashed in home fallout shelters, at least 1,500 of which had been built by 1960. "By all means provide some tranquilizers to ease the strain and monotony of life in a shelter," it urged. "A bottle of 100 should be adequate for a family of four." The narrator reassured listeners that drugs were safe and not habit forming. Stanley Kubrick's acclaimed dark comedy, *Dr. Strangelove or: How I Learned to Stop Worrying and Love the Bomb,* presented tranquilizers as yet another part of daily life in the atomic age. In one sardonic scene, Major T. J. King Kong inventories the survival kit and finds lipstick, condoms, pep pills, a combination Russian phrase book and Bible, and tranquilizers: enough for a "pretty good weekend in Vegas." Released after the Cuban missile crisis at the height of America's cold war paranoia, the film nevertheless managed to depict tranquilizers as an integral part of America's tool kit for surviving—with alacrity, no less—impending doom.[18]

If the politics of anxiety containment helped paved the way for Miltown's acceptance so too did the era's rampant consumerism. The benefits of the post–World War II prosperity in John Kenneth Galbraith's *Affluent Society* were not spread equally. But the expansion was broadly based and long-lasting enough to secure the United States the highest standard of living in the world. In the 1950s the GNP rose by a whopping 50 percent.[19]

Buoyed by extra income, Americans went on an unprecedented buying spree. Partly this reflected the postwar baby boom, a sharp spike in the fertility rate that added 76 million more people to the country's population between 1946 and 1964, all needing shelter, clothing, and food. Americans bought houses and cars en masse. By 1960, 60 percent of American households owned homes and 75 percent owned cars. The growing legitimacy of conspicuous consumption, what Liz Cohen has called the "consumer's republic," encouraged many Americans to spend beyond their means using credit cards, another commercial convenience that came of age in the 1950s. Private debt more than doubled during the decade, as people borrowed heavily to acquire cars, swimming pools, and an assortment of labor-saving gadgets such as electric washers and dryers, garage-door openers, lawnmowers, even electric pencil sharpeners. As giant supermarkets began to dot suburban landscapes, Americans filled their shopping carts with TV dinners that could be stashed in their new freezers and prepared on demand. The construction of a modern highway system, abetted by the Interstate Highway Act of 1956, quickened the pace of suburbanization even as it generated a corollary of goods and services: gas stations, motels, and drive-through eateries. A noteworthy example of this nouvelle cuisine was McDonald's, where a family of four could eat hamburgers, fries, and milkshakes for less than $2. On the surface, McDonald's fifteen-cent hamburgers and Wallace's ten-cent Miltowns had little in common. Yet both were part of the tide of new material and social comforts. Consumer convenience was trumpeted as a particularly American answer to a peculiarly American set of woes.[20]

Just as Americans counted on aspirin to reduce fever and penicillin to treat infections, millions unhesitatingly turned to tranquilizers to quell frayed nerves. A 1957 time capsule recently unearthed in Tulsa, Oklahoma—a Plymouth Belvedere filled with artifacts the capsule's creators considered typical of the time—included a woman's purse packed with bobby pins, gum, loose change, a compact, cigarettes, an unpaid parking ticket, and a bottle of tranquilizers. That tranquilizers were just another accessory of modern middle-class life was, presumably, the point. Antibiotics, cortisone, the Salk vaccine: why shouldn't an antianxiety pill be next? Different from penicillin, it was a variation of the same pharmaceutical theme: a modern medical marvel that worked quickly, reliably, and efficiently.[21]

Compounding Miltown's allure was its bargain price, which remained ten cents a tablet throughout the 1950s. Psychoanalysis, a therapeutic encounter that put the individual's identity and personal history on center stage, remained an attractive option in the 1950s. But psychoanalysts remained in short supply, and the time commitments and costs of therapy remained, for many Americans, prohibitively steep. Miltown, in contrast, was cheap, about the same price as a can of tomatoes or a roll of toilet paper at the neighborhood Safeway. It was convenient. And like the teenage crew at McDonald's, it delivered the goods in a few short minutes.[22]

Miltown thus meshed easily with the convenience mentality of the 1950s, the therapeutic ethos that sanctioned changing oneself rather than the world, and the sociopolitical uncertainties that kept Americans on edge. Another popular (but vastly more expensive) quick-fix medical triumph in the 1950s was the facelift, a surgical trend driven by plastic surgeons' need for new markets (most war-related surgery had been reconstructive rather

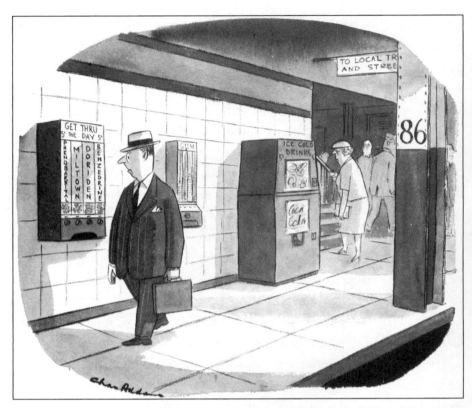

Commuter Drugstore. This 1956 *New Yorker* cartoon satirized America's dependency on drugs to "get through the day," suggesting that the pills were as ubiquitous and irresistible as an ice-cold cola. *New Yorker,* August 11, 1956. Copyright © Charles Addams. Reproduced with permission of the Tee and Charles Addams Foundation.

than cosmetic) but also by a middle-class culture that promised liberation in the form of scientifically sanctioned conveniences effecting immediate, individual change. As politicians sang the praises of endurance, parents everywhere complained of exhaustion. The era's exodus to suburbia and the baby boom meant restless nights with crying children, the animated din at the dinner table, and hushed conversations about how to feed so many new mouths. The very act of moving from city to suburb—in the 1950s more than 18 million did—caused an upheaval that historian Elaine Tyler May has aptly described as a rootlessness: a sense of disconnect from time-worn traditions and community networks. Breadwinners were foot soldiers in a period of sustained economic growth even as they battled pressures that equated success with consumption.[23]

A survey published in a 1956 edition of *Ladies Home Journal* highlighted what Americans worried about—an issue that was clearly a national concern. One respondent noted the "inability to be articulate and graceful when meeting people or loved ones," while another fretted about "money, the insurance premium, the atom and hydrogen bombs." One respondent confessed to fears of "loneliness and old age" and another admitted that "my only real worry is the thought of a physical disability which would end my earning power and make me a financial burden to my family. This is a real horror."[24] When journalists and scientists announced the availability of a drug to curb everyday nerves, they spoke to a society already primed by a compelling cultural, economic, and political rationale for their use. In the absence of an organized antidrug lobby, the question in many Americans' minds in the 1950s may have been: Why *not* take a tranquilizer?

Men on Miltown

The millions who found no reason to demur included women, children, and especially men: executives, athletes, doctors, and countless others who wanted to experience for themselves what the drug journalists and movie stars were raving about. Because anxiety was regarded as the root cause of many disorders (one psychiatrist suggested that "60 percent of all the patients who go to private physicians suffer not from organic diseases but from psychoneurotic conditions"), Miltown had a broad therapeutic range. Stress, anxiety, and tension were problems in their own right. But in the medical parlance of 1950s America they also explained disorders such as asthma, arthritis, bedwetting, colitis, dermatitis, headaches, insomnia, premenstrual tension, frigidity, *and* nymphomania.[25]

Partly for this reason, tranquilizers were used by overworked businessmen harried by office deadlines, virgin brides nervous about their honeymoons, petulant toddlers and teenagers, Americans fearful of nuclear annihilation, and a young farm housewife from Beaver Dam, Kentucky (population 1,349). Her peace pills, she said, gave her a coveted relaxed feeling in an era she considered to be "too fast." Long before Ritalin was prescribed to children to treat hyperactivity and garrulous behavior, parents and pediatricians relied on tranquilizers to achieve the same result. A Palo Alto dentist used Miltown on children prone to fear or egregious hostility: the kind of kid who "wouldn't think twice before biting off the dentist's digit." He instructed mothers to medicate aggressive children with Miltown an hour before the appointment. A Louisville truck driver, a self-professed "excitable type," counted on Miltown to control the road rage he would experience whenever another driver cut in front of him. In the old days, he would retaliate: "cuss out the driver and perhaps run into his car." But since he had been on Miltown, he had become a new man and a better driver: calmer, more controlled, and accident-free.[26]

This diversity in tranquilizer demography in the 1950s is an essential part of the Miltown story that has often been disregarded. The outpouring of critical newspaper and journal articles, television broadcasts, congressional investigations, and patient testimonials in the 1970s and 1980s encouraged many scholars to rewrite history according to a familiar heroes and villains narrative. Often the victims in this narrative of corporate greed and patient passivity are suburban housewives. "Mother's little helpers," wrote psychiatrist Peter Kramer in his important and acclaimed *Listening to Prozac,* were pills "popular and widely available in the fifties and early sixties that were used to keep women in their place, to make them comfortable in a setting that should have been uncomfortable, to encourage them to focus on tasks that did not matter." Others have echoed this view, depicting tranquilizers as a medical technology hatched by men chiefly to pacify women—a less invasive but no less insidious measure of control than earlier "heroic" somatic treatments such as electroconvulsive therapy or lobotomy.[27]

A deeper look at the historical record shows that although a gendering of the tranquilizer market was clear by the late 1960s, when women accounted for two-thirds of the consumer market, it was not obvious to doctors, pharmaceutical executives, or patients in the 1950s. A focus on the overmedicated woman, an artifact of a different generation, has caused us to neglect how tranquilizers were initially marketed to and used by men. Pharmaceutical firms had no financial incentive to confine these drugs to women. Indeed, the surest path to profit was to position them as a panacea for *all* anxious Americans. In fact, at least in the beginning, tranquilizers were very much a

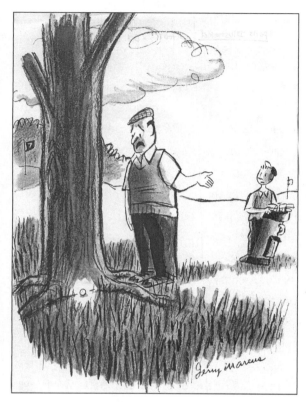

My Nine-Iron and Another Miltown. Miltown was considered as much a natural fixture of the male universe in the 1950s as a game of golf, as this *Sports Illustrated* cartoon reveals. *Sports Illustrated*, October 15, 1956. Copyright © Jerry Marcus Foundation. Reproduced courtesy of Julius Marcus.

man's drug.[28] Miltown's fanatical following among businessmen in this decade earned it the nickname Executive Excedrin. Moreover, in popular and cultural representations, the picture of the typical user was male. In the Academy Award–winning film *The Apartment*, the male lead, C. C. "Bud" Baxter, a business associate in a New York office, takes prescription sedatives to ensure he is well rested for his day job. "How can I be efficient in the office if I don't get enough sleep at night?" he asks. (The fact that Fran Kubelik, the emotionally distraught elevator operator, tries to overdose on Baxter's pills does not detract from the fact that they were prescribed to Baxter and routinely used by him.) From the male patient's perspective, there was no reason to feel embarrassed about taking tranquilizers or other prescription medicines. In the 1950s and beyond, the stigma of "mother's little helper," linking the feminization of prescription drug taking and societal decay, had not yet taken hold. In such a gender-neutral milieu, men remained avid users and often outspoken proponents, critical to stoking demand.

Miltown offered men a way to attenuate unpleasant symptoms. But it also represented something else: a technological fix for a malaise that countless novelists, philosophers, and social critics portrayed as the emotional predicament of the times. Auden's majestic and critically acclaimed *The Age of Anxiety*, published in 1947, captured the foiled attempts of individuals to find meaning in a modern world where the rules of sociability and mobility had changed, where disorder meant there was no longer "one-to-one correspondence between a [man's] social or economic position and his private mental life." A spate of self-help books written primarily for men—*Relax and Live, How to Control Worry, Cure Your Nerves Yourself*—vilified anxiety while casting it as the emotional epicenter of middle-class male life. As the efflorescence of self-help guides tacitly suggests, the national nervous breakdown was never regarded as a lost cause, for the triumph of a therapeutic culture had created a psychological vocabulary of self-improvement, predicated on the belief that Americans were *entitled* to happiness and self-fulfillment. Paradoxically, charges that man's individuality was being stifled by the totalitarian weight of mass conformity, a fear articulated in some of the decade's canonical works, including David Riesman's *The Lonely Crowd* (1950), William Whyte's *The Organization Man* (1956), and Sloan Wilson's *The Man in the Gray Flannel Suit* (1956), legitimated male autonomy and ambition. As a cultural marker, anxiety was thus a double-edged sword. Riesman wrote in *The Lonely Crowd* of the diffuse anxiety experienced by the man who lived for the approval of others, but anxiety was also associated with the trailblazing achiever, the very personality type (in a culture increasingly preoccupied with personality types) critics exalted as an antidote to the quotidian conformist. Reisman extolled the virtues of inner-directed men: "ambitious, energetic, self-reliant men engaged in transforming physical nature, instituting large-scale formal organization, and revolutionizing technology." Whyte wrote of the "executive neurosis" that befell the businessman who followed his self-instincts and drive; in this sense, anxiety was the unavoidable upshot of man's capacity to break free from the herd mentality. Like neurasthenia in the late nineteenth century, anxiety signaled American achievement and advancement; unwanted and uncomfortable, it was

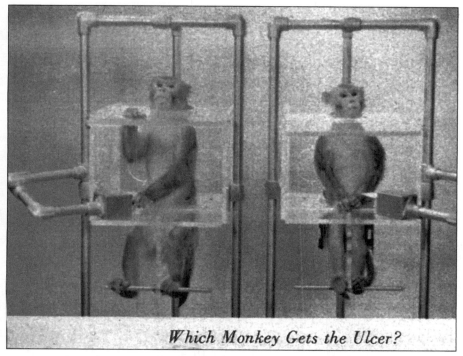

Which Monkey Gets the Ulcer?

Which Monkey Gets the Ulcer? In a series of tests, scientists at the Walter Reed Army Institute of Research determined that the "executive monkey," burdened by the responsibility of protecting his peer, suffered the most. Further research suggested that tranquilizing the executive monkey improved his health and mood. What worked for executive monkeys presumably worked for men. *Fortune*, May 1957.

the inevitable price of success. It was no wonder that society's most brilliant leaders and creative artists experienced it.[29]

Leading the pack of tranquilized men was the business executive. In the mid-1950s, scientists at the Neuropsychiatric Division at the Walter Reed Army Institute of Research conducted what became known as the executive monkey experiments. Researchers placed two monkeys at opposite sides of the same cage and administered electric shocks to their feet every twenty seconds. The monkey on the left, the executive monkey, could shield both monkeys from the shock if he pressed the lever on his side every twenty seconds. That responsibility put a lot of stress on the monkey, and researchers were unsurprised to discover that in test after test, it was the executive monkey who developed the ulcer, became demonstrably agitated, and died first. When the executive monkey took a tranquilizer, however, he did his job better.[30]

Researchers assumed that tranquilizers would offer the same benefits to businessmen. Few questioned the ubiquity of anxiety among the male managerial class. For these upstanding citizens, a good day's work meant doing one's job and earning a good salary, but also playing a social role: making decisions and completing tasks while maintaining confidence and control. Maintaining the persona was as taxing as the job.

Researchers disagreed about which professional men were most anxious (one study found newspaper editors to be the most and university administrators to be the least), but no one doubted that anxiety was potentially injurious. Physician reference manuals published by tranquilizer manufacturers underscored the serious consequences of untreated anxiety among businessmen while imparting the message that the men who needed them most were also America's most industrious. As Carter-Wallace's Henry Hoyt insisted, Miltown was a drug intended for "active, productive people" who "normally work under pressure." Wallace Laboratories urged doctors to prescribe Miltown to shield the white collar worker from ulcers, high blood pressure, and heart disease. *Aspects of Anxiety,* a manual produced by Roche Laboratories, catalogued the many stresses confronting the male breadwinner. "In today's competitive society, where masculinity and even virtue are so often equated with success, the American male can rarely afford to relax. . . . To win recognition . . . he must advance, make money, go up fast." When this virile drive caused acute stress, Roche recommended tranquilizers. "Since it is usually almost impossible to change the conditions of employment," the book concluded, "the physician [must] attempt to change the patient's outlook on life and attitudes to his worth through 'pharmacotherapy.'" J. B. Roerig and Company distributed a film, *The Relaxed Wife,* advocating the tranquilization of breadwinners who returned home too keyed up to enjoy the affections of a loving spouse or children.[31]

A 1957 national survey on tranquilizer use among executives found that one-third of respondents used them. Half of these were habitual users. Seventy-two percent of respondents reported that minor tranquil-

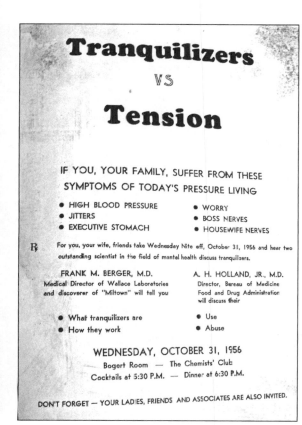

Tranquilizers

VS

Tension

IF YOU, YOUR FAMILY, SUFFER FROM THESE
SYMPTOMS OF TODAY'S PRESSURE LIVING

- HIGH BLOOD PRESSURE
- JITTERS
- EXECUTIVE STOMACH
- WORRY
- BOSS NERVES
- HOUSEWIFE NERVES

℞ For you, your wife, friends take Wednesday Nite off, October 31, 1956 and hear two outstanding scientist in the field of mental health discuss tranquilizers.

FRANK M. BERGER, M.D.
Medical Director of Wallace Laboratories and discoverer of "Miltown" will tell you

A. H. HOLLAND, JR., M.D.
Director, Bureau of Medicine Food and Drug Administration will discuss their

- What tranquilizers are
- How they work
- Use
- Abuse

WEDNESDAY, OCTOBER 31, 1956
Bogert Room — The Chemists' Club
Cocktails at 5:30 P.M. — Dinner at 6:30 P.M.

DON'T FORGET — YOUR LADIES, FRIENDS AND ASSOCIATES ARE ALSO INVITED.

Tranquilizers Versus Tension. At New York City's Chemists' Club, founded in 1898 by a group of chemists to promote the advancement of chemical science, members and guests were invited to convene at the elegantly appointed Bogert Dining Room. Here, they could enjoy cocktails, dinner, and a presentation on the use of tranquilizers to treat a range of disorders, including "executive stomach" and "boss nerves." Reproduced courtesy of the Berger Family.

izers improved job performance. Users liked how tranquilizers promoted relaxation, sleep, and personal relations. A haggard newspaper executive too weary from insomnia to perform his job got Miltown before a publisher's convention, with good results. "I could stop taking them tomorrow," he reported. "But I don't want to. They make me happy. I still have my worries, but now I don't worry about my worries." In another instance, the president of a Madison Avenue advertising agency produced a large bottle of Equanil and invited colleagues to "join in." They did. According to one observer, "the meeting went off with less argument than it had in years."[32]

One psychiatrist recounted the case of a thirty-six-year-old salesman with acute job-related stress. The man's anxiety forced him to quit his job and consult the psychiatrist. Apparently the patient "could not sit still for more than a few minutes without having to get up and pace."

Other medications failed to help, but when the psychiatrist prescribed meprobamate, the results were instant and miraculous. The salesman "telephoned to cancel further appointments, saying that for the first time in his life, he was free from a constant feeling of shaking and tension and that he was going back to work."[33] Here was a true American success story: with a little pharmaceutical help, the neurotic salesman resumed his place among the productive citizenry. Tranquilizers kept corporate America functioning.

They also helped sustain the U.S. government's top executive of the early 1960s, President John F. Kennedy. He took as many as eight medications a day to treat his various illnesses (including Addison's disease and colitis) and help him cope with the unrelenting tension that came with being commander in chief. Kennedy's medical records reveal that the suave and youthful-looking king of Camelot took codeine, Demerol, and methadone for pain, Ritalin for energy, barbiturates for sleep, and meprobamate and Librium for anxiety.[34]

Physicians, 95 percent of whom were male in the 1950s, were also no strangers to chemical tranquility. In Beverly Hills, a busy psychiatrist affirmed that he popped Miltown to prepare for the nerve-wracking drive home. "I wish the government would subsidize tranquilizer slot machines on every corner," he joked in 1957. In 1966, the *New York Times* named physicians "the most devoted users of the tranquilizers they prescribe." They were enabled by the common practice among pharmaceutical firms of sending doctors free drug samples in the mail. One North Carolina doctor admitted that popping samples got him through his day. "I became sort of a one-man testing station of each new tranquilizer as it came along," he recalled. "I couldn't see any patients until the mailman came. Where other doctors read their mail, I ate mine."[35]

Members of the military took tranquilizers to handle the stresses of duty. An air force study of 1,100 military personnel at the Orlando air force base in Florida found that meprobamate helped curb insomnia among pilots, who "tend to refly each mission at night." Tranquilizer use among aviators became so common that in 1957, the air force surgeon general sent out instructions to all commands to halt the practice of unauthorized tranquilizer procurement; their unregulated use could cause reckless behavior and accidents. Colonel James Nutall, air force chief of aviation, explained that pilots were under the false impression from "articles in popular magazines" that the new drugs were harmless. Flight personnel were henceforth instructed to obtain pills exclusively from flight surgeons. In addition, General Maxwell D. Taylor, the army chief of staff, signed a special order grounding pilots for four weeks after taking meprobamate or "any of the newer mood-ameliorating, tranquilizing or ataraxic (calming) drugs." Indiscriminately mixing tranquilizers and military maneuvers was not a good idea.[36]

With such precautions in place, the U.S. military remained one of meprobamate's most reliable and largest buyers. Between January 1958 and February 1959, the Military Medical Supply Agency paid over $1.7 million to acquire 84,440 bottles (with 50 tablets per bottle) of meprobamate. Mild tranquilizers were also widely distributed to veterans at Veteran Administration (VA) hospitals. Between July 1959 and August 1960 the VA spent a further $1.4 million on meprobamate.[37]

Tranquilizers also enhanced the performance of male athletes.[38] In the 1950s, doctors prescribed minor tranquilizers to professional athletes not only to calm nervousness but also to combat spasms, sore muscles, and inflammation. Reno Bertoia, a twenty-two-year-old third baseman for the Detroit Tigers, seemed to have a promising career until his jitters got the better of him. Tigers trainer Jack Homel was distressed to see Bertoia consumed by nervous worry, to the point where Bertoia "couldn't hit and sometimes bobbled fielding plays that should have been easy." In 1957 the Tigers were ready to send Bertoia back to the minors. Instead, they put him on meprobamate. Homel described Bertoia's miraculous metamorphosis:

Perhaps part of it was a psychological lift, but he stopped holding himself in. He's a different man on the bench—talking and joking—and much more relaxed. He had the skill. Pills won't make a ball player out of someone who hasn't got it. You can't make chicken salad out of chicken feathers.[39]

On Miltown, Bertoia was the dynamic player his team needed, "pounding the ball in tremendous fashion." The year he started Miltown marked Bertoia's personal best, with a .398 batting average that put him at the top of the American and National Baseball Leagues. [40]

Other athletes and trainers also used meprobamate. In major league baseball, the drug's use was publicly endorsed by team physicians for the Philadelphia Phillies and the Cincinnati Redlegs for muscle spasms, pain, and "difficulty sleeping on trains." In professional football, meprobamate helped wide receivers Dorne Dibble and Jim Doran, and defensive halfback Bill Stits. Boxing legend Sugar Ray Robinson, world middleweight champion, used tranquilizers to help him sleep and box his way through the pain of injured ribs. Speed skater Bob Snyder would get stomach upsets before big races. Meprobamate attenuated his nervousness, enabling him to claim the North American speed skating champion title. [41]

Therapeutic success stories such as these encouraged widespread tranquilizer use among athletes of all ages and stature, a phenomenon that sparked commentary and occasional concern. Homel conceded that a disquieting effect of Bertoia's publicized experience was a fascination with tranquilizers as "athletic enhancers" among high school athletes and minor league clubs. Others wondered how the tranquilization of ball players had altered the dynamics and virtuosity of the game. Sports journalist Oscar Fraley warned New York fans that while they may be as excitable and frustrated as ever, "due to wide use of the prescription drug in major league camps the players may be the most relaxed athletes in history." If firebrands "Russ (The Mad Monk) Meyer or mercurial Bobby Bragan calmly shrug off bad calls, don't be trapped with your eyebrows up. There's a reason. Miltown!" [42]

Tranquilizers for All

Clearly the excitement surrounding Miltown was infectious, but not everyone believed antianxiety agents were the answer to the challenges of life. Throughout the 1950s, psychoanalytically trained doctors championed their treatment methods over pharmacotherapy, while others counseled that the drugs had become a crutch rather than a cure. A few physicians warned that their clinical experience suggested a potential for addiction to tranquilizers that rivaled the increasingly discredited barbiturates.

But such cautionary remarks were largely eclipsed by the hyperbole of the pharmaceutically minded. Indeed, the most persistent public criticism of minor tranquilizers attacked neither their medical nor social hazards, but their inaccessibility for lower-income families. Pharmaceutical firms' high profit margins had not translated into lower prices, politicians and mental health activists contended, and many strove to make tranquilizers available to *more* Americans. In January 1960, Senator Estes Kefauver's Subcommittee on Antitrust and Monopoly made national news with piercing allegations that the country's top tranquilizer manufacturers, Carter Products, American Home Products (whose subsidiary, Wyeth, sold Equanil), and Smith Kline & French, manufacturers of Thorazine, were fixing prices and hoarding profits. The price of a bottle of fifty tablets of 400 mg of Miltown in the United States had stayed constant since 1955, costing American druggists about $3.25. Meanwhile, consumers in other countries reaped the benefits of cheaper prices, for an identical bottle cost druggists $1.77 in Italy, $1.48 in Great Britain, and $0.69 in Germany. The Kefauver hearings drew attention to corporate profits, but the inquiry confirmed an unshakable belief in the importance of reducing prices and diffusing tranquilizers to a *wider* segment of the population: "In selling to sick people, why do you charge so much? . . . You are not selling a luxury; you are selling a necessity, something that people have to have." In Kefauver's view, all Americans should have equal access to tranquilizers.[43]

People took to tranquilizers in a remarkable way. Yet the history of psychopharmacology in general and mild tranquilizers in particular unfolded in a context that differed from the one that would frame a subsequent generation's response to them. In the 1950s, contemporaries evaluated the drugs' value not only to individuals but also to the perceived needs of society as a whole. Tranquilizers seemed to smooth over cultural fissures that, left unattended, threatened to widen into more serious chasms. They coaxed unemployed men back into the workplace.

They made breadwinners, artists, and writers more productive. They softened the complaints of exhausted mothers. They improved batting averages. They made juvenile delinquents less edgy and soothed crying babies. Minor tranquilizers were at once medically innovative and culturally conservative. There would be no tranquilizer problem in the public eye until this important link between tranquilizers and social stability, forged in the 1950s, was unbound.

(6)

Corporate Choreography and Molecular Play

Miltown's resounding popularity launched a tranquilizer boom that whetted the commercial appetites of rival pharmaceutical companies. Many, still struggling financially, were hunting for reliable "round-the-clockers," drugs for chronic disorders such as hypertension, arthritis, and hypothyroidism. Miltown's success suggested that anxiety might figure on this coveted list. Eager to cash in on the craze, pharmaceutical companies instructed their top scientists to invent drugs that would outperform Miltown pharmacologically and commercially. In 1960 and again in 1963 Hoffman-La Roche struck gold with Librium and Valium, respectively, the first of a new class of antianxiety agents, the benzodiazepines ("benzos" for short).

Unlike mephenesin, the precursor to meprobamate whose tranquilizing properties were discovered by serendipity, and meprobamate, which was only reluctantly brought to market, Librium was the product of a global race to create a drug that would outsell all others. The commercial angle to the discovery of benzodiazepines sets them apart from other drugs of the era, whose development was driven by university researchers and government grants, the emblems of impartial science. Texas psychiatrist Irvin Cohen, who ran clinical trials on Librium, later observed that the benzodiazepines were a "model of how a therapeutic agent is conceived and brought forth by an enterprising pharmaceutical manufacturer who simply seeks to find a drug superior to others already in the marketplace." Years later, this aspect of their history would inflate critics' charges that tranquilizers were created to boost corporate profits rather than eradicate human suffering. In its day, however, Librium was hailed as a path-breaking innovation that materialized because its quixotic inventor, Leo Sternbach, had eschewed faster research trajectories for the painstakingly slow and unpredictable methods of trial and error.[1]

Fritz Hoffman founded Hoffman-La Roche (often referred to as Roche) in 1896 in Basel, Switzerland. A dynamic entrepreneur, Hoffman came from an established merchant family with close ties to the silk ribbon trade, the mainstay of the Basel economy since the seventeenth century. From the start, the name Hoffman commanded respect. So too did La Roche, a venerable family with long-standing community ties. When Fritz Hoffman and Adele La Roche married in 1895, they followed Swiss tradition and adopted a single, hyphenated last name. Hoping to benefit from the confluence of several developments—rising consumer demand for standardized and easy-to-take medications, advances in drug synthesis, an established commercial infrastructure in Basel, and growing concerns among physicians and pharmacists about patent medicines—Hoffman-La Roche began operations the following year. It was a modest-size manufacturer of drugs, principally finished pharmaceuticals retailed to doctors and pharmacies. Fritz Hoffmann-La Roche was the sole shareholder, his father a silent partner. Even now, descendants control half the company shares.[2]

Hoffman-La Roche quickly made a name for itself, thanks to its supply trade, specializing in glandular and medicinal plant extracts. In 1898 it launched Sirolin, an over-the-counter guaiacol cough syrup whose commercial success (sales rose from 700 bottles in 1898 to 78,000 in 1900) stemmed in part from aggressive advertising. Newspaper ads peddled the orange syrup as a sweet-tasting panacea that would banish coughing fits and the concomitant indignities of illness. Digalen, a digitalis-based preparation for heart troubles, followed in 1904. Buoyed and emboldened by escalating profits, the company established subsidiaries in Grenzach

(Germany), Milan, New York City, and London. In 1910, it established its first subsidiary in tsarist Russia, where agents in Moscow, Odessa, Rostov, Kazan, and Saint Petersburg helped create the company's largest and most lucrative market. By 1914 its products included not only Digalen and the ever popular Sirolin, but also the bromide sedative Sedabrol (used to treat epilepsy and nervous disorders). It also manufactured an array of hormone extracts, as well as digitalis, ergot, and opium preparations.[3]

World War I and the Russian revolution dealt the company a devastating blow. Germany boycotted Hoffman-La Roche's products, and the war temporarily halted operations at the Grenzach plant in Germany, which after 1910 had come to manufacture most of Hoffman-La Roche's products. As executives wondered how the company would weather these setbacks, its prospects became even bleaker. In 1917 the revolutionary forces that swept across Russia froze Roche's Russian assets and destroyed the company's most important market. On the brink of bankruptcy, it scaled back its operations and transformed itself into a self-financed joint-stock company.[4]

Hoffman-La Roche's languishing fortunes began to reverse in the 1920s with the development of barbiturates and analgesics, which found a wide market, especially in the United States. But the real secret to Hoffman-La Roche's renewal was its pioneering work on synthetic vitamins. In the 1920s and 1930s, scientists identified the chemical structure and physiological effects of several vitamins (a deficiency of vitamin C could cause scurvy; of vitamin D, rickets), and popular magazines were awash with articles on the health benefits of supplementation. Hoffman-La Roche was one of many pharmaceutical companies that entered the vitamin business, and its quick success in isolating, synthesizing, and mass-manufacturing a wide array of micronutrients reaped it huge profits. In 1933 the Zurich-based scientist Tadeusz Reichstein, who would later share a Nobel Prize for his work on cortisone, demonstrated a technique for creating vitamin C in the laboratory identical to naturally occurring ascorbic acid. Capitalizing on Reichstein's work, Roche proudly unveiled Redoxon in 1934, the first mass-manufactured synthetic vitamin in history. While other companies teetered on the cusp of bankruptcy during the Depression, Roche thrived. Emboldened by the successful vitamin C breakthrough, Roche scientists went on to synthesize vitamins A, B1, B2, E, and K. By the mid-1940s, it had reinvented itself as the world's largest vitamin manufacturer.[5]

As war engulfed Europe, Roche chairman Emil Christoph Barrell made the momentous decision to transfer the company's headquarters from Basel to its American subsidiary in Nutley, New Jersey, for the war's duration. Barrell announced his decision on May 21, 1940, shortly after Germany launched its western offensive and German tanks had reached the English Channel. The company had already lost over 70 percent of its staff to military duty, forcing managers to scramble for new workers (pulled chiefly from the ranks of youth and women) and new sources of raw material to offset war-related shortages. Government regulations also required the company to provide its own antiaircraft defense in case of attack and to destroy production facilities if Switzerland were invaded. Germany's successful offensive jeopardized the safety of the company's Basel operations. Some projected that a German takeover of Switzerland was imminent.[6]

In comparison, New Jersey seemed a safer bet. Elmer Bobst, head of Roche in Nutley, had made successive overtures to Barrell to smooth the way for a transnational relocation. The Nutley branch was located on a twenty-three-acre plot of land fifteen miles west of Manhattan, where Hoffman-La Roche had established its first U.S. facility in 1905. The Nutley corporate campus was a modest affair when it began operations in 1929, employing a total of 165 workers. The influx of Roche's top executives and researchers transformed Nutley into a research and manufacturing hub. Roche built two new factories and a state-of-the-art laboratory facility in 1942 and more than doubled its Nutley personnel between 1940 and 1942. Among those who joined Nutley's staff was Leo Henryk Sternbach, who, along with other promising Jewish scientists, had been relocated to the United States in 1941 for their own protection.[7]

Sternbach was born in 1908 in Abbazia, a seaside resort on the Adriatic coast, whose temperate climate and physical beauty made it a popular tourist destination. Sternbach's father, a pharmacist, did a brisk trade at the family's main street pharmacy, popular with tourists and spa goers. As a child, Sternbach helped mind the store, an apprenticeship that spawned a keen interest in chemistry. There was no fighting in Abbazia during World War I, but the friendly Italian troops who occupied the city later gave Sternbach and his friends "many rounds of carbine (rifle) shells," an unusual gift that fueled his lifelong passion for chemical experimentation. Sternbach would open the shiny brass cartridges and empty out the nitro cellulose gunpowder before exploding it in elongated glass tubes. "I just loved chemistry," he told me in 2005, "every facet of its detail, every aspect of it." None of the schools he attended had their own chemical laboratories. Undeterred, Sternbach used available materials to construct makeshift labs, damaging and destroying several windowsills as he experimented.[8]

Deferring to his father's wishes, Sternbach studied pharmacology at the University of Krakow in Poland. His school grades had been mediocre, but because the program gave preferential status to the children of pharmacists, he landed one of the program's thirty coveted spots. He earned his degree in 1929 and stayed on as a doctoral student in organic chemistry, studying dyes and synthesizing several substances known as benzheptoxdiazines, which would be critical to his later work on benzodiazepines. After receiving his Ph.D. in 1931, he continued to work as a research assistant and lecturer. A colleague remembered him as a "possessed" chemist who "worked all hours on a variety of projects, running from one set of flasks to another. No one but Leo knew what was in any of them. And he was obsessed by the process of crystallization. 'It crystallizes so beautifully.' That was perhaps his most pleasurable statement."[9]

Universities in Europe in the 1930s weren't bastions of academic and religious freedom, however. In 1937, Sternbach's adviser, Professor Karol Dziewonski, told his protégé he would have to leave. Krakow University did not abide Jews readily and Sternbach's parents were Jews, albeit not particularly devout. They celebrated Rosh Hashanah and Yom Kippur (only his mother fasted) but rarely attended synagogue. Sternbach had no interest in Judaism. A lifelong atheist, he regarded religion as "senseless and negative." All the same, he resolutely refused to conceal his heritage. As a child in a predominantly Christian elementary school, he experienced firsthand the cruelties of anti-Semitism when classmates called him disparaging names. Now rising anti-Semitism at the university led to a clear administrative mandate: Sternbach's post must be filled by a Polish Christian, and soon. Sternbach's adviser held off as long as he could before transferring his prized pupil to safer regions. After securing a prestigious scholarship funded by Jewish textile magnate Feliks Wislicki, Dziewonski sent Sternbach to Vienna in 1937.[10]

After a brief stint at a Vienna laboratory, Sternbach moved to Zurich in October 1937 to work with Leopold Ruzicka, a distinguished chemist (who in 1939 won the Nobel Prize for his research on sex hormones) at the Federal Institute of Technology, Switzerland's equivalent of MIT. Ruzicka was a Catholic and a fellow Croatian who had earned a reputation for protecting and mentoring young Jewish scientists from Eastern Europe. Sternbach thrived intellectually at the institute, although he knew his post would end once his fellowship did. His fellowship gave him only $60 a month, enough to eat, pay bills, and rent a room in a local pension. In 1940 he accepted a position as a research chemist at Roche's Basel headquarters, where he started work on the synthesis of vitamin B2, also known as riboflavin. Among Swiss chemical companies, Roche alone resisted political pressure to "Aryanize" its workforce. Jews and foreign workers were not only recruited but protected from deportation to German or Polish labor camps.[11]

A more permanent outgrowth of Sternbach's formative Zurich years would be the relationship he established with Herta Mia Kreuzer, his landlady's daughter. Twelve years younger than Sternbach and only a teenager when they met, Herta looked after the household while her mother, a divorcee with three children, worked at a local silk company. Herta fell in love with the new boarder, and in 1940 she and Sternbach married. It was a plucky thing to do. She was a Christian, and marrying a Jew, even in Switzerland, jeopardized her security. In addition, Swiss law required her to forfeit Swiss citizenship and take her husband's Polish citizenship. Indeed, no sooner had she married than she received word from the police that she was now a "tolerated foreigner" and would be expected to leave Switzerland soon.[12]

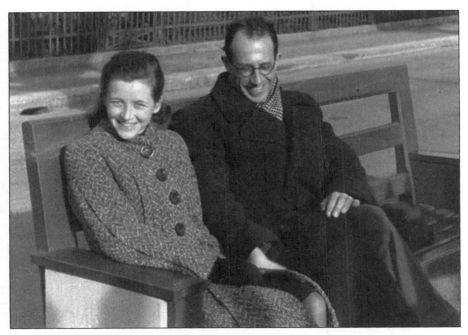

Leo Sternbach and Herta Kreuzer. Leo Henryk Sternbach with Herta Mia Kreuzer, shortly before Hoffman-La Roche relocated the couple from Zurich to its American campus in Nutley, New Jersey. Reproduced courtesy of the Sternbach Family.

Hoffman-La Roche agreed to relocate the newlyweds to New Jersey. Sternbach's scientific training earned him a visa; Roche insisted that Sternbach's expertise in vitamin synthesis made him indispensable to America's war effort. The Sternbachs began life in the New World in the residential enclave of Upper Montclair, a few miles from the company's expanding Nutley campus. In time, the campus's towering research building would be known as "the house that Leo built" in recognition of Sternbach's invention of Librium and Valium, the most profitable drugs in Roche history. In the 1940s, however, Sternbach was but one of many scientists (officially a senior chemist, "the lowest level of the Ph.D.s") organizing the laboratories and working on vitamins, which remained Roche's commercial stronghold.[13]

Sternbach's first breakthrough was the synthesis of B7 (biotin), a vitamin that breaks down fatty acids and carbohydrates. Even today, it is a staple ingredient of multivitamins. Along with benzodiazepines, it's the

achievement Sternbach valued most. In the mid-1950s, as profits for synthesized vitamins declined in the wake of patent expirations and increased
competition, Roche gave its chemists a new imperative: develop a drug
that will outsell Miltown and Thorazine, now the bestselling major tranquilizer. The new tranquilizers, particularly Miltown, were the envy of the
ethical pharmaceutical trade: every company wanted in on that market. It
was, in the words of one journalist, the time of the "Great Tranquilizer
War." Sternbach remembered the corporate ambience of those years as one
of great uncertainty and high expectation. "We chemists were asked to
submit proposals for the synthesis of tranquilizers which we then could
follow up," he recalled. "So I submitted something." The proposal seemed
sufficiently promising to the research director, who reassigned Sternbach
to Roche's tranquilizer team.[14]

Ensconced in his Nutley laboratory, Sternbach considered how best to
formulate a compound that would satisfy Roche's management. A medicinal chemist has several options for creating new compounds. One is to
synthesize natural medicinal products. Roche had already done this with
vitamins, and other companies were beginning to do this with hormones.
Another approach is molecular modification, sometimes disparagingly
called molecular manipulation. It is this chemical tinkering that underlies
the phenomenon of "me-too" drugs with a similar therapeutic and chemical profile to those already available. Today they represent an astounding
77 percent of new prescription drugs on the American market. Zeroing
in on a profitable therapeutic, chemists tweak its molecular structure to
create a drug that is not particularly innovative but new enough to secure patent protection and thus higher prices. Pharmaceutical firms
often time the launch of me-too drugs to coincide with the end of the
patent life of a blockbuster medication. For example, when the patent
protection on the popular allergy pill Claritin was scheduled to expire in
2002, Schering-Plough refigured Claritin's active metabolite and
patented the new compound as Clarinex. The new drug hit the pharmacy shelves just as Claritin was poised to go generic. In these cases and
others, company chemists create me-too drugs hoping to extend a
blockbuster's profits.[15]

More often, as physician and writer Marcia Angell notes, chemists are asked to modify the structure of *other* companies' drugs to capture a piece of a competitor's market. Sternbach could have pursued this strategy, creating me-too drugs modeled after Smith Kline & French's Thorazine or Carter's Miltown. In fact, his superiors had asked him to pursue just this tack, which they saw as the quickest road to success. Beginning with Miltown's chemical family, the meprobamates, he could "change the molecules a little. Make them different enough to avoid violating Wallace's patent, but similar enough to produce a tranquilizer." Sternbach balked. Molecular modification struck him as superlatively boring, and he assumed researchers in other companies would be doing the same. Sternbach wanted to be different. The management's suggestion "did not appear to be very promising," he remembered. "If you work with modifications of old drugs," he once contended with gentle disdain, "you can only find drugs which are similar to those."[16]

Sternbach's suspicions proved prescient. In 1955, at the start of the tranquilizer war, there were three pharmaceutical companies marketing three tranquilizers. By 1957 ten companies shared the tranquilizer market. By 1959 there were nineteen. Within a four-year span, the pharmaceutical industry had concocted a fusillade of minor tranquilizers, new drugs reengineered from old chemistry. None was as profitable as meprobamate.[17]

Sternbach held steadfast to his desire to invent something pharmacologically novel. Rejecting molecular modification, he pursued a riskier strategy: the random pharmacological screening of chemicals. His objective was to identify a compound with previously unknown tranquilizing properties. This approach was vastly more time-consuming than molecular modification. Since the 1990s, much of this labor-intensive work, historically carried out by bench chemists (who literally worked on a bench, experimenting with molecules), has been automated. Laboratories now use computers to generate many molecules simultaneously, and robots scan them to determine which may have the desired characteristics. The age of bench chemistry and the sequential testing of new compounds has yielded to computer-generated combinatorial chemistry and high-throughput screening. Smaller pharmaceutical outfits often shun these

capital-intensive screening procedures, precisely because of the low probability that random screening will yield a marketable (never mind profitable) drug. When the strategy does bear fruit, however, the payoff can be
huge. "People say the chances are very small," Sternbach averred. "But
then, if you find something, it will be something completely new." Such
was the case with Librium.[18]

Sternbach revisited the benzheptoxdiazines, compounds he had
worked with as a postdoctoral assistant at the University of Krakow in the
early 1930s. At the time, he had hoped to identify new dyestuffs. That
search had failed. But the benzheptoxdiazines had other advantages that
made them well suited for Sternbach's current mission. They were accessible, easily synthesized, and chemically malleable. Twenty years after
Sternbach had worked with them, they remained relatively obscure. They
crystallized well, which meant that it was possible to generate quickly a
large batch of compounds. The benzheptoxdiazines had never been tested
for biological activity, but in Sternbach's mind, their molecular weight
suggested that they might produce biologically active agents. Did he believe they would produce tranquilizers? Not initially. "I didn't have any
idea," he admitted. But they seemed like a good place to begin. His section chief at Hoffman-La Roche, Wolf Goldberg, was less confident that
Sternbach's exploration would identify tranquilizing compounds. But he
gave Sternbach his consent.[19]

Scrawling on his blackboard and poring through his notes, Sternbach
began his benzheptoxdiazines experiment. The chemistry fascinated him.
Ever the tinkerer, he tested multiple combinations, altering the tempera-
tures at which they were mixed, changing the method by which they were
dissolved. A scientist who rejected theory-based hypotheses in favor of intuition and gut feelings, he once likened his zeal for chemistry to an artist's
irresistible but inexplicable love of his craft. On a hunch, he synthesized
some of the compounds with a chlorine in the side chain (a part of the molecule attached to the core structure) and reacted them with various secondary amines. (Amines are members of a family of nitrogen-containing
organic compounds derived from ammonia. They are classified as primary,
secondary, or tertiary depending on how many of the hydrogen atoms—

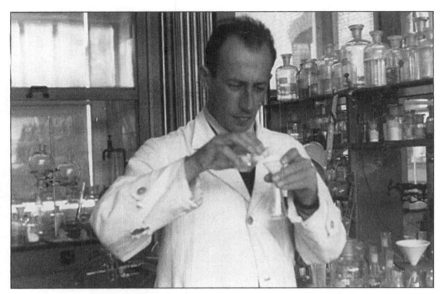

Leo in the Lab, 1941. A self-described "chemist's chemist" who rejected theory-based hypotheses in favor of instinct, Sternbach was more interested in working in his laboratory than in creating a blockbuster medication. It was during a laboratory clean-up that Sternbach stumbled on Librium, a compound he and coworker Earl Reeder had forgotten to submit for pharmacological testing. Reproduced courtesy of the Sternbach Family.

one, two, or three—have been replaced by organic compounds.) Harking back to that moment, he remembers that inventing a blockbuster medication was not uppermost in his mind. "I wasn't interested . . . in helping the whole world," he said. "I was interested in working in the laboratory."[20]

Sternbach synthesized some forty new benzheptoxdiazine derivatives. Each was submitted for testing to Dr. Lowell Randall, Roche's new chief of pharmacology. To Sternbach's chagrin, each proved pharmacologically inert, totally devoid of tranquilizing attributes. Roche executives were frustrated too, and in 1956 they reassigned Sternbach to antibiotic research, chiding the chemist for failing to produce something useful. Before Sternbach concluded his tranquilizer experiments, however, he and coworker Earl Reeder treated one of the derivatives with methylamine, a primary amine (given that secondary and tertiary amines had produced consistently negative results). He labeled the result Ro 5–0690 and shelved it for later evaluation.[21]

By 1957, the most remarkable feat Sternbach could claim in his antibiotic work was the clutter he and his coworkers had created in the laboratory. It was, he remembered, a chaotic and hopeless situation. Laboratory benches were "covered with dishes, flasks, and beakers—all containing various samples and mother liquors. The working area had shrunk almost to zero, and a major spring cleaning was in order." It was during the April cleanup that Earl Reeder drew his attention to the untested sample, the white crystalline powder he and Sternbach had created the year before. The two debated whether they should throw it out. Reeder encouraged Sternbach to submit it, the last of the benzheptoxdiazine derivatives, for pharmacological evaluation. Sternbach sent the sample to Randall on May 7, 1957. It was Sternbach's forty-ninth birthday.[22]

A month earlier, the *New York Times* had reported Roche's entry into the mental health market. The drug of note was iproniazid, trade name Marsilid. It was one of two potent drugs Roche had developed in 1951 for the treatment of tuberculosis, still the world's deadliest scourge. Doctors observed unexpected and remarkable psychological changes in TB patients on Marsilid: they gained weight and became energetic and cheerful. Psychiatrists took notice. Nathan Kline, director of research at Rockland State Hospital, proceeded to test the drug on hospitalized schizophrenics and private-practice neurotics. As Kline told colleagues at the annual meeting of the American Psychiatric Association, the drug produced remarkable mood improvement among both groups. The results suggested that the drug would be effective "with severely depressed patients who are sometimes made worse by the tranquilizers." Roche wasn't sure how to market Marsilid. In 1957 scientists were beginning to discuss chemical explanations for depression, but there was as yet no market for antidepressants. The company's research had focused exclusively on the hunt for a tranquilizer. Marsilid was clearly no tranquilizer. "Marsilid increases what doctors call psychic energy whereas the tranquilizers reduce energy," one report explained. Roche latched onto this descriptor, initially marketing Marsilid as a psychic energizer. Although Roche withdrew the drug in 1961 because of adverse effects on the liver, its success in launching what would later be considered the first MAO inhibitor helped advance the company's legitimacy in the field.[23]

With Ro 5–0690, Randall applied the standard protocol to assess whether experimental compounds had tranquilizing attributes. In what is known as the inclined screen test, mice were fed the experimental compound and placed at the bottom of a tilted screen. Undrugged mice scramble to the top without difficulty. Tranquilized mice, on the other hand, eventually slide, as if commanded by gravity, in a relaxed stupor to the bottom. Remarkably, although the mice in Randall's test slid to the bottom of the screen—proof of the agent's muscle relaxant and anticonvulsant properties—they remained alert and active. Mice hung limply when held by one ear but were able to walk when prodded. The compound also passed the industry-wide "cat test." Medicated cats held by the nape of the neck hung flaccidly and without struggle; those that had once been considered "mean" became both amenable to handling and "contented, sociable, and playful." Randall tested the properties of Ro 5–0690 against meprobamate, chlorpromazine, and phenobarbital, drugs used widely in clinical practice. He released the results to his superiors on July 26, 1957. Randall's words became part of the benzodiazepine legend. "The substance has hypnotic, sedative, and antistrychnine effects in mice similar to meprobamate," he reported. But it was vastly more potent. It was also less toxic and sedating than any tranquilizer on the market. Indeed, it was the most interesting antianxiety compound Randall had seen. Through luck, intuition, and the long process of trial and error, Leo Sternbach had landed Roche a winner. The company christened Ro 5–0690 Librium, from the last syllables in "equilibrium."[24]

Sternbach discovered something else. Mapping the molecular structure of Ro 5–0690, he learned that he had unwittingly created chemicals unrelated to the structure of his forty previous derivatives. A step in Sternbach's synthesis—what he might later have dismissed as a chemical error had it not portended success—had unintentionally created a new class of chemicals, the benzodiazepines. Presently there are dozens of benzodiazepines on the global market, but Ro 5–0690, generic chlordiazepoxide, was the first. Benzodiazepines share a chemical structure that consists of a benzene ring of six carbon atoms attached to a seven-membered diazepine ring.[25]

Scholars debate who or what should get credit for the discovery of a new technology. Does innovation spring from the inventor, from the community and collective actions that lead to its discovery, or from the long pedigree of ideas that readied the way? What counts as a breakthrough? How do we distinguish genuine innovation from pedestrian improvement? The birth of the benzodiazepines highlights these complexities. Had Miltown not been a commercial success—had patients and physicians not come to understand anxiety as meriting pharmaceutical treatment—there surely would have been no tranquilizer war to inspire Sternbach's hunt. Miltown's triumph laid the commercial and cultural topsoil that created an enabling environment for the invention of benzodiazepines. But benzodiazepines also sprang from the acts and predispositions of a number of individuals: Leo Sternbach's determination to create a new rather than a me-too compound and the chemical misstep that generated Ro 5–0690, Earl Reeder's discovery of the shelved sample and his insistence on testing it, and Lowell Randall's recognition and determination of the pharmacological properties of benzodiazepines. Librium's genesis was nested in the confluence of diverse factors, personalities, and events. Over time, however, the birth of the benzodiazepines came to be known to the public as Leo Sternbach's heroic achievement as well as his lucky break.[26]

Official clinical trials of Ro 5–0690 began in 1958, but Sternbach conducted the first unofficial trial on himself. This was not an uncommon practice among psychopharmacologists in the 1950s. At a time when results from randomized clinical trials were increasingly being counted as objective evidence of a drug's effects, many succumbed to the desire to know what drugs felt like, firsthand. Roche did not condone self-testing in the 1950s, and now it strictly forbids researchers from serving as "two-legged rats." Sternbach did it anyway, on the sly. He swallowed 50 mg of Librium in the fall of 1957. (Today, 10–40 mgs is considered an appropriate onetime dose for anxiety relief.) The time was 8:30 A.M. By 10:00, he wrote in his journal, he was starting to feel "slightly soft in the knees." By the afternoon, he felt drowsy, and by 6:00 P.M. the effects had passed. In the spring of 1958 he applied for a patent on the compound. The application described the novelty of the benzodiazepine and the methods for producing it. But it made no mention of its therapeutic applications, which clinical trials were only beginning to demonstrate.[27]

Premarket trials provided the company with ammunition for creating a novel niche in the robustly competitive tranquilizer market. The clinical uses of tranquilizers had hitherto been divided into two therapeutic spheres: meprobamate for mild anxiety and antipsychotics such as chlorpromazine (phenothiazine derivatives, also known as the major tranquilizers) for severe disorders. Neurotics had their own class of tranquilizers, psychotics another. But what if one pill could alleviate anxiety in patients in both diagnostic camps, as well as those who fell into the diagnostic borderlands? If such therapeutic versatility could be demonstrated, Roche would have itself a blockbuster.[28]

Scales and questionnaires to measure the severity and extent of a person's anxiety were just coming into use. This was part of a larger impetus in medicine to recognize only clinical data that could be impersonally collected and quantified. Together with randomized clinical trials and diagnostic screening tests, anxiety scales signified a growing trend toward discounting subjective experience and standardizing variability. Scientific claims about a person's health or a drug's efficacy would henceforth be based on the putative objectivity of aggregate numbers. People's experience of nervousness—what might previously have been dismissed as an atypical but normal bump in the road—was reread as an objective medical condition. In 1959 London-trained psychiatrist and statistician Max Hamilton created the Hamilton Anxiety Rating Scale (HARS), a fourteen-item questionnaire that provided clinicians with a tool for quantifying the severity of patients' anxiety symptoms. Each of the fourteen items, which included fears, anxious moods, and muscular complaints, was assigned a value ranging from 0 (not present) to 4 (severe). Hamilton's was not the first anxiety scale, but it proved particularly popular. Together with its cousin, the Hamilton Rating Scale for Depression (devised in 1960), it demonstrated rising enthusiasm for psychometrics and facilitated the transformation of isolated symptoms into proven pathology. This process was critical for the medicalization of anxiety. In the 1960s and 1970s, it also provided doctors and pharmaceutical companies with a scientific justification for the clinical use of benzodiazepines. This changeover did not happen overnight, of course. The title of a chapter in Roche's 1965 physicians' manual, *Aspects of Anxiety*, "Can Anxiety Be Measured?" suggests the absence of a consensus that it could. Still, the codification of anxiety into medical pathology had begun.[29]

Miltown's popularity had fueled doctors' interest in the pharmaceutical treatment of anxiety while marking the drug—at least in some psychiatrists' minds—as insufficiently potent for what could now be "objectively" defined as chronic or severe cases. As Irvin Cohen, a psychiatrist and professor at the University of Texas-Galveston, explained, the most frequently encountered psychiatric patient in the late 1950s was the "ambulatory psychoneurotic." These were not the Hollywood celebrities or television personalities who popped Miltown for fun. Indeed, Miltown's reputation for recreational use only amplified its association with mild and transient anxiety. Psychoneurotics fell into a different category. In such patients, anxiety was debilitating enough to necessitate regular medical monitoring but insufficiently acute to warrant hospitalization. Treating psychoneurotics was a pharmacological challenge. Meprobamate was often too weak, whereas the phenothiazines were frequently too strong. The phenothiazines, Cohen recalled, also "had too many side effects and potential complications to warrant regular use." Doctors were intrigued by the possibility of a compound whose potency fell somewhere in between.[30]

Roche enlisted Cohen and other researchers to conduct trials of Librium on adults in prison, hospital, outpatient, and office settings. The diversity of treatment sites and patient populations was strategic. Roche hoped that the trials would reveal Librium to have a wide therapeutic range, applicable to patients with an array of medical disorders but also divergent "social addresses." This would give the company the data it needed to market Librium as a drug suitable for a broad patient population: an expanded diagnostic category that warranted more tranquilizer users. In this way, Hoffman-La Roche was able to shape the contours of the future Librium market even before the FDA approved the tranquilizer. The profiles of trial participants ran the clinical and social gamut and included outpatient neurotics, narcotics addicts, college students, geriatric patients, alcoholics, and psychiatric patients recently discharged from a New Jersey hospital. In Aberdeen, South Dakota, researchers tested Librium on more than two hundred patients at the city's mental health center and in private practice, including a group of premenopausal farm women with phobic anxiety states who were purportedly obsessed with menopause.[31]

Trial participants also included male prisoners at the psychiatric treatment center of the Texas Correctional System in Houston. Included were inmates in a high-security penitentiary with psychopathic personalities and a history of antisocial behavior. These were not the worried well of Miltown fame but men prone to violent or erratic outbursts. Distributing a tranquilizer to dangerously unruly state prisoners was thought to be a true test of its clinical reach; if Librium could calm these individuals, surely it could calm anyone. But the recruitment of prisoners also reflected the widespread practice of using incarcerated convicts as medical subjects in the 1950s and 1960s, a practice that declined only in the 1970s following the adoption of new federal guidelines. Across the country, federal and state prisoners were utilized for studies on cancer, influenza, malaria, syphilis, pain tolerance, and chemical warfare. As historian David Rothman and others have shown, the gilded age of research in postwar American medicine was marked by the categorical belief that prisoners—abundant, cheap to use, easily monitored, long-term and, as one pharmaceutical company researcher put it, "guaranteed to show up"— were ideal research subjects. As Roche had hoped, clinical studies revealed Librium to be an effective and safe tranquilizer that reduced anxiety, agitation, and aggression. It was more potent than meprobamate and did not have the same complications or side effects as Thorazine. Equally important, as Cohen reported, Librium's "calming action was accomplished . . . without clouding consciousness or interfering with intellectual acuity." Librium soothed but did not sedate.[32]

Thus even before a single prescription had been written, Roche had amassed vast data on Librium's clinical performance and a research pedigree that framed how the tranquilizer could be marketed. In the new drug application (NDA) submitted to the FDA and approved on February 24, 1960, the company confined its analysis to 1,163 patients. In reality, the drug had been tested on some 20,000 subjects (a discrepancy partly explained by regulations that allow companies to choose which trial data they submit for review to the FDA). Because NDAs are private documents, the media discussed the exponentially higher figure Roche made available to the public when it reported trial results. Newspaper articles waxed enthusiastic about trials involving 2,000 physicians, more than a dozen "leading institutions," and upward of 20,000 patients.[33]

The scientific allure of aggregate numbers was matched by the rhetorical power of anecdote. In journals, researchers enthusiastically recounted their Librium success stories. A college student with "long-standing anxiety neuroses" showed an immediate improvement after he began taking 25 mg of Librium three times a day. His nightmares stopped, he became more affable and relaxed, and his grades improved. A fifty-one-year-old depressed woman with both "menopausal distress" and anxiety about her son (who had recently dropped out of college to pursue a singing career) improved dramatically on Librium after just six days. Her electroconvulsive therapy was canceled in favor of a maintenance drug regimen. A sixty-one-year-old male physician who had begun to complain of "increasing anxiety with insomnia and belching" had reduced his patient load, certain that work stress was to blame. After eight weeks of Librium, he resumed his practice without further complaint. During a trial involving German American women from strict backgrounds who had married farmers and feared going insane, harming their children, or losing their husbands to other women, researchers coined a new term: "frustrated farmer's frau syndrome." All but one made a quick recovery. The improvement had been so consistent among the more than two hundred patients enrolled in the trial that the researcher proclaimed Librium "the most significant advance to date in the psychopharmaceutical treatment of anxiety states."[34]

The prison trials affirmed the drug's worth as a tool of social control and prompted researchers to ponder its potential for managing other disruptive groups. One obvious target was disorderly children. Texas researchers discussed Librium's value for treating conduct disturbances in children and adolescents. The *New York Times,* in turn, relayed this suggestive finding to millions of readers. Roche would subsequently promote the use of tranquilizers in children and college students experiencing isolation, aggression, learning difficulties, and apathy.[35]

In the 1950s and 1960s, mental health researchers frequently faced a litany of criticism, including the subjective nature of psychiatric illness and the related concern of how to evaluate objectively improvements in a class of disorders whose etiology and expression were individual and unique. Efforts to objectify the findings of psychiatric trials were further complicated by their varied settings. If psychiatry recognized the importance of the environment in causing and curing disorders, how could the effects of a reduced workload or a less restrictive regimen for prisoners be disassociated from the workings of a drug?

What helped make the Librium studies so compelling was the unanimity of the results. Irrespective of where the trials had been carried out or on whom, Librium had consistently proved therapeutic. It calmed outpatient neurotics as well as agitated prisoners. Researchers had even found Librium useful in the treatment of eczema and epilepsy, and in allaying anxiety associated with childbirth and operations. By the time Librium hit the market in March 1960, the drug's efficacy and safety were the subject of over a dozen medical reports, including a clinical note in the prestigious *JAMA.*[36]

In 1960 Roche scientists and executives were still in the dark about how benzodiazepines worked or why they worked differently from other sedatives such as barbiturates and meprobamate. They only knew that they did. As it turned out, that was enough to position Librium as the country's newest ethical blockbuster.[37]

Roche had amassed a number of key selling points for the promotion of Librium. The marketing campaign, masterminded by Manhattan's McAdams advertising agency, made the most of them. McAdams had been established in 1926 by Chicago journalist William Douglas McAdams; its other clients included Glaxo, Amgen, and Hoechst-Rouseel Pharmaceuticals. McAdams promoted Roche's new drug aggressively, spending over $2 million in Librium's inaugural year. Detail men showered doctor's

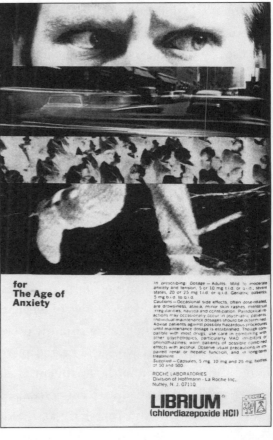

Librium for the Age of Anxiety. Hoffman-La Roche marketed Librium, the first benzodiazepine, as the perfect panacea for cold war frights and phobias. Tellingly, the face of anxiety pictured in this 1964 advertisement was male. *Archives of Internal Medicine* 114 (1964).

offices with the *Roche Record Report*, a pamphlet containing five long-playing records on which physicians discussed their clinical successes with Librium. The McAdams agency sent forty mailings to doctors in a few months and published eight-page ads in dozens of medical journals. The promotion's objective was stunningly ambitious, as novel as Librium itself. Instead of trying to corner a niche in one sphere of the polarized tranquilizer market, Roche decided to conquer both therapeutic halves.[38]

The campaign trumpeted two main points. The first was Librium's status as a new chemical agent and not a manipulated molecule. In a commercial milieu in which most of the roughly four hundred new drugs introduced each year were variants of older drugs, Roche showcased this distinction. While journalist naysayers decried the slowed pace in the production of radically new drugs, Roche trumpeted its tranquilizer as unique.

The refrain most frequently found in advertising copy boasted that "Librium is as different from the tranquilizers as they were from the barbiturates." The drug's package insert described Librium as "completely unrelated chemically, pharmacologically, and clinically to any tranquilizer . . . [currently] used in medical practice."[39]

The second strand of Roche's campaign emphasized Librium's versatility in the treatment of a multiplicity of anxiety states. After two years of clinical trials, Roche determined that Librium could help patients whose anxiety ranged from mild to moderately severe. In 5 mg doses, Librium was branded "effective in mild to moderate anxiety and tension, tension headache, pre- and post-operative apprehension, premenstrual tension and menstrual stress, behavior disorders in children, and whenever anxiety and tension are concomitants of gastrointestinal, cardiovascular, gynecologic or dermatologic disorders." In doses of 20 mg, Librium was "of value in the more severe anxiety and tension states, chronic alcoholism, agitated depression, and ambulatory psychoneuroses (e.g., acute and chronic anxiety states, phobias, obsessive-compulsive reactions and schizoid behavior disorders). In addition, Librium may be useful in certain types of acute agitation, such as delirium tremens, hysterical or panic states, paranoid states and acute stages of schizophrenia." Librium was thus both chemically unique *and* therapeutically versatile. Roche recognized the risks of its promotional strategy, acknowledging that "any attempt to aim at both halves of the market entailed a risk of failing to capture either." Instead, Librium swept the market, rendering other tranquilizers commercially obsolete.[40]

When Librium was introduced, five tranquilizers dominated the trade: Equanil, Compazine, Thorazine, Miltown, and Stelazine. Their combined sales accounted for 70 percent of the market. Three months after its commercial debut, Librium had become the bestselling and most frequently prescribed of the bunch, effectively dethroning the others. Once established as the market frontrunner, Librium stayed there. By October 1960, newcomer Hoffman-La Roche had ensnared 20 percent of the tranquilizer market with a drug rightly described as the runaway ethical drug of the year. Doctors were writing more than 1.5 million new prescriptions for

Librium every month.[41] Other compounds, particularly me-too tranquilizers, could not compete. In August, Merck, Sharpe & Dohme launched Striatan, a manipulated molecule related to the meprobamate family. It never stood a chance. Doctors and patients remained infatuated with Librium, a tranquilizer in a class by itself.

Within the beige walls of his laboratory in Nutley, Leo Sternbach was largely shielded from the marketing hype. According to Sternbach, Roche chemists were not involved in the machinations behind the promotion or sale of their drugs. Librium's patent acknowledged Sternbach as the inventor, but patent rights and profits were the exclusive province of Hoffman-La Roche. As did most pharmaceutical scientists, Sternbach sold his patent to Roche for $1, the going rate. "Most chemists at that time were all hired under that type of proviso," he recalled. The company rewarded Sternbach with a bonus of $10,000, a mere pittance next to the drug's sizable profits. A few years later, Hoffman-La Roche would give Sternbach the same amount—a $1 patent sale and a $10,000 bonus—for the invention of Valium.[42]

Although the two blockbusters earned the company billions, Sternbach never felt bitter or even shortchanged by what he got out of the deal. "I am not," he later contended, "a victim of capitalistic exploitation. If anything, I am an example of capitalistic enlightenment. . . . I was grateful to the company for bringing us over from Europe, for providing my family with a certain security." The trappings of material success held no appeal. (Whether this general contentment with his lot in life and passion for chemistry made Sternbach different from other chemists is unknown, but it is intriguing that chemists in the United States have the lowest divorce rate of any professional group.) "I have never made money the major objective of my life. It has always been chemistry. Herta and I—we don't have any especially expensive hobbies. You see, we were brought up modestly, and I never developed any expensive hobbies, since chemistry was my hobby and I could live from my hobby by getting paid for it. . . . We don't want any more houses. One house gives us enough work." Asked in 1976, three years after his retirement, if he might like to own shares of Hoffmann-La Roche stock, Sternbach replied, "Not particularly. What I would like to see in terms of medicinal chemistry are some drugs which would lower blood pressure and keep it low and some anti-inflammatory drugs which would keep arthritis in check. Those are the things which interest me—not villas, not yachts, not shares of Hoffman-La Roche stock. I am really a very simple man."[43]

Sternbach's modesty did not keep him from taking pride in his achievements. He knew that the corporate world was replete with research chemists who worked for decades and invented nothing the company deemed valuable. Librium's success also secured him new opportunities and instant prestige: "I made the compound [but] it also made me." Executives at Hoffman-La Roche who had previously disparaged his laboratory output treated him with renewed respect, even awe. He was promoted to senior group chief, overseeing the work of several laboratories. "People were listening more to what I was saying," he recalls. "I was a very happy scientist." His son Michael remembers how his dad got very emotional about Librium, the drug that "buried Equanil [and] Miltown." But the best part for Leo Sternbach was how Librium's commercial success freed him to continue to work in his lab.[44]

Sternbach's next big project was to create a better benzo, more potent with fewer side effects, and without Librium's bitter aftertaste. Librium had been the fortuitous outcome of Sternbach's trial-and-error screenings. No one questioned its innovative character. Now, however, Sternbach reversed course. He turned to molecular modification, setting his sights on other members of the benzodiazepine family, a class of chemicals he had created but insufficiently explored. "You always look for something better," he explained to justify his altered direction. "You go on to cover the whole area of your patent. You don't want to have ten compounds patented and then have somebody come along with the eleventh. You explore the whole area to see how much you can change the molecule without losing the tranquilizing activity."[45]

Sternbach would go on to patent other benzodiazepines, including flurazepam (trade name Dalmane) and clonazepam (trade name Klonopin). But the one that brought him fame and had the widest impact was made on October 26, 1959, just months before the FDA approved Librium's sale. The compound had a cumbersome chemical name: 7-chloro-1,3-dihydro-1-methyl-5-phenyl-2H-1,4-benzodiazepin-2-one. A member of the Hoffmann-La Roche advertising team named it Valium, for the Latin word *valere,* meaning to be in good health, to fare well. Thanks to Librium and Valium, Roche handily won the tranquilizer war. As we shall see, however, not all users of these and other tranquilizers were as convinced as Roche management that they fared well under their chemical spell.[46]

(7)

Suffering Amid
the Silence

In 1960 Hoffman-La Roche invited Leo Hollister, a Stanford professor and physician at the Palo Alto Veterans Administration hospital, to a meeting in Princeton, New Jersey, to discuss the launch of Librium (chlordiazepoxide). Although he lacked formal training in psychiatry and pharmacology, Hollister had become a major figure in the development of both fields, renowned for his carefully crafted and documented clinical trials of psychiatric drugs. Hollister's impressions of the meeting gave him pause. Despite his enthusiasm for pharmacotherapy, he became increasingly wary of the company's zeal. Did the hype match the reality? "If this drug is as good as these people say," he remembered thinking, "it's going to be abused." Medical studies since the early 1950s had documented the addictiveness of barbiturates, and reports on similar problems associated with meprobamate had begun to trickle in. Hollister wondered if Librium, poised to be the next pharmaceutical sensation, might also cause problems. He decided to investigate.[1]

For several months, Hollister administered high doses of Librium to thirty-six hospital patients and then abruptly switched eleven to placebo. Ten suffered withdrawal reactions: insomnia and agitation, decreased appetite, and nausea. Two patients had seizures. Hollister's study suggested

141

that it was possible to become physically dependent on high-dose Librium. This finding effectively countered Roche's claims that its new and improved tranquilizer was not habit forming.[2]

Hollister relayed the bad news to Roche. "I wasn't trying to kill their drug," he recalled. But he thought patients needed to know about the documented withdrawal reaction *before* the drug was marketed so they could be informed that after "long-term use of the drug they [should] taper it as they stopped." According to Hollister, Roche was not very happy with the discovery. Hollister's results were published in 1961 in *Psychopharmacologia*, the first article to document withdrawal reactions to benzodiazepines. A few years later, Hollister published findings demonstrating a comparable withdrawal reaction to Valium (diazepam), Roche's second benzo blockbuster.[3]

Concern about benzodiazepine dependence failed to find a wide audience, however. Prescription drug addiction in general and tranquilizer dependency in particular would not become front-page news until the 1970s and 1980s. Even among physicians cognizant of the problem, the benefits of a drug that soothed crippling anxiety and smoothed social relations often outweighed the risks of individual dependence. Enthusiasm for tranquilizers remained rampant. In this milieu, patients kept demanding them, doctors kept prescribing them, and the media stayed mum about a problem as grim sounding as "prescription addiction."

That respected doctors prescribed tranquilizers to some of the nation's most upstanding citizens helped, in the short run, to shield the drugs from critical censure. Moral panics about drugs and alcohol were nothing new in American culture, yet the perennial links between illicit drugs, deviant behavior, and socially marginal groups didn't hold in the case of tranquilizers; they were prescription-only medications used by America's finest. In the nineteenth century, working-class immigrants had been the public face of middle-class moralists' crusade against demon rum. In the twentieth, campaigns against heroin, cocaine, and marijuana were permeated by a vitriolic racism, xenophobia, and class prejudice. Headline-hungry journalists invoked racially charged stereotypes to spin sensationalist tales of African American miscreants crazed on cocaine raping white women, and Mexican migrants, wild on weed, crashing cars for the sheer thrill of it.[4]

This inflammatory reportage created a climate of paranoia, kindling anxieties about the dangerous addict and his sinful, drug-bound culture. It also divided the world into artificial realms of vice and virtue: the addict on the street hived off from law-abiding Americans cocooned in the protective confines of an abstemious home. In such a falsely compartmentalized world, the idea of a successful executive or suburban housewife addicted to prescription tranquilizers had limited political salience.

It took a sea change in American culture to recast addiction to prescription medications as a problem warranting sustained public scrutiny. During the interlude, when the politics silenced the science, millions of people around the globe took Librium, Valium, and other tranquilizers. Their enthusiasm, augmented by rising acceptance of the biochemical basis of anxiety, catapulted Hoffman-La Roche into the pharmaceutical stratosphere, making it the most profitable drug company in the world.

But the silence surrounding the drug's safety left tranquilizer users in the dark. Often uneasy, sometimes confused, patients and their caregivers contacted friends, family, doctors, and agencies for guidance and support. The paper trail they left for posterity is a poignant tribute to the personal costs of medical uncertainty. Sadly, by the time the habit-forming potential of tranquilizers became common knowledge, untold numbers had already experienced the private anguish addiction can bring.

Writing for Answers

In 1957, a concerned woman wrote the FDA about Miltown. Her niece was taking the tranquilizer and the aunt, a book dealer in Mount Vernon, New York, was worried. She was not convinced that her niece's fondness for this drug "for settling the nerves, is a wholesome thing." The niece's doctor had promised his patient that Miltown was not habit forming, but the aunt wanted the FDA's position. "I will never be completely at peace till I have an opinion from such an authority," she contended.[5]

In the 1950s and 1960s, hundreds of women and men penned similar missives, chronicling their experiences and soliciting the agency's counsel on tranquilizers. These letters, often written with touching candor, captured the

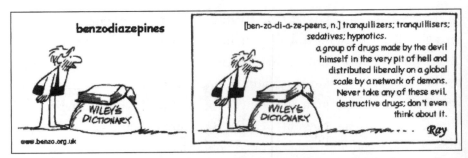

Benzos Defined. Activist organizations such as benzo.org.uk were among the first to collect and circulate information on the hazards of benzodiazepine use. Reproduced courtesy of benzo.org.uk.

profound faith Americans had in the FDA as the country's most trusted source of pharmaceutical information. In today's information age, when details about prescription drugs are accessible online and in reference books, it is difficult to appreciate the obstacles our predecessors faced attempting to educate themselves about medications. Yet at a time when patient package inserts were not yet available to inform consumers about possible side effects, in an age when the mainstream media celebrated the wonders of new drugs, countless Americans turned to the FDA for objective and reliable advice.[6]

Their letters also reveal nagging and growing doubts about the veracity of media claims and the reliability of doctors' judgment. Over time, these reservations—Is my niece's physician right? Is this drug really safe? Why am I having these problems if it is?—helped galvanize the fledgling consumer and women's health movements and fueled a political backlash against tranquilizers and other prescription drugs. Accounts of private experience were an integral part of the activist movements that made the side effects of medications part of the public domain. From the 1950s until the 1970s, however, patients, friends, and families were left to sort out the pros and cons of tranquilizers largely on their own.

The doubts that prompted these letters gave them a palpable edge. A man from Braintree, Massachusetts, wrote in 1956 asking if meprobamate was addictive. Like the doctor treating the book dealer's niece, his physician had insisted it was not. The man had done some independent reading, however, and discovered a few articles refuting his doctor's claim. He wanted a decisive answer. "What I want to know,' he asked the FDA, is "is it a so-called habit forming drug? Is there a definite opinion on it? Would two tablets [of 400 mg each] once a day create tolerance for it or a craving for it later or over a period of time for larger amounts?"[7]

FDA officers fielded these questions with discretion and diplomacy. Under section 502(d) of the Federal Food, Drug, and Cosmetic Act, non-narcotics (such as tranquilizers) did not have to be labeled habit forming unless they contained a derivative of barbituric acid. The act made no provision for exemptions from this requirement, even when the *possibility* of addiction existed. The FDA's responses tenuously balanced the latest clinical evidence and assessed drug responses among a general population, while upholding doctors' preregoatives to evaluate individual patients' needs and risks. Communicating research findings, the FDA steadfastly supported physicians' professional authority and redirected correspondents to them. By law, manufacturers were obligated to furnish doctors (but not consumers) with information on the proper dosage, use, possible side effects, and contraindications of tranquilizers. This, presumably, was enough. As the director of the Bureau of Medicine's Division of New Drugs explained to one correspondent in 1961, "We believe that these drugs can be used safely by the physician with this labeling available to him." This stance, which took little heed of a patient's "right to know" (the subsequent rallying cry of the consumer and women's health movements), made doctors the final arbiters of prescription decision making. Only physicians were capable of judging whether tranquilizers were appropriate, given the complex variables in play.[8]

The FDA's response to the inquiry from the Braintree man typified its handling of these inquiries. "It is difficult to give you a direct yes or no answer to your question," the FDA official wrote. "Certainly, meprobamate is not in a class with the opium derivates insofar as its habituating tendencies are concerned, and it is not one of those drugs which is required by law to be labeled with the legend: 'Warning—may be habit forming.'" But the official also acknowledged that "it cannot be said unequivocally that the drug cannot in any circumstances be habit forming in certain individuals who have a tendency to overuse or misuse any drug which has a pleasurable effect." The patient was encouraged to talk to his doctor. "If your physician has advised you that there is no danger of habit formation in your case, we certainly have no reason to question his judgment."[9]

Unfortunately, information furnished by manufacturers to doctors would later be proven incomplete. When a physician published a case study asserting Librium addiction (evidenced by escalating dosages and withdrawal symptoms when the drug was discontinued), Roche's s medical director published a response suggesting a very different interpretation: an intensification of the disorder that required higher dosages and the recurrence of preexisting symptoms once the drug was stopped. The company steadfastly championed this position—that tranquilizers were rarely habit forming—in other communications. The literature that Carter-Wallace and Roche sent to doctors about Miltown, Librium, and Valium, for example, acknowledged that discontinuation symptoms had occasionally been reported. But it emphasized that this problem was most likely to occur in addiction-prone individuals or patients who had taken excessive (nontherapeutic) doses for extended periods of time.[10]

The diplomacy apparent in FDA correspondence in the 1950s and 1960s was partly attributable to the murkiness of addiction science in this era. Research on prescription sedatives and hypnotics was still in its infancy, and current-day distinctions between addiction, habituation, and psychological and physical dependence, pleasure-seeking behavior, therapeutic misuse, tolerance, and withdrawal reactions upon abstinence were still being debated and refined. The fuzziness of addiction research was compounded by the absence of clear scientific answers to several questions. Was everyone equally susceptible to addiction or was there significant individual variability? Did the likelihood of addiction inhere in an individual (the so-called addictive personality) or was the drug mainly to blame? Did the dosage or duration of use affect dependence? When Senator Estes Kefauver's subcommittee reprimanded Carter-Wallace in 1960 for failing to disclose "reservations about the habit forming characteristics of the drug," Frank Berger's reply hinted at some of the crosscurrents of contemporary ideas about addiction. Berger urged policy makers to assess the addictive properties of meprobamate in a comparative context. "Alcohol, when used improperly, can be habit-forming [too]," he contended. "But you don't find a warning to that effect on a bottle of beer." Berger's rejoinder sought to soft-pedal meprobamate addiction by equating it with other accepted habits. Americans were dependent on alcohol, coffee, and tobacco, he told *Vogue,* but "most people don't think of these as addictions. There are some people who just get addicted to things—almost anything." By the same token, "There is no warning on scalpels—this is sharp—don't cut yourself."[11]

Berger's argument—that when addiction existed, the problem was tied to the person rather than the drug—did little to silence meprobamate's growing chorus of critics. The safety of tranquilizers, first meprobamate, then benzodiazepines, had been grounded on a series of contrasts. When meprobamate was marketed in 1955, no evidence suggested it was habit forming. Compared to barbiturates, which produced colossal casualties, meprobamate appeared *relatively* safe. As the exchange between Berger and the committee suggests, however, by the late 1950s studies had begun to show that, among some users, meprobamate caused physical and psychological dependence. Less toxic than barbiturates, meprobamate was nevertheless something other than the "non–habit forming" drug its manufacturer originally claimed. Although death rarely resulted from a meprobamate overdose, studies showed that it was possible. Concerns about meprobamate's addictiveness, in turn, paved a receptive path for Librium. Chemically different from meprobamate, benzodiazepines seemed (and in the long run were proved) safer too, as long as safety was measured by a drug's lethality in overdoses. As Librium buried meprobamate as America's tranquilizer of choice, Leo Hollister's cautionary report on withdrawal reactions to benzodiazepines remained on the back burner.[12]

As benzodiazepines swept the country, ordinary Americans were thus left to their own devices to discern the risks of the newest tranquilizers. In the early 1960s, the FDA's handling of the thalidomide disaster gave countless patients added incentive to seek the agency's counsel. The tragedy, which caused at least 10,000 children to be born with severe abnormalities, stoked patient doubts about prescription medications even as it strengthened respect for the FDA's role in protecting Americans from harm.[13]

Developed by the German pharmaceutical firm Grunenthal, thalidomide was used widely in Western Europe between 1957 and 1961, chiefly
in Germany. It was prescribed for insomnia, nervous tension, and as an
antiemetic for morning sickness among pregnant women. Drug regulation
in postwar Germany was more decentralized than it was in the United
States (partly a reaction to the Nazi regime, which had banned the manufacture of new drugs and limited pharmaceutical expenditures on sick or
"degenerate" citizens), and the German system gave pharmacists, doctors,
and health insurers significant control over the pharmaceutical market. In
this regulatory environment, Grunenthal zealously marketed thalidomide
as a nonaddictive and safe alternative to barbiturates that would not cause
death upon overdose. Advertisements for thalidomide pictured tranquil
nature scenes and touted its benefits as an antidote to workplace stress. By
1960, thalidomide had become the country's bestselling sedative, used regularly by about 700,000 Germans of all ages; indeed, its use in restless
children earned it the dubious nickname of "West Germany's baby-sitter."
Although by 1960 Grunenthal was marketing thalidomide in over forty
countries, its sale was blocked in the United States by a newly appointed
FDA reviewer, Frances Oldham Kelsey.[14]

Kelsey was a mother of two who held undergraduate and master's degrees in pharmacology from McGill University and M.D. and Ph.D. degrees from the University of Chicago. She joined the FDA in August
1960, a month before the U.S. licensee, William S. Merrell, Inc., submitted its application to sell thalidomide under the brand Kevadon. Merrell
wanted Kevadon on the U.S. market by Christmas, when holiday stress
historically delivered sedative manufacturers their largest sales. Given the
drug's global popularity, FDA approval was expected to be straightforward
and simple. Partly for these reasons Merrell's application was assigned to
Kelsey, the bureau's newest recruit.[15]

When she joined the FDA, Kelsey was one of only seven full-time
and four part-time physicians in charge of drug applications. Unknown
to Merrell, she had a long-standing interest in drugs and fetal safety. As
a graduate student, she had studied how quinine, used to treat malaria,
was metabolized differently in pregnant rabbits and observed how the

drug passed the placental barrier from mother to fetus, a view that challenged prevailing pharmacological wisdom that drug use in pregnancy was inherently safe. Reviewing Merrell's thalidomide application, she found its data on toxicity, absorption, and excretion woefully inadequate. She asked the company to submit additional data in a new application. It did. Kelsey remained unconvinced. The scientific evidence seemed incomplete, "more like testimonials than the results of well-designed, controlled studies," she remembered.[16]

Frustrated by this unexpected female bottleneck, Merrell's representative, Dr. Joseph Murray, tried to influence Kelsey with personal appeals. When phone calls and office visits failed to exact their desired effect, he contacted Kelsey's superiors. He complained that the female rookie was "unreasonable and nit-picking," and that she was stubbornly delaying the drug's approval. Kelsey was unmoved by the company's admonitions. "I think I always accepted the fact that one was going to get bullied and pressured by industry," she recalled, about what her FDA work would entail.[17]

While Kelsey stood firm, medical reports from Europe began to document an alarming phenomenon: a wave of miscarriages, stillbirths, and deformed babies. The common link was women's use of thalidomide during pregnancy. The drug would soon be associated with severe birth defects, including phocomelia—a condition previously considered so rare that it wasn't even listed in many medical dictionaries—in which children are born with extra appendages (such as toes appended to the hip or fingers attached to the shoulder), abnormally short limbs, or no limbs at all. Thalidomide was also associated with eye and ear abnormalities and malformed internal organs. Thousands of thalidomide babies, about 40 percent German-born, died in childhood.

In late 1961 German health officials took the drug off the market. Other countries soon followed suit. In March 1962, Merrell finally withdrew its sixth application, a testimonial to Kelsey's caution and concern. As a full accounting of thalidomide's horrors became known, Kelsey found herself thrust into the spotlight. "Heroine of FDA Keeps Bad Drug Off of Market," ran the headline on the front page of the *Washington Post* on July 15, 1962. "This is the story," author and acclaimed journalist Morton

Mintz began, of "how the skepticism and stubbornness of a Government physician prevented what could have been an appalling American tragedy, the birth of hundreds or indeed thousands of armless and legless children." Public response to the drug-related calamity helped propel the passage of stronger regulations to protect medical consumers. In 1961 Senator Estes Kefauver, who had spearheaded a multiyear investigation of the pharmaceutical industry, had proposed a bill to reduce drug prices. Initially blocked by the American Medical Association and drug manufacturers, Kefauver's crusade was reenergized by the thalidomide disaster and President Kennedy's entreaties to Congress to support regulatory reform. The political momentum converged in the 1962 Kefauver-Harris amendments, which gave the FDA greater control over clinical trials and required firms to demonstrate a new drug's efficacy (in addition to its safety). For the first time, the FDA was empowered to monitor the accuracy of manufacturers' promotional claims. The amendments, which also extended FDA oversight of drug approval and marketing, were passed unanimously in the Senate and House on August 7, 1962, only a few weeks after the *Post* ran the story. President John F. Kennedy awarded Kelsey the medal for Distinguished Federal Civilian Service, the highest civilian honor.[18]

Kelsey's actions inspired not only politicians and lawmakers but also ordinary citizens who turned to her for tranquilizer advice. The thalidomide scare had popped the bubble of unbridled confidence in the safety of pharmaceutical panaceas. Pictures of thalidomide babies published in magazines and newspapers around the world paid silent tribute to the potential hazards of all medications, reminding American consumers of their vulnerability to the machinations of industry and the inadvertent ignorance of well-intentioned physicians. Paradoxically, the thalidomide disaster also confirmed the value of America's regulatory exceptionalism in the global pharmaceutical market, based on a centrally controlled review process that would be strengthened in the years after thalidomide. (Ironically, during the AIDS crisis, activists contended that the FDA's measured handling of new drug applications, far from protecting patients, was condemning countless people to die.) In a world where drugs could hurt as well as heal, the FDA had bucked other countries' regulatory trend and kept its citizens safe. Soon Americans of all ages and backgrounds wrote Kelsey, as they would a family member or friend, for honest answers about the country's newest pharmaceutical sensations, Librium and Valium.[19]

"I am writing you in regards of [sic] a new tranquilizer my doctor gave to me just a few weeks ago," wrote one sixty-three-year old woman. "It is called Valum [sic]." She was nervous that the drug might be proven hazardous. "I am writing you asking if this drug is OK to take, has it been proven safe, or is it like the one I read about? I am afraid of these new drugs. How do we know they are safe?"[20] "Honorable Dr. Kelsey," began another letter from a public assistance worker in Puerto Rico,

> I read about the great service you rendered our country in keeping the drug thalidomide out of the market. Congratulations; ORCHIDS on you. Along with the presidential award comes to you the recognition and eternal gratitude of we American parents who will praise forever the 'woman doctor who saved thousands.' As the use of tranquilizers and sleeping pills is widely spread and with little or scarce medical data or info at hand, I'll appreciate your knowful [sic] orientation in regard to the LIBRIUM caps.[21]

A Vermont woman applauded Kelsey's vigilance but urged the FDA officer to devote equal time to reviewing the safety of other approved medications, "drugs which the doctors are giving without knowing too much about them." She even volunteered to help. "If I can be of any help in any way, how I would love that!" she exclaimed. In the meantime, "Do you know anything about the drug LIBRIUM?"[22]

Kelsey or one of her assistants responded to each inquiry, thanking correspondents for their compliments. But the letters upheld the spirit and limits of previous communications: the information communicated was largely formulaic. Similar to the advice dispensed on meprobamate, FDA correspondence on benzodiazepines charted a fine line between judging the overall safety of benzodiazepines and respecting physicians' prerogatives to ascertain their suitability for individuals. Understandably, consumers wanted information directly relevant to them. Instead, the FDA's letters, nested in a broader

complex of ethical obligations and political limitations, stopped short of offering private medical advice. Hence the woman from Vermont was apprised
that Librium had been approved under the terms of the Federal Food, Drug,
and Cosmetic Act, based on careful scientific review of "clinical investigations showing it to be safe for use in the conditions for which it is offered in
its labeling." Her personal physician, rather than the FDA, was best positioned to advise her. FDA officials found it perfectly consistent to acknowledge the variability of patients' needs while affirming the FDA's resolve to
pull benzodiazepines off the market or change how they were labeled if sufficient evidence proved them hazardous to a broad population. A woman
from Long Island, New York, apprehensive that her use of Librium during
pregnancy might harm her fetus, was advised that the FDA had no information "which conclusively establishes a causal relationship associated with the
use of 'Librium' and birth deformities," but that appropriate action would be
taken if "future data establishes a direct relation between birth abnormalities
and the use of a particular drug." Until such time, she should assume that the
drug was safe to be used as her doctor saw fit.[23]

Although we cannot know if tranquilizer users were comforted by the
FDA's feedback, what seems likely is that they fared no better seeking information from manufacturers. In June 1963, a few months before Valium
came on the market, a Florida man contacted Roche. He wanted to know
the side effects and safe dosage margins of the "turquoise colored, small
tablets" a psychiatrist had dispensed to his son during a clinical trial. "I believe the proper name is Valium," he wrote. He enclosed a tablet for chemical analysis so the company could corroborate its identity. George W.
Wyllie, Roche's associate director of professional services, responded, thanking him for writing Roche directly. However, he noted, "at the present time
I can simply point out that this is still a rather new product . . . available only
to selected clinicians through our clinical research and medical investigation
departments. These physicians, of course, are making observations on the
use of the product so that information concerning its beneficial effects and
limitations will be readily available to other physicians when the product is
eventually distributed for their regular prescription use." The father became
irate. He wrote again, demanding immediate answers. He got none. Echo-

ing the FDA's refrain, Wyllie encouraged the man to contact his son's physician, who was in "a position to evaluate it objectively in terms of a particular patient's individual requirements and response."[24]

Benzodiazepine Blockbusters

While patients and their caregivers pondered and puzzled, for Hoffman-La Roche, these were happy times. Librium remained the nation's most frequently prescribed drug until 1968 when Valium, released November 15, 1963, overtook it. While Librium had been unexpectedly lucrative, Valium was astronomically profitable. More potent than Librium and lacking its unpleasant aftertaste, Valium was the first $100 million brand in pharmaceutical history, and between 1968 and 1981, the most widely prescribed medication in the Western world. Valium rapidly became a staple in medicine cabinets, as common as toothbrushes and razors. In Auden's age of anxiety, Westerners had found their favorite chill pill.[25]

At Roche's Nutley plant, three giant pill-stamping machines spat out tablets at a rate of four hundred per second. In fifteen hours, the factory's assembly lines generated a whopping 30 million of them: enough to satisfy global consumption for five *days*. Roche's commercial coup reflected the fact that they were sitting on two bestsellers. Interestingly, Valium did not render Librium obsolete but increased net tranquilizer sales at a time when they already claimed a huge portion of the prescription drug market. In 1973, when Valium topped the sales charts, Librium held firm in fourth place behind oral contraceptives and painkillers. Between them, Librium and Valium cornered the mushrooming tranquilizer industry, accounting for $200 million of Roche's $280 million sales in 1971 and 81 percent of America's total tranquilizer sales in 1974. *Fortune* called the benzodiazepine blockbusters "the greatest commercial success in the history of prescription drugs."[26]

Their triumph fanned the fortunes of the Swiss-based company. The benzodiazepine boom spurred a meteoric rise in company sales that escalated as Valium swept the global market. Within a few years, Roche's economic viability became inseparable from its tranquilizer trade, which by 1968 accounted for a whopping 62 percent of the company's prescription drug revenue. The triumph of benzodiazepines made the company the world's largest and most lucrative pharmaceutical manufacturer, not only the "undisputed world market leader in psychopharmaceuticals," according to *Fortune*, but also "one of the most profitable enterprises on earth." By 1972, a single share of Hoffman-La Roche cost $73,000, making it the most expensive stock in the world.[27]

Benzodiazepines thrust Roche into the pharmaceutical super leagues while increasing the company's vulnerability to the financial vagaries of the psychotropic market. In the vernacular of the business world, Roche was at risk of becoming a flamingo business standing on one leg because of its overdependence on a single product group. The company tried to protect itself from the inevitable financial downturn that would follow once the "money spinners" went off patent by developing new benzodiazepines, several of which, including Klonopin, were commercially successful. It also continued to research treatments for fungal and tropical diseases, chemotherapy for cancer, and cardiovascular drugs.[28]

Despite its diverse portfolio, most Americans viewed Roche as a tranquilizer firm. Carter-Wallace and other firms continued to manufacture tranquilizers, but the success of Librium and Valium caused Carter-Wallace's profits to tumble (dropping 16 percent the year after Librium was introduced) and cemented Roche's tranquilizer identity. The company cultivated this identity among practitioners through a marketing campaign coordinated by the McAdams advertising firm. With McAdams's prodding, the company redirected most of its revenue into product promotion, reserving only a fraction of sales income for benzodiazepine manufacture and distribution. In 1975 Roche spent an estimated $400 million on Librium and Valium promotion.[29]

The pitch was slick but professional. The 1960s were marked by rising concern about the truthfulness and scientific accuracy of drug promotion, a concern reflected and furthered by the passage of the Kefauver-Harris amendments. At the same time, pharmaceutical advertising increased and medical advertising agencies thrived. Marketing research became more sophisticated as agencies began auditing purchases of prescription drugs, systematically tracking the relationship between doctors' medical journal readerships and drug-prescribing preferences, and establishing physician focus groups to gauge doctors' visceral responses to proposed ads.[30]

Roche was part of this marketing expansion, as pharmaceutical firms increasingly allocated larger sums of money for detailing, advertisements, samples, and physician education programs. Doctors and medical institutions were courted by Roche detail men, who were coached to hype Valium's unique action and therapeutic versatility. Valium was cast as a one-of-a-kind drug, superior to other benzodiazepines, even Librium. FDA tests in the 1960s *had* demonstrated that Valium was five times more potent as a tranquilizer and muscle relaxant than Librium and ten times as strong as an anticonvulsant. Roche beseeched sales representatives to hammer home this message, employing visual aids to augment their verbal pitch. These included glossy brochures left in offices for review that explained why "all benzodiazepines are not alike," and how to "select a benzodiazepine."[31]

The one thing detail men did not leave behind was samples. Hoffman-La Roche supplied them but only by mail, and only when doctors returned a prepaid postcard requesting them. The company adopted this strategy in 1973 to make the company's campaign appear more detached and professional after critics complained of the company's penchant for showering doctors' offices with samples. As the company's president and CEO boasted in 1979, "technically . . . we [no longer] give out any samples." In practice, the bureaucratic loophole made little dirt on the unfettered traffic of free Valium. In 1978 the U.S. market in samples to doctors' offices was estimated to be 15 million tablets. The company also donated free tranquilizers to medical institutions. In Canada, Hoffman-LaRoche gave away 82 million Valium samples, valued at $26 million, to hospitals in a single year.[32]

Hoffman-La Roche also promoted Valium and Librium in a spate of glossy ads. Psychotropic drug advertising had mushroomed in the 1960s and 1970s. The April 1978 issue of the *American Journal of Psychiatry*, for example, contained an astounding sixty-four pages of advertisements.

Because psychiatrists represented a minority of doctors prescribing tranquilizers (with an estimated 97 percent of general practitioners prescribing them, there was no need to consult a specialist for a script), the McAdams agency placed most ads in mainstream medical journals. Ads by themselves, of course, do not tell us if or how they influenced practitioners; what they do best is reveal the workings and aspirations of marketers. Roche ads encouraged the use of its benzodiazepine blockbusters for the "relief of tension and anxiety alone or whenever somatic complaints are concomitants of emotional factors." Given that emotions were thought to affect or contribute to many, if not most, physical disorders, Valium could be prescribed for almost anything; it soon became known in the trade as Valium the Versatile. Roche also promoted the drug for alcohol withdrawal and as an adjunct in the treatment of convulsive disorders and skeletal muscle spasms caused by inflamed muscles or joints and cerebral palsy.[33]

Advertisements covered a wide pathological spectrum. As women's activists rightly insisted, many depicted Valium as a quick fix for the problem of simply being female. Ads championed Valium as a remedy for neurotic singles, worn-out moms, exhausted businesswomen, and irritable menopausal women, such as Sally Wilson, a fictional character featured in one ad. "Sally Wilson has lost her reputation," it began. But there was good news. After only a week on 5 mg tablets of Valium, *four times a day,* her reputation as an "unpredictable grouch" had melted away. The menopausal misfit finally relaxed: "She's less tense and taut; she's more friendly and cheerful and wants to be part of her world." Another equally disturbing ad recommended Valium for Jan, an archetypal thirty-five-year old single woman whose inability to find and marry a man as good as daddy was the primary culprit behind her twinned spinsterhood and psychoneurosis.[34]

Tranquilizer ads consistently championed pscyhotropics as an antidote to "transgressive" female behavior: being single in a world where women were expected to get married, getting cranky or tired juggling the dual demands of caregiving and breadwinning. Social functionality was pivotal to the drug's putative success; the real winners in these narratives, it seemed,

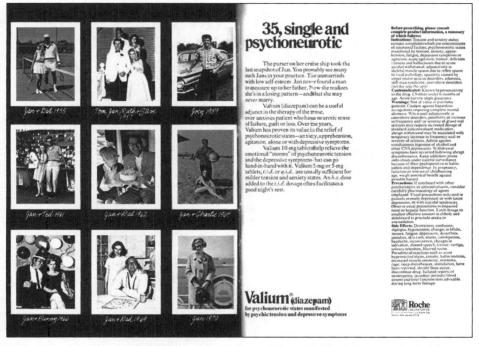

Thirty-Five, Single, and Psychoneurotic. This Valium ad chronicled Jan's downward spiral into a state of agitation and depression after the attractive go-getter fails to find a man good enough to measure up to daddy. The presumption that being single in an age when women were expected to marry could cause psychoneurosis suggests how ideas about women's proper place shaped psychiatric diagnosis and psychopharmacology. *Archives of General Psychiatry* 22 (1970).

were less the tranquilized women than the children, husbands, coworkers, and friends who had suffered at their hands. In one Valium ad featuring a formerly tense schoolteacher, Mrs. Raymond, pupils do a delighted double take when the medicated and mollified instructor returns to the classroom "trim and smartly dressed the way she was when school began." The ad pictured the teacher, coiffed and elegantly appointed, applying lipstick in front of an open compact held by manicured nails to her flawless face. The teacher-student relationship, bounded by proper appearances and good behavior, had been pharmaceutically restored. [35]

Men too appeared in Roche ads for benzodiazepines. This mirrored a broader pattern. One study examining sex differences in pharmaceutical advertising from 1968 to 1972 found that a majority—52 percent—of patients were male.[36] But men's anxieties were more likely to be characterized as

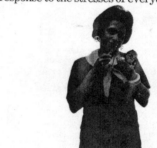

Mrs. Raymond's pupils do a double-take

And with good reason. She's trim and smartly dressed the way she was when school began.

Valium (diazepam) has helped free her of the excessive psychic tension and associated depressive symptoms accompanying her menopause.

Now she's poised and cheerful again.

Like many patients on Valium, Mrs. Raymond has tolerated it well. Such commonly reported side effects as drowsiness, fatigue and ataxia have not bothered her. Nevertheless, her physician is observing all the precautions and warnings summarized on the opposite page.

Whenever you need an effective adjunct to hormonal therapy for tense, menopausal patients, consider Valium...to help encourage a calmer response to the stresses of everyday living.

Mrs. Raymond. Pharmaceutical advertising in the 1960s and 1970s consistently promoted tranquilizers to counteract deviant female behavior. This ad pathologized menopause while vaunting Valium's ability to restore a teacher's proper appearance and conduct. *Archives of Internal Medicine*, November 1970.

somatic, a hidden but contributing cause of duodenal ulcers, heartburn, and cardiovascular disease. Because men's anxiety was experienced inwardly through organic illnesses rather than emotional outbursts, their problems were less debilitating to others but more incapacitating to them. A 1968 Roche manual, *Aspects of Anxiety*, encouraged physicians to regard men as different from women but no less in need of tranquilizers:

Like women, men are under particularly heavy stress during periods of major adaptive efforts. For adult males, these typically include leaving the parental home, serving in the armed forces, marrying, becoming a father, getting ahead in business, growing older, and retiring. Men's problems, however, are compounded by an unspoken obligation to live up to society's concept of ideal masculinity. This concept requires the adult male to 'act like a man' in difficult situations or actual crises. Whatever occurs, a man must be 'stronger' and 'better controlled' than a woman would be. Which may be one of the reasons he dies earlier than his wife [sic]. Men—according to one point of view—dam up their feelings and develop ulcers and high blood pressure. Women, being feminine, are irrational, complaining, given to tears.[37]

The challenge faced by the typical American man, the manual maintained, was that he could rarely afford to relax. Reinforcing the gendered stereotypes of the 1950s, ads pitched anxiety and its accompanying discontents as the natural but injurious cost men paid for their success.[38]

Tranquilizer ads presented a picture of male anxiety replete with stock characters of overachievement: exuberant athletes, successful executives, and stridently individualistic bachelors unable to forge meaningful familial relationships. The athlete who pushed too hard on the basketball court or the football field and the overwrought businessman grappling with gastrointestinal disorders were glorified as social achievers with physical disorders that Valium could heal. "Have you heard the one about the traveling salesman?" one Roche ad began. "The strain of tracking down customers and living out of a suitcase—the family matters left unsolved at home—no joking matter to a man emotionally overreactive to stress and vulnerable to duodenitis." Tranquilizers wouldn't remove the cause of male anxiety. But in easing its pain and physical consequences, they helped deal with the psychological fallout.[39]

Roche's focus on the pathology of success was furthered by a three-year program, inaugurated in 1979, on the effects of stress and the benefits of tranquilizer therapy. Designed to educate physicians and the public on the management of stress, it was funded by a $4.8 million educational grant from Roche and was supported by visiting faculty lectures, audiotapes and brochures, and a three-hour closed-circuit broadcast televised in twenty-six cities and viewed by nearly 10,000 general practitioners and psychiatrists. The consumer phase of the program involved seminars for journalists writing on health topics and included the epidemiology of stress, its diagnosis, psychological and psychosomatic expressions, and the role of pharmacological intervention in its management, particularly the use of Valium. Physician attendees received continuing education credit, an added incentive to participate.[40]

The program's newsletter, *Clinical Roundtables,* highlighted the causal connection between stress and organic disease. Roche's program was developed at a time when many medical problems, including asthma, allergies, ulcers, and migraine headaches, were considered largely the result of "stress." (Physicians today dispute the view that one's mental well-being can single-handedly cause or modify physical disease, although few would deny that mental states may encourage a person to engage in behaviors—such as smoking or alcohol consumption—that increase one's risk for disease.) Stress possessed tremendous explanatory power. Impossible to define as a distinct entity, it was that much more impossible to dismiss. Tranquilizers fit neatly into this disease paradigm. However tenuous the evidence regarding causality, no one could disprove scientifically (in part because stress is impossible to measure precisely) that stress is harmful. In this diagnostic gray zone bounded by science, speculation, and semantics, manufacturers such as Hoffman-La Roche worked to expand their market. Acknowledging the difficulties defining the relationship between stress and disease, one edition of the newsletter nonetheless recommended the judicious use of tranquilizers to allay its incontrovertible hazards.[41]

Other initiatives also gave benzodiazepine a timely boost. One took place during the Carter administration under the leadership of Dr. Peter Bourne. Bourne was a British-born and American-educated psychiatrist who had served in a neuropsychiatry unit in Vietnam and as the director of Georgia's office of drug abuse when Carter was governor. As Carter's special assistant for health issues and director of the Office of Drug Abuse from 1977 to 1978, he spearheaded many medical initiatives, but the one that garnered perhaps the most attention was his campaign to restrict access to barbiturates. Despite the popularity of tranquilizers, barbiturates were still among the most widely used drugs in the United States in the 1970s ($21 million of barbiturates were sold wholesale in 1975 and more than 3 million prescriptions were written the following year). Their popularity perpetuated the devastating cycle of addiction and death that had begun in the early twentieth century. Indeed, their dangers became front-page news again as Americans mourned the barbiturate-related deaths of several cultural icons, including Marilyn Monroe, Judy Garland, and Elvis Presley. Obviously most victims were not rich and famous. According to Bourne, "more persons die from barbiturates than all drugs put together— suicides, accidental deaths of children who get them in medicine cabinets, inadvertent overdoses." A self-identified liberal who had publicly advocated a more forgiving policy toward marijuana use, Bourne held fast to his proposal that doctors limit barbiturate use to hospitalized patients. Outpatient users were encouraged to talk to their doctors about the "availability today of other, safer drugs to ease tension and promote relaxation."[42]

Bourne's initiative spurned an immediate and incendiary response from angry users. One woman lambasted Bourne's scheme as nothing short of horrendous. There was, she fumed, "a vast difference between people who pop 20, 30 or so pills a day . . . and someone like myself who has had a series of very tragic incidents in my life, or a business man under great pressure, who takes a sleeping pill every night under a doctor's prescription." If a doctor felt comfortable prescribing a sleeping pill so that a patient could get a good night's sleep, who was Bourne to take that authority away from him? Bourne's staff reassured the irate constituent that the objective wasn't to remove sedatives from the market but to replace barbiturates with "alternative, safer medications."[43]

These, of course, included benzodiazepines. Studies showed that the number of deaths related to the exclusive use of benzodiazepines was small; most fatalities involved mixing tranquilizers with alcohol or other drugs. Marketed as suicide-proof, Valium was considered safe, even when taken in excess. This claim was tested in very public ways. When Robert McFarlane, Ronald Reagan's national security adviser, tried to kill himself during the Iran-Contra scandal, he downed between twenty and thirty 5 mg tablets, far exceeding the maximum approved daily of dose of 40 mg. The attempt was futile. He woke up days later in the hospital, embarrassed but very much alive.[44]

The exchange between Bourne and his constituent also revealed something else: a growing acceptance among patients and practitioners that anxiety was a serious medical matter warranting pharmacotherapy. Neither

Bourne nor the angry constituent contested the therapeutic value of psychotropic drugs; at issue, rather, was which drug was best. By the 1970s and 1980s, drugs had become the gold standard in the treatment of mental illness. The widely discussed case *Osheroff v. Chestnut Lodge* illustrated the extent to which patients had come to regard pharmacotherapy a medically essential, individual right. The plaintiff, a physician named Dr. Rafael Osheroff, was admitted to Chestnut Lodge psychiatric hospital in Maryland on January 2, 1979, following a two-year bout with anxiety and depression. For more than four decades, Chestnut Lodge had been a leading center for psychotherapy and psychoanalysis. Hospital staff diagnosed Osheroff with severe depression and a narcissistic personality disorder. He was treated exclusively with individual psychotherapy four times a week. But his condition worsened and he became agitated, paced incessantly, developed insomnia, and lost forty pounds. Alarmed by his physical and mental deterioration, his family demanded that the hospital review and modify Osheroff's treatment. Chestnut Lodge ceded to the first request but continued to trumpet psychotherapy as Osheroff's best hope for recovery. After seven additional months of psychotherapy yielded no sign of improvement, the family transferred Osheroff to a hospital in Connecticut, where he was given a combination of phenothiazines and antidepressants. In a few weeks, his symptoms improved. Osheroff was discharged three months later to resume his medical practice with outpatient medication and psychotherapy.[45]

In 1982, Osheroff filed suit against Chestnut Lodge, claiming medical malpractice. Had the center not withheld drug therapy, Osheroff and his lawyers contended, his condition would have improved sooner. "I lost a whole life," Osheroff avowed. "I had a million-dollar medical practice. I lost that. I lost my status in the medical community. I lost the respect of my patients, I even lost contact with my children."[46] Osheroff won an out of court settlement.

Osheroff v. Chestnut Lodge provoked widespread debate in medical, lay, and legal circles. The case raised several key points. One was the resistance of some psychiatrists and hospitals to pharmacotherapy. Far from being foisted on resistant patients, drugs had been deliberately withheld at

Chestnut Lodge in favor of talk therapy, a treatment that a growing numbers of psychiatrists now considered outdated and ineffective. Osheroff had suffered because drugs had been denied. Were other doctors similarly undermining their patients' well-being through dogmatic stubbornness? Would they too be sued? *Osheroff* illustrated the steep price of refusing to prescribe psychotropics at a time when they had become medically sanctioned and routine.

The perceived seriousness of anxiety and its status as a recognizable medical problem were tied up with the issue of the subjectivity of psychiatric evaluation and treatment. In 1979, when Osheroff was admitted to Chestnut Lodge, the American Psychiatric Association's reigning diagnostic guide remained the second edition of the *Diagnostic and Statistical Manual of Mental Disorders* (DSM), published in 1968. The first DSM, issued in 1952, was the product of American military psychiatrists' frustration with existing psychiatric nomenclature, catalogued in the American Medico-Psychological Association's *Statistical Manual* (initially drafted to allow the Bureau of Census to collect uniform data on the institutionalized population). It proved woefully inadequate for the range of cases doctors encountered in World War II, particularly servicemen afflicted with combat-related disorders. DSM overhauled existing guidelines in an effort to expand and standardize psychiatric diagnosis in ways that acknowledged reigning psychodynamic and psychoanalytic models while recognizing the various mental health problems of the noninstitutionalized population. Particularly influential were the ideas of William C. Menninger (brother of the equally well-known psychiatrist Karl Menninger), who served as chief of the Army Medical Corps psychiatric division during World War II, and Adolf Meyer, a professor of psychiatry at the prestigious Johns Hopkins University medical school who helped groom the leadership of American psychiatry during the interwar years. DSM-I meshed the tenets of prevailing psychoanalytic theory with Meyers's related and influential conviction that mental illness is best understood in terms of specific reactions stemming from the individual's incapacity (the result of a person's life history) to adapt successfully to his or her environment. Psychiatry's goal, wrote Meyer, must be to explain "how the observed maladjustment came about." In DSM-I, anxiety was considered the chief characteristic of psychoneurotic disorders; how a person handled anxiety denoted the type of reaction.[47]

The DSM-II, written by the psychoanalytically dominated APA in 1968, expanded the number of listed diagnoses from 106 to 182 but maintained the discipline's etiological emphasis. Reactions were reframed as neuroses, the bread and butter of psychoanalysis. Until DSM-III came along, the clinician's charge was, in the words of one psychiatrist, to "understand the meaning of the symptom and undo its psychogenic cause, rather than manipulate the symptom directly."[48]

Published in 1980, DSM-III was hailed as a revolution in biological psychiatry and the beginning of the end of psychoanalysis. DSM-III abandoned the etiological orientation of the first and second editions in favor of diagnostic criteria based on descriptive psychopathology. Suffering that had at times defied words was classified by committees of psychiatrists, chaired by Columbia University's Robert Spitzer, into a laundry list of 265 mental illnesses defined by symptoms rather than causes. To buttress claims of objectivity, DSM-III's nomenclature was subjected to extensive clinical field tests in which psychiatrists assessed its reliability and utility. In the words of Harvard psychiatrist Gerald Klerman, a proponent of the new manual, DSM-III represented "a strategic mode of dealing with the frustrating reality that, for most of the disorders we currently treat, there is only limited evidence for their etiologies." Hypotheses and theories abounded, but for most disorders "the evidence is insufficient and inconclusive."[49]

The third edition of the diagnostic manual found a dedicated following almost immediately and put the American Psychiatric Association (APA), not yet a globally respected authority in 1952 at the time of the first DSM, on the international map. Indeed, DSM-III became one of the world's most used and respected diagnostic reference tools, eventually superseding the World Health Organization's competing *International Classification of Disease* series. Two years after its publication in February 1980, DSM-III had sold more than 240,000 copies. Klerman remembers what a thrill it was to track its reception in Western Europe, Scandinavia, the Middle East,

China, and Japan, where "it was a delight to see leading Japanese psychiatrists, particularly the professors, carrying around the mini-DSM-III and studying it with characteristic Japanese vigor."[50]

DSM-III was ostensibly atheoretical. For the first time, the identification and alleviation of symptoms took pride of place over theories of pathogenesis. The APA hailed the latest revision as an important step in the discipline's march toward scientific perfection. In DSM-III, enthusiasts insisted, field trials and objective markers of illness had triumphed over unproven theories and unverifiable clinician intuition. But DSM-III was nevertheless steeped in assumptions. Its radical retooling merely demonstrated how psychiatric diagnosis and treatment reflected the ideas of its time. As Leo Hollister put it, DSM-III ought to be regarded as less a definitive guide than a representation of "the thinking of some experts at a particular period of history . . . [and] not immutable." Just as psychiatry is an imperfect science, so too are psychiatric diagnoses, "often imprecise and seldom limited." Although the caveats Hollister flagged were debated, DSM-III's emphasis on alleviation of symptoms quickly prevailed.[51]

The manual's rhetoric and findings were ineluctably yoked to biological psychiatry, particularly the views of a new breed of psychopharmacologists who believed that clinicians could and should use drugs to treat patients' symptoms. Under DSM-III, the symptoms denoted the illness. The commercial and clinical success of pharmaceutical treatments cemented this biomedical identification. Chlorpromazine, meprobamate, benzodiazepines, and antidepressants: the very fact that these drugs improved patients' symptoms encouraged biological explanations for mental illness while providing practitioners with a broader mandate to treat it pharmacologically. No one claimed that chlorpromazine *cured* schizophrenia. But if psychopharmacology made the illness less devastating, how could doctors ethically exclude it from their therapeutic domain?[52]

Ultimately the DSM-III both mirrored and encouraged the prevalent prescription of anxiolytics. In the early 1950s, when psychoanalysis ruled American psychiatry, advertisements for Miltown had gingerly introduced the drug as an adjunct to psychotherapy. By the late 1970s, manufacturers confidently promoted anxiolytics as stand-alone compounds useful for treating a range of disorders. As one contemporary observed in 1975, advertisements for benzodiazepines cast anxiety as a medical problem, making "individual brain chemistry, rather than social conditions, the target for intervention."[53]

Expanding research on neurotransmitters and benzodiazepines gave scientific weight to the view that anxiety is a biochemical disorder of the brain amenable to pharmacotherapy. Neurotransmitters are chemical substances that transmit nerve impulses across a gap (synapse) that separates one nerve cell from another. These chemical messengers communicate information between neurons and the brain. One of the tenets of modern neuroscience is that our thoughts and feelings are produced when billions of neurons in our brain simultaneously communicate with one another.[54]

There are different types of neurotransmitters. Researchers studying the effects of drugs had concluded that benzodiazepines, like barbiturates, meprobamate, and alcohol, affected the neurotransmitter gamma-aminobutyric acid (GABA). It is the brain's chief and most prolific inhibitory neurotransmitter. GABA produces a calming effect by slowing the rate of neuronal firing, decreasing the nerve membrane's excitability. By the 1960s, scientists had already determined that alcohol, barbiturates, and other agents potentiated GABA's inhibiting effects on animal subjects. But because benzodiazepines were markedly less sedating than other agents, researchers began to explore the mechanisms that would explain benzodiazepine's selectivity of action.[55]

In 1973, scientists published research demonstrating the existence of opiate receptors in the brain, proteins located on the surfaces of nerve cells to which opiates such as morphine and heroin attach. They suggested that opiate drugs work by mimicking the natural workings of opiate-like molecules. The discovery of opiate receptors prompted researchers to look for benzodiazepine receptors too. Like opiates, benzodiazepines are both potent and selective in action. In April 1977, Richard Squires, a scientist at a small drug company in Denmark (Ferrosan), and his graduate assistant Claus Brestrup published an article in *Nature* reporting the results of experiments on rats. Like previous work on opiate receptors, Squires found that benzodiazepines also attach to specific brain receptors. A few months later, a team of researchers headed by Hans Mohler of Roche published similar findings in *Science*. Subsequent research revealed that the highest concentration of benzodiazepine receptors is in the amygdala, part of the brain's limbic system that plays a vital role in the regulation of emotions. Just as opiates relieve pain by mimicking natural opiate-like molecules (the opiate receptors), benzodiazepines appear to exert their soothing effects by potentiating GABA receptors that modulate the emotional states associated with anxiety. This research not only helped identify the molecular workings of benzodiazepines but paved the way for a synaptic theory of anxiety disorders.

The 1977 identification of benzodiazepine receptors further enhanced the scientific and clinical legitimacy of anxiolytic therapy. Whatever its cause, anxiety clearly involved biochemical processes that benzodiazepines and other drugs attenuated. Psychiatrist Donald Klein's experiments on the tricyclic antidepressant imipramine, for instance, had demonstrated that the drug relieves panic attacks without altering chronic anxiety, suggesting that a panic attack is more than an intensification of chronic anxiety. Findings such as these helped reposition anxiety from a problem bequeathed by one's past to a neurobiological disorder responsive to pharmacotherapy. DSM-III permanently dropped neurosis as an organizational category. Anxiety was split and reclassified into separate, ontologically distinct disorders: panic, obsessive-compulsive, posttraumatic stress, social phobia (or social anxiety disorder), specific phobias, and generalized anxiety. Although the precise contribution of Miltown and benzodiazepines in driving this change is impossible to quantify, patient enthusiasm for tranquilizers helped engineer the new paradigm shift embedded in DSM-III. Their undeniable efficacy provided strong evidence of anxiety's biomedical moorings. Jerilyn Ross, the founder of the Anxiety Disorders Association, regarded benzodiazepines as "the first weapons in our arsenal for fighting anxiety disorders." Indeed, the scientific argument for anxiolytics in the 1970s and 1980s was reinforced by patients' decades-old experiences with pharmacotherapy. A 1981 study found that a majority of tranquilizer users regarded anxiety as a biophysical disorder that requires medication rather than a social problem that a person's behavior can fix. Anxiety, like the flu, is "caused by changes in the body's chemical structure."[56]

With this in mind, the Osheroff case served as a timely reminder not only that psychotropic medications worked, but that patients increasingly expected and demanded them. Freud and talk therapy were more than unfashionable and their exclusive use could result in lawsuits. Since the 1950s, millions of Americans had taken tranquilizers, evaluating their therapeutic worth through the prism of private experience. By the 1970s, this history, much of it affirmative, had become part of the therapeutic matrix that made prescription drugs an integral aid to psychiatric wellness.[57]

The medicalization of anxiety contributed to the social veiling of what had, for some Americans, once been a quasi-public experience. In the 1950s, Miltown was chic and neurosis was fashionable. By the 1970s, this earlier whimsy had been eclipsed by a medical gravitas that unwittingly stigmatized and privatized anxiety. In this new milieu, anxiety was less a sign of achievement or an invitation to experiment than a problem to be medicated and concealed. Public figures still took tranquilizers, of course. But they were less likely to talk about it with the legendary candor and enthusiasm of Milton Berle or his contemporaries. Instead, Americans in the 1970s and 1980s typically learned about celebrity tranquilizer use when deaths or rehab visits made private prescription habits a matter of public record. It was only after superstar Elvis Presley died of a heart attack on August 16, 1977 that coroners and journalists revealed that the idol had consumed the equivalent of six hundred doses per month of prescription drugs, including titanic quantities of Valium. The shift from candor to secrecy was, of course, neither linear nor clear-cut. Even in the 1950s and 1960s, many Americans were reticent about disclosing their tranquilizer use. While Berle bragged about his, John F. Kennedy's was concealed from the public. Presumably, such an act of discretion was framed by the conviction that American citizens expected a different degree of mental acuity from their commander in chief than from their television entertainers. Still, the cultural shifts made anxiety more of a private medical issue.

Taking tranks was no longer standard cocktail fare and anxiety was, increasingly, no laughing matter.[58]

There *were* still occasional laughs and jabs. One of the more amusing occurred in the 1979 Hollywood film *Starting Over* starring Burt Reynolds as Phil Potter, a downtrodden thirty-something struggling to regroup after his cool and collected Manhattan wife, Jessica (Candice Bergen), leaves him and tries to launch a singing career. Phil moves to Boston where he meets Marilyn (Jill Clayburgh), a quirky nursery school teacher getting her master's degree. The two hit it off and in short order Marilyn moves in. Shopping for the perfect couch at Bloomingdale's, Phil suddenly finds himself unable to breathe and perspiring heavily. He curls up, panting, on a showroom bed, the ever attentive Marilyn stroking his shoulders, while a crowd gathers to watch. Phil's brother Michael, a psychiatrist, is called to the scene, and quickly determines that Phil is in the throes of a panic attack. Michael asks the crowd if anyone has Valium. Shoppers dig into their pockets or purses and cough up dozens of vials; apparently everyone but Phil is on it. Michael gives Phil two and tells him to breathe into a paper bag. The panic attack is Phil's cue to give his relationship with Jessica one last try, which he does before calling it quits and starting a new life with Marilyn.

But scenes such as these were increasingly the exception to the rule. Barbara Gordon, the television producer and author of the bestselling tranquilizer memoir, *I'm Dancing As Fast As I Can,* remembers that her friends in the 1970s kept quiet about Valium, even those who used it. "People just didn't talk about Valium the way they talked about Miltown," she told me. "We talked about other things. Watergate. Politics. Producing television shows. Travel. It just wasn't a hot topic of conversation."[59] Privacy concerns meant that people generally experienced the best and worst effects of tranquilizers on their own.

For myriad users, tranquilizers were a welcome boon. One study found that the vast majority of Valium users (over 95 percent) believed it helped them either a "great deal" or "some." Fewer than 5 percent of respondents thought that Valium helped only a little or not at all. When asked by researchers or journalists directly, patients credited tranquilizers with allowing them to lead fuller and more productive lives. One woman suffered from debilitating panic attacks until she took Valium. "I was too scared to leave the house, let alone get a job, and spent my days doing crossword puzzles and going off my head," she reported. Eventually she saw her doctor who gave her a prescription. When she took the pill, the panic disappeared. She rarely needed Valium again. The reassurance that came from knowing that the drug was on hand kept her anxiety at bay. "I made the first prescription—for ten tablets—last nearly a year. But by that time my life had been transformed." She went on to university and became a lawyer. She believed that anxiety was an immutable, biological disorder that occasionally required pharmaceutical modulation. "I was born with an anxious disposition and nothing is going to change that," she insisted. "Diazepam is part of my armory."[60]

Other patients credited occasional tranquilizer use with helping them face an unexpected crisis, insomnia, or the occasional rough day. A family physician in Louisville admitted not only to prescribing Valium but to taking it too. "It is a good drug," he proclaimed in 1975. "I take it myself to relieve unavoidable tensions and overwork—but I mostly use making love with my wife, tennis, and music for that."[61]

The Trouble with Tranquilizers

Benzodiazepines claimed legions of beneficiaries. But in the absence of sustained public discussion about their hazards, those who experienced side effects, which could range from bewildering to overwhelming, typically suffered alone. In one case, a man found that his 5 mg daily dose of Valium caused impotence. "After a period of time of taking the tablets, I don't recall how long, I detected that I could not have an erection and enjoy the sexual relationship," he complained to the FDA. His internist was of no help. When the distraught man asked if Valium might be to blame, the doctor admitted he wasn't sure. The man went off Valium and was thrilled by the results. "One night my wife and I were together in bed, just playing around and all at once I became normal, like old times, and everything worked out in fine order," he gleefully admitted. In another instance, a woman prescribed 10 mg of Librium four times a day after a hysterectomy had "gone wild" with excitability.[62] Users catalogued other complaints including weight change, dizziness, sluggishness, mental confusion, depression, headaches, and nausea.

More alarming, perhaps, was the anguish patients experienced when they stopped using the drug. Hollister's findings—that stopping cold turkey can be psychologically and physically excruciating as well as dangerous—are now widely recognized. Today, patients withdrawing from benzodiazepines have recourse to helpful information in print and on the Internet, such as the tapering regimen and compassionate advice offered at www.benzo.org.uk. In an earlier age, the challenges of withdrawal were often compounded by confusion and social solitude. One man who had been on various tranquilizers since the late 1950s stopped taking them altogether in October 1974. "By February 1975 I was not sleeping and in general felt horrible," he complained. "Sometimes I thought I would die and other times wished I had." The man who rediscovered the pleasures of matrimonial passion went back on the drug after six weeks of feeling "weak, nervous, and fearful." In another case, a woman was prescribed 10 mg of Librium four times a day to ease her anxiety about her baby's ill health. After a few months, she complained that the medication was no longer effective (what doctors today would likely identify as tolerance). Her physician upped the dose to 25 mg four or five times a day. A year or so later, the mother was hospitalized for surgery, her Librium abruptly discontinued. She began to hallucinate, hearing French horns and other orchestral sounds. After surgery, she started to have convulsions. Her family physician was surprised by what had happened, given the manufacturer's claim that Librium was "safe, harmless, and nonaddicting."[63]

After *Ms.* magazine published a pathbreaking story in 1975, "Do You Take Valium?" on the downside of its use, readers contacted the editors to share experiences of their own. One complained that her doctor had prescribed a 10 mg dose for depression, instructing her to take the little blue pills "as needed." When her depression worsened, she took more. She assumed, as did many patients at the time, that upping the dose was harmless, since her doctor had given her carte blanche permission to use the pills as needed. At some point she realized that Valium was failing to improve, and may indeed have been worsening, her malaise. She stopped taking it, not anticipating her withdrawal reaction. "I can't begin to describe the physical and mental anguish that accompanied my withdrawal," she ruefully wrote.[64]

Another woman was more upbeat about the drug's uses but equally damning of its potential to cause dependence. She had been taking 10 mg of Valium a day. "Since it's played up to be such a widespread and harmless drug," she explained, "I saw no danger in increasing the dosage." She did so when the regular dosage stopped alleviating her anxiety and insomnia. Locked in a cycle of escalating dependency, she decided to taper down to the originally prescribed amount. "My withdrawal symptoms are a double-dose of the anxiety, irritableness, and insomnia I used to feel." She admitted that the temptation to reach for her "little yellow pills," a quick fix for the withdrawal symptoms but one that would undo her progress, sometimes "seems unbearable."[65]

These patients were profoundly unsettled by such suffering. Meanwhile, the FDA had reason to suspect that hundreds, if not thousands, of patients were already or would soon face similar problems. By the mid-1960s, the FDA had amassed numerous reports of benzodiazepine dependence. Especially among patients who had taken high dosages of the drug for prolonged periods, abrupt withdrawal was marked by rebound anxiety and insomnia, and often tremors, headache, irritability, sleep disturbances, and agitation. More rarely, convulsions, delirium, and paranoia had been observed. In 1966, the agency launched a comprehensive investigation of the "potential for abuse of the drugs Librium and Valium." While witnesses disagreed about the probability of dependence and withdrawal among patients, the final report, issued April 7, 1967, concluded that sufficient evidence existed to demonstrate that these drugs had enough potential for abuse "as to require controls comparable to those imposed on amphetamines and barbiturates" as specified in the Drug Abuse Control amendments of 1965.[66]

Hoffman-La Roche countered these claims. Its executives insisted that Valium was safe and effective when properly used, and that addiction, while possible, was extremely rare. The matter remained bogged down in legal proceedings until July 1975. Only then did the Justice Department order that benzodiazepines be classified as Schedule IV drugs under the 1970 Controlled Substances Act. Schedule IV status allowed consumers to refill an original prescription no more than five times before consulting a physician for a new prescription. (In contrast, Schedule I drugs such as heroin and cocaine were deemed too addictive to be legal; Schedule II drugs, including opium, morphine, and barbiturates, were legal but deemed to have such a high abuse potential that refills were simply banned; Schedule III drugs, including anabolic steroids and certain painkillers, were subjected to extensive monitoring and refill limits.)[67]

The new scheduling status tacitly communicated the drug's hazards to patients by impeding their access to them. But only doctors received updated information about side effects and withdrawal reactions, and that information was the result of a protracted but largely covert skirmish between the FDA and pharmaceutical executives over the language and accuracy of specific claims. Tranquilizer users in the late 1970s were no less at the mercy of manufacturers' claims and doctors' ignorance than they had been for decades. Ordinary Americans were, in short, still in the dark.[68]

As an FDA officer admitted in 1979 to a California woman who complained of a Valium withdrawal that lasted over a year, the history of tranquilizer safety and regulation was replete with uncertainty, confusion, and concealment. Those who suffered most were tranquilizer users. "When first introduced on the market, Valium (and other drugs within the same class), [were] thought to have little potential for producing dependency," the officer admitted. Since then, "evidence of this potential started to appear." Physician labeling had been revised and new regulations had increased the likelihood that their long-term use would be medically monitored. He earnestly hoped that in the near future a patient package insert, like those already available for oral contraceptives, estrogens, and some medical devices, will "provide [Valium] users the kinds of information they needed to assure proper use of the drug and to provide caution against the drug's potential for dependence, as well as other warnings."[69]

As the FDA officer had hoped that time finally came, but it did so almost two decades after Leo Hollister had established the science of benzodiazepine dependence in his California trials. As Hollister told a Senate subcommittee in 1979, surging political interest in tranquilizer addiction may have made for good press, but for people who had suffered for years, it had come too late.[70]

Mother's Little Helpers

O n May 22, 1978, some 17 million viewers of the NBC evening news broadcast learned the medical misfortune of Cyndie Maginniss, a prescription drug addict. Like millions of other American women, the thirty-two-year-old college-educated wife and mother of three struggled with the challenges of a busy life. When she discussed her difficulties with her doctor, he prescribed Valium. When her problems got worse, he prescribed more. Maginniss soon discovered that she had become a prisoner of prescription pills, taking increasingly higher doses to keep calm. Breaking her tranquilizer habit proved difficult. "My body was completely out of whack," Maginniss told the NBC reporter. "Why did you wait so long before seeking help?" the reporter asked. "I thought I was taking medicine," Maginniss replied.[1]

Maginniss's story, broadcast on NBC and recounted in 1979 in a special government hearing on women's dependency on prescription drugs, was among the thousands of tranquilizer narratives recounted in newspapers, magazines, courtrooms, government investigations, and television studios across the United States in the 1970s and 1980s. Although the circumstances varied, these narratives offered a chilling account of prescription drugs and middle-class mothers veering out of control.[2]

Only a few decades earlier, researchers, journalists, and doctors had hailed Miltown as a triumph of American pharmaceutical science. By the

1970s, however, minor tranquilizers had been recast as dangerous drugs—recklessly prescribed, aggressively promoted, and carelessly consumed, especially by housewives—a commercial bonanza achieved at patients' expense. Senator Edward Kennedy opened a 1979 hearing on the use and misuse of benzodiazepines by warning that tranquilizers had "produced a nightmare of dependence and addiction, both very difficult to treat and recover from."[3]

What caused this seismic shift in perceptions of tranquilizers? By the late 1970s, ingesting tranquilizers was routine, and the chemical properties of benzodiazepines hadn't substantially changed. Nor had evidence of the drugs' potential to cause dependence been newly unearthed; indeed, by the time Kennedy's hearing began, studies of withdrawal reactions had been in print for over a decade.

What had changed, in short, was not the fact that Americans took tranquilizers (about 800 tons in 1977) or that, like Cyndie Maginniss, many had a tough time when they stopped. What was new was that Americans were for the first time politically unnerved by their prescription behavior. The backlash against tranquilizers was the by-product of a particular historical moment in which assessments of the drugs' value to society were framed by a constellation of concerns. Among them were the views being expressed by the consumer and women's health movements, mobilized around the issue of patient self-education and empowerment. There were political worries too, notably the nation's preoccupation with the counterculture, whose open and often defiant use of recreational drugs was widely derided. So seamless was this web of influences that teasing apart the different strands of protest may be impossible. Admonitions against wanton tranquilizer use were inextricably linked to denunciations of reckless youth, the paternalism of the male medical establishment, and the atomization of suburban life. What *was* clear is that amid rising discontent, nothing vexed pundits and policy makers more than the finding, first exposed by researchers in the late 1960s, that the group most likely to use tranquilizers was middle-class mothers. As journalists spun apocryphal tales of the chemical takeover of apple pie suburbia, critics pondered the changing identity of a drug whose vast female market had seemingly turned tranquilizers into mother's little helpers.[4]

Addiction by Prescription

In 1963, when Valium debuted on the market, Betty Friedan published her trailblazing *The Feminine Mystique.* The bestseller, often credited with igniting the second-wave feminist movement (so called to distinguish it from the "first wave" of feminism in the late nineteenth and early twentieth centuries) suggested that women, especially homemakers, had been snookered into thinking that happiness can be found in the material trappings and decorative roles of suburbia. Promises of personal fulfillment, propelled by a powerful postwar back-to-the-kitchen ideology sustained by advertisers, conservative educators, sociologists, and psychiatrists, had nudged women into the soul- and mind-numbing confines of the home, what Friedan famously called a "comfortable concentration camp." Television shows such as *Leave It to Beaver* and *Ozzie and Harriet* had projected normative images of apolitical self-sacrificing wives and mothers. Women's magazines had shored up this creed. An advice column in *Better Homes and Gardens* insisted that the two biggest steps a woman must take are to "help their husbands decide where they are going and use their pretty heads to help them get there." Women who strayed from this script were branded deviant. As *Newsweek* warned, a good education offered nothing more to American wives than a dangerous temptation to reject the tried-and-true adage that "anatomy is destiny" and devalued their most important role as gracious, charming housewives. *Esquire* labeled working wives a "menace." In one California hospital, women wanting abortions were given shock treatments on the grounds that rejection of their natural procreative role indicated a serious disturbance. Historians have questioned the extent to which this domestic blueprint for female success represented a monolithic ideal; many films, books, and articles offered alternative representations of womanhood from which women could draw. Yet there is little question that the glorification of domesticity was a salient ingredient of postwar mass culture.[5]

Legions of women became trapped in the interstices between domestic myth and reality. Friedan, a Smith College graduate who lost a job to a returning war veteran, was among them. "Gradually, without seeing it clearly for quite a while, I came to realize that something is very wrong with the way American women are trying to live their lives today," she wrote. According to Friedan:

> I sensed it first as a question mark in my own life, as a wife and mother of three small children, half-guiltily and therefore half-heartedly, almost in spite of myself, using my abilities and education in work that took me away from home. . . . There was a strange discrepancy between the reality of our lives and the image to which we were trying to conform, the image that I came to call the feminine mystique.[6]

Friedan noted that women often took tranquilizers to assuage their inner turbulence. The drugs did not provide answers, but they quieted the malaise. "Just what was this problem that has no name?" Friedan wrote about the psychological split between the promise of fulfillment and the reality of a stifled life.

> What were the words women used when they tried to express it? Sometimes a woman would say, "I feel empty somehow . . . incomplete." Or she would say, "I feel as if I don't exist." Sometimes she blotted out the feeling with a tranquilizer. Sometimes she thought the problem was with her husband, or her children, or what she really needed was to redecorate her house.[7]

Friedan couldn't say how many women sought pharmaceutical solutions for their private pain. But she guessed it was a lot. In her estimation, suburban housewives were popping tranquilizers like cough drops. "You wake up in the morning, and feel as if there's no point in going on another day like this. So you take a tranquilizer because it makes you not care so much that it's pointless."[8]

In 1968, five years after *The Feminine Mystique* gave voice to the festering discontent of scores of women, sociologist Hugh Parry confirmed the prevalence of tranquilizer use among suburban women in one of the first user studies in the United States. While studies on the sale and manufacture of tranquilizers abounded, researchers had neglected the everyday use of psychotropics, focusing instead on the so-called glamorous hard drugs (such as cocaine) or psychedelics (such as LSD and mescaline). Parry was particularly interested in elucidating patterns of prescription drug taking among everyday (that is, noninstitutionalized) Americans. His study, drawn from two national surveys and in-depth investigation of drug use in a California city, sought to redress this gaping lacuna.[9]

What Parry found was alarming. Women were twice as likely to use tranquilizers as men. Most users were white and educated; fully two-thirds had graduated from high school or attended college. Subsequent studies confirmed Parry's results. Regardless of age or region, women were twice as likely as men to take tranquilizers, and among both sexes tranquilizers like Valium were more frequently used than stimulants, antidepressants, or major tranquilizers.[10]

These findings fueled apocalyptic claims about the chemical corruption of mainstream America, claims that reflected the nation's anxieties about drugs' relationship to broader social unrest. The tranquilizer epidemic was not America's first drug panic, but before the 1970s the drug problem had been propagandized as something foisted on upright citizens by foreign heathens (such as the nefarious German plot during World War I, unveiled by the *New York Times,* to spike toothpaste with addictive substances to pacify America for a quick-and-easy takeover) or by criminal elements from within. Typically, the villains in these oft told tales were marginalized men: the unemployed, political radicals, and criminals. This characterization conveniently swept under the carpet a long history of women's use of drugs, from the potassium bromide pills taken by Charlotte Perkins Gilman and other neurasthenics, to the opium- and cocaine-laced elixirs (many advertised as soothing tonics for children) that proliferated on the patent medicine market. Still, drug panics have historically privileged the politics of exclusion—the problem lies without—to the more troubling and awkward admission that sometimes the problem resides within.[11]

Moral sanctimony also framed the establishment's vilification of countercultural drug experimentation. The language of this campaign mirrored the politics behind it. The rhetoric of an oppositional culture comprised of young people perceived as misguided, reckless, or dangerous spoke volumes about the need to cleave off drug users from ordinary citizens. Potheads and bra-burning feminists, draft dodgers, disgruntled veterans, and psychedelic hippies: the labels that branded these groups as different conveyed the trenchant message that they had no place in middle-of-the-road America. The political left was sharply divided on whether drug use could be regarded as a form of meaningful dissent. Many urged restraint. Herbert Marcuse, the influential author of *One-Dimensional Man*, linked pill taking and psychotherapy with an alienated and unhappy capitalist order, while Malcolm X feared that drugs would cloud the thinking of African Americans and discredit the black nationalist movement as a whole. Yet many who rebelled against the social system regarded drugs as a legitimate form of protest, and just enough protesters used them to make the stigma stick. Thus did drug use in the 1960s and 1970s become intertwined in the public imagination with assaults on materialism, consumerism, and the political leadership that had dragged the country into Vietnam.[12]

Hippies living in communes dropped acid and decried the tyranny of property ownership. Angry Vietnam veterans sometimes returned to the United States with an unwanted heroin addiction (by 1971, half of the army's enlisted men had tried it) and barbed words about American imperialism in Southeast Asia. In January 1967, thousands of young people gathered in San Francisco's Golden Gate Park for the first human be-in. They swayed to the music of the Grateful Dead and Jefferson Airplane, listened to Beat poet Allen Ginsberg's Buddhist mantras, and heard Timothy Leary, a psychologist who had abandoned a promising career at Harvard to promote the psychedelic cause ("LSD is more important than Harvard"), admonish the crowd to "turn on, tune in, drop out." Drugs were illicit not only because they were illegal but also because the social contexts in which they were used threatened the political order. When the *New York Times* reported Jane Fonda's arrest for smuggling drugs from Canada into the United States, it reminded readers that "Miss Fonda has been an outspoken critic of the Vietnam War and has been active on behalf of the Black Panthers, American Indian claims, and G.I. rights." Enough said. That Fonda's detention in jail forced her to cancel a college speaking engagement was icing on the political cake.[13]

Imagine, then, the revulsion kindled by the discovery that these same drugs were being used by mainstream America: pendant-winning athletes, the nurtured offspring of upper-middle-class families, respectable businessmen, even God-fearing Republicans. "Pot smokers and LSD trippers may still be the exception in high school," proclaimed one journalist in a 1967 exposé, "but they no longer represent the misfits, the oddballs, the disturbed; they are just as likely to be the intellectuals, the politically and socially concerned, the quiet ones, the youngsters parents have rarely had to worry about."[14]

Americans from all walks of life, it seemed, were hooked on getting high. In the wealthy enclave of Belle Haven in Greenwich, Connecticut, an eleven-year-old girl, egged on by her teenage brother, became intoxicated inhaling an aerosol spray sold to frost cocktail glasses. In tony East Hampton, the police busted a back-to-school bash where students, "some bearded and in tight, dirty slacks" were high on heroin, marijuana, hashish, and LSD. At a Thanksgiving party in Houston, the expensively coiffed wife of a dress shop owner and the other guests—a computer expert, a lawyer, and a toy store manager—gathered around the table to eat turkey, play improvisational word games, and smoke marijuana joints. "You make them too thin," complained the stylish wife of the dress shop owner. An affluent retailer in North Carolina, southern-born and Republican, credited five LSD trips for helping him to divine the sanctity of life and to transform him into an outspoken critic of Vietnam.[15]

Widespread use of mind-altering prescription medications in offices and homes collapsed distinctions between illegally peddled and doctor-prescribed drugs. The bloodstreams of businessmen were coursing with chemical enhancers, "respectably labeled" prescription drugs, to be sure, but potent pharmaceuticals all the same. The functionality of prescription junkies often masked the severity of their dependence. Take the case of Norman, a self-described "uptight Wall Street stockbroker." The thirty-eight-year-old wasn't looking to get high when he got his first pill, "some kind of barbiturate." Like other drug users, he just wanted to cope with the rigors of his job. Barbiturates and alcohol helped him unwind. When he needed to "be up" for a meeting, he'd take amphetamines. Alcohol and sedatives allowed him to relax on demand. In no time, his roller coaster of uppers and downers had made him pill dependent. Getting a steady stash of drugs was easy. "If a doctor didn't want to renew a prescription, [my] immediate reaction was to go to another." Norman finally joined Pills Anonymous, an offshoot of Alcoholics Anonymous established in 1974 to help addicts with polysubstance abuse. Members "don't walk around stoned," explained Norman. "Most of us are from middle-class backgrounds, had to be high achievers early in life . . . doctors, judges, models." The message of this cautionary tale was clear: even respectable people could be addicts. Businessmen scurrying to work with a marijuana joint—a "tuned-in, turned-on modern executive's afternoon snack"—tucked in their coat pocket, schoolteachers who popped prescription sedatives to relax: this was the troubling face of modern drug culture.[16]

The medicine cabinet and the corner pharmacy, rather than the drug peddler on the street, had given rise to what Republican vice president Spiro Agnew called America's "collective national 'trip.'" In this drug-fueled world, it no longer made sense to talk of prescribed medicines as politically sacrosanct or socially benign. America, railed Democratic senator Thomas Dodd, was home to a "virtual epidemic of nice-drug addiction." Prescription drugs had brought addiction and its concomitant ills—escapism, apathy, recklessness, and protest—into the very heart of white America— Junction City (KA), Pagedale (MN), Woodford (VA), Plymouth (MI)— "places with apple pie smells and wind-snapped flags." Even President Richard Nixon joined the chorus, insisting in a 1971 address to the AMA that there existed a clear and toxic link "between the inappropriate use of drugs within the medical context and the abuse of drugs outside that context. . . . We have created in America a culture of drugs. We have produced an environment in which people come naturally to expect that they can take a pill for every problem—that they can find satisfaction and health and happiness in a handful of tablets or a few grains of powder."[17]

In this environment, where drugs of all sorts were newly scrutinized and politically demonized, tranquilizers came under fire. Valium and its chemical cousins were sold not via shady transactions on dimly lit street corners to hippies and vets, but to affluent Americans at respectable pharmacies with the scripted endorsement of the medical profession. Previously lionized for their ability to patch social fissures and keep the economy functioning, tranquilizers were now disparaged as culturally disruptive and politically dangerous. Like Timothy Leary's disciples, tranquilizer takers were "tuning out" the realities of the world. The fact that users got their drugs from doctors rather than street peddlers made them no less pernicious. Indeed, it made the tranquilizer problem seem that more ominous, for it meant that mind-altering agents had wormed their way, undetected, into the inner sanctum of middle-class suburbia. The tranquilizer epidemic breathed life into the cinematic perils presented in *Invasion of the Body Snatchers*, in which a doctor cocooned in the imagined safety of a small town discovers that his patients, family, and friends have been taken over by emotionless, human-duplicating pods from outer space. Much like the pod takeover, Valium had invaded sacrosanct domains, leaving those it ensnared emotionally numb. In an interesting twist, however, it was doctors, not aliens, who shared the blame for the chemical hijacking of Middletown.[18]

The Chemically Dependent All-American Woman

In this cacophony of concern, most disquieting was the realization that stay-at-home moms, sentimentalized symbols of wholesome family values, were the biggest users of tranquilizers. In just a few decades, the billion dollar tranquilizer trade had been feminized and domesticated; stay-at-home mothers, it appeared, drove its success. This revelation, as well as the cultural malaise it heralded, was popularized by the Rolling Stones' hit, "Mother's Little Helper." The song chronicles a housewife's despair over the tedium of life, relieved only by the little yellow pill, Valium. Set to an upbeat tune, the song is, upon closer inspection, a woman's death narrative. The little yellow pills deliver a calming shelter to the

flummoxed mother, forced by circumstance to battle unruly kids, an oner-
ous husband, tedium, and one too many dinner disasters. They help her
endure busy days and boring nights but can't reconcile the emptiness of a
prosaic life. She begs the doctor for another refill before drugging herself
to death. Mick Jagger later claimed that he and Keith Richards penned
the lyrics to remind listeners that ordinary people, not just rock stars, had
drug problems and breakdowns too.

The feminization of tranquilizers precipitated a sensationalistic media
campaign that dramatized the pathology of the overmedicated woman. A
Connecticut panel called the epidemic the "housewives' disease"; the
Washington Post noted that women's drug dependency had become a coun-
trywide epidemic. Images of pill-popping suburbanites upended the more
reassuring vision of mothers as the last bulwarks against encroaching
chaos. In the politically charged 1960s and 1970s, Friedan's chemically
pacified women were no longer doing their part to maintain domestic
peace. They were subversive or, as in the case of the Rolling Stones song,
burning frozen steaks and then dying. In addition, many commentators
active in the burgeoning field of drug and alcohol research cautioned that
tranquilizers had become gateway drugs for other illicit compounds: One
researcher warned that evidence was mounting that a number of suburban
housewives "have experimented with marijuana."[19]

The tone of jeremiads in mainstream magazines was equally menacing.
McCalls exposed disturbing details about "The Over-Medicated Woman."
Good Housekeeping offered readers "The Complete Book of Women and
Pills," and the *Ladies Home Journal* chronicled the horrors of "Housewives and
the Drug Habit." "The typical woman who uses drugs to cope with life is not
a fast-living rock star, nor a Times Square prostitute, nor a devotee of the
drop-out-and-turn-on philosophy," proclaimed one exposé. "She is an adoles-
cent, confused by the stresses of impending adulthood. She is a newlywed, by
turns anxious and depressed by strains of adjustment to a new relationship
and new responsibilities. She is a once-busy housewife, her youngsters grown,
who finds her days increasingly empty and her thoughts obsessed with the in-
exorable passing of the years." She was, in short, "an average, middle-class
American—one of the folks next door. She could even be you."[20]

While these magazines raised interest in the problem of female drug dependency, a curious coalition of interest groups converged to turn women's use of tranquilizers into a mainstream political issue. Some were social conservatives who blamed both the drug and lax government regulations for allowing it to flourish and to sully the sanctity of the home. "The abuse of these 'little helpers,'" complained one man to the FDA, "has torn families apart, completely changed personalities, and made vegetables out of many." If the FDA and government officials "would devote their efforts to something as vital as this, instead of worrying about rats drinking 80 gallons of soft drinks sweetened with saccharin [a reference to the FDA's ongoing investigation of the safety of saccharin] we would be much better off."[21]

This man may have identified with votaries of "pharmacological Calvinism," a term coined in 1970 by psychiatrist Gerald L. Klerman to explain the peculiarly American propensity to demonize as bad drugs that made them feel good. This mind-set, which had once driven opposition to coffee and tobacco, idealized chemical abstinence. For true believers, nothing less than America's virtue was at stake. If the United States was to prosper it must do so on the back of hard work, individualism, and independence. Pharmaceutical concoctions were nothing more than chemical crutches that compromised citizens' free will and political autonomy. As such, they were as ruinous to individuals as to the nation's moral health. One survey found that 40 percent of Americans in 1973 agreed that it was better to use "willpower than tranquilizers" to solve problems. As early as 1967, Stanley Yolles, then the director of the National Institutes of Mental Health, had sounded the alarm about the political liabilities of tranquilizer use. In a land where citizens were chemically pacified, he asked, "would Yankee initiative disappear?" This argument turned on its head the earlier political case for tranquilizers as chemicals to promote a calmer, more productive and efficient America, a precondition of cold war political supremacy, and substituted it with a more somber, at times evangelical, antidrug zealotry that presaged Nancy Reagan's "Just Say No" crusade of the 1980s.[22]

The foiled assassination of President Ronald Reagan in 1981 by John W. Hinckley Jr. illuminated how much was at stake in the debate. The troubled twenty-six-year-old had been undergoing psychotherapy and taking 15 mg of Valium a day before he fired a revolver six times at Reagan as the president left the Washington, D.C., Hilton Hotel, a violent act allegedly intended to win the affection of actress Jody Foster, with whom Hinckley had become obsessed. At his trial, psychiatrists debated the degree to which Hinckley's capacity to act freely had been compromised by his drug use and psychiatric problems. Hinckley was found not guilty by reason of insanity and committed to St. Elizabeths Hospital for treatment. Stunned that an outpatient on Valium could be freed of the responsibility of standing trial for attempting to assassinate a president, several states rewrote their insanity defense laws, modifying the use of psychiatrists and psychologists as expert witnesses.[23]

Others who sounded the alarm were activists in the fledgling consumer and women's health movements, which shared common ground in their suspicion of pharmaceutical and medical interests and their demand that patients be apprised of the risks of *all* medical technologies, including drugs. Both movements drew from the larger protest impulses of the 1960s that focused national attention on injustices in American society and provided an ideology of oppression and grassroots activism that activists could identify and appropriate as their own. In 1965, Ralph Nader's *Unsafe at Any Speed,* a damning indictment of General Motors' flawed and improperly tested Corvair, helped stimulate a movement predicated on the belief that American consumers were being hurt, physically and financially, by corporate greed and inadequate regulation. Disciples of Naderism called on consumers to empower themselves through economic self-determination and decision making informed by unbiased data. The automobile fracas was just the beginning of the assault on rapacious corporatism. Activists also tackled water pollution, the airline industry, nursing homes, and the pharmaceutical industry, lobbied for consumer protection laws, and established a group of watchdog organizations, including Public Citizen and the Public Citizen Health Research Movement, dedicated to promoting safer drugs and public health.[24]

Revived interest in the women's movement, particularly important in shaping responses to tranquilizer use, was also animated by contemporary political campaigns. Angered by the mistreatment of women and the neglect of gender issues in the civil rights, New Left, and antiwar movements, women banded together to demand a cause of their own: women's liberation. Through an impressive network of new organizations, second-wave feminists called for an end to occupational segregation and egregious pay disparities. They also lobbied for unfettered access to higher education, a national system of child care, an Equal Rights Amendment, and the decriminalization of abortion. Second-wave feminism involved much more than group activism, of course, and feminists didn't necessarily agree on what the end goal should be. Like any social movement, feminism struggled with competing claims of universality—the rhetoric of universal sisterhood was often at odds with the diversity of female experience. Yet one benefit of variegated approaches and ideas was the multitude of activities they sparked on the ground: marches, sit-ins, day care cooperatives, and consciousness-raising groups, where women's articulation of private, often painful experiences catalyzed political action, solidifying the movement's creed that the personal was political.[25]

Women's health care activism grew out of this fervor, fusing complaints about systemic injustices with women's private concerns. There were plenty of issues around which women could mobilize. The thalidomide tragedy was followed by public debates and disturbing disclosures about the safety of oral contraceptives, the poorly designed Dalkon Shield, the nation's most popular intrauterine device, and the synthetic hormone DES. In the 1960s, oral contraceptives, which the FDA had approved in May 1960, constituted, alongside tranquilizers, the largest female drug market and one of the pharmaceutical industry's most profitable. Democratic senator Gaylord Nelson's hearings on the safety of the Pill, held in early 1970, well intentioned in principle, turned out to be a political debacle. Nelson had read Barbara Seaman's pioneering book, *The Doctor's Case Against the Pill,* which documented the Pill's health risks so persuasively that it established Seaman as the "Ralph Nader of the birth control pill." Nelson decided to hold a government inquiry to investigate the matter further, but he won few feminist fans when he refused to allow women activists to testify before the all-male committee in the first round of hearings, notwithstanding the fact that feminist organizations had petitioned to be heard. The televised hearings—watched by an estimated 87 percent of women between twenty-one and forty-five—captured for posterity women's anger at being callously ignored. On the first day of testimony, members of D.C. Women's Liberation, a group formed in 1969 that promoted feminist health care and safe and legal abortions, disrupted the meeting with angry shouts. Nelson tried to restore order but made matters worse when he referred to the demonstrators as girls, reproached them for their unruly behavior, and implored them to sit down and be silent.[26]

Equally disheartening were the paternalistic proclamations of committee members debating the advisability of patient inserts to educate women about the Pill's side effects. Committee member Bob Dole, then the junior senator from Kansas, wondered if informing women about the drug's potential hazards would make them unduly anxious. "I would guess they may be taking two pills now," he joked. "First a tranquilizer and then the regular pill."[27]

Such boorish proclamations incited women to action—not drugged passivity. Energized and angry, they wrote letters to the FDA and elected officials demanding that women be informed of all drug risks. Wrote one: "I DEMAND—that as a woman, having the option to take the pill or not, I have *all* facts in front of me!"[28]

By the time the Nelson hearings began, the feminist health care movement, which provided an organizational and collective conduit for women's protests, was already mobilized. In 1969, twelve young feminists had established the Boston Women's Health Book Collective to educate women about health and sexuality and to challenge conventional models of medicine that pushed women into passive roles. In 1970, the collective published its landmark *Our Bodies, Ourselves,* which went on to sell almost 4 million copies in twelve languages. It encouraged women to educate themselves about everything from miscarriage, birth control, and menstruation to childbirth practices performed for the convenience of doctors rather than women (such as unnecessary episiotomies). The book's popularity ignited the grassroots-based health movement, anchored in personal experience, self-education, and the critical questioning of doctors and traditional Western medicine. By 1974, more than 1,200 women's groups provided alternative, female-focused health care. The National Women's Health Network was founded in 1975. A nonprofit organization that served as an information clearinghouse to educate policy makers and women about drugs and devices, it became an important agent of health activism.[29]

In January 1973 reproductive rights activists claimed victory in the Supreme Court's decision in *Roe v. Wade,* which made first-trimester abortion a private matter between a woman and her physician. But the next year brought bad news. In 1974 the FDA withdrew the Dalkon Shield from the domestic market. Its flawed design caused over 200,000 infections, miscarriages, hysterectomies, and other gynecological complications, and buttressed activists' charge that women were systematically being denied—by doctors, industry, and a lax regulatory environment—the facts they needed to make competent medical decisions.[30]

By the mid-1970s, then, the enthusiasm and scientific optimism of an earlier age had yielded to a skepticism seasoned by the time-worn realization that drugs and devices could be dangerous, even deadly. In the aftershocks following thalidomide, oral contraceptives, and the Dalkon Shield, women scrutinized tranquilizers with a hard-earned cynicism. Many felt that the male and pharmaceutical establishments had bamboozled them into taking dangerous and unnecessary drugs. Feminist psychologists such as Phyllis Chesler, a cofounder of the National Women's Health Network and author of the landmark *Women and Madness,* characterized tranquilizers as a tool of social control, thwarting opportunities for lasting social change by putting women in chemical straitjackets, encouraging them to interpret anger and anxieties created by a sexist world as isolated problems. Others, outraged by the paternalism of the Pill hearings, demanded that women be properly apprised about tranquilizers too. One librarian called on the FDA to pressure "Roche Laboratories to advertise all the side effects of this drug . . . in order to protect the consumers who are paying the bills for prescriptions [and to] . . . make health education information available to young people, especially women."[31]

Women's public testimonials invigorated the Valium panic. By the late 1970s, patients from all walks of life were sharing their trank tales with journalists, television and radio hosts, and congressional committees. Some wrote letters to advice columnists such as Ann Landers, published and read by thousands in syndicated newspapers. Of the many tranquilizer confessionals that occupied this new political landscape of pharmaceutical concern, none were more powerful or influential than those of former First Lady Betty Ford and television producer Barbara Gordon.[32]

Ford's came first. In April 1978, a few days after her sixtieth birthday, the former First Lady checked herself into the Long Beach Naval Hospital's alcohol and drug rehabilitation unit. Her statement was short and forthright: "Over a period of time I got to the point where I was over-medicating myself. . . . It's an insidious thing and I mean to rid myself of its damaging effects."[33]

As the Republican First Lady, the mother of four had been both praised and disparaged for her trademark candor. A strong and spirited supporter of women's rights, she had advocated the legalization of abortion and the proposed Equal Rights Amendment during her husband's presidential term. She earned the wrath of the far right for her tolerant attitude toward young people who smoked marijuana or engaged in extramarital sex, subjects she openly discussed on CBS's *60 Minutes*. After the episode aired, a few party militants demanded her resignation, disdainfully calling her "No Lady." In 1974, Ford painfully discussed her breast cancer and mastectomy. Now, four years later, she tackled her drug and alcohol problem with the same characteristic grittiness that the public had come to expect and, for the most part, admire.[34]

At first, Ford had resisted the mere suggestion she had a problem. For fourteen years, she had taken various doctor-prescribed medications—pain pills and mild tranquilizers, including Valium—for a pinched nerve, arthritis, muscle spasms, tension, and insomnia. "I took pills for pain, I took pills to sleep, I took mild tranquilizers." She drank, but never in secret: "I'd never hidden bottles in the chandeliers or the toilet tanks." Neither did she drive under the influence, "I worried about my children too much to risk taking them anywhere in a car when I'd been drinking," or consume alcohol before the afternoon hours. Indeed, at social gatherings, "I would look at friends who knocked back Bloody Marys in the morning, and I would think, isn't that pathetic?"[35]

Still, there were warning signs of her growing dependence: slowed speech, memory lapses, and a precipitous fall in the bathroom that left her with three cracked ribs. Mixing alcohol with pills exacerbated the depressant effects of each, leaving Ford groggy. In the fall of 1977, she accepted an invitation to narrate *The Nutcracker* ballet in Moscow. The televised event showed the First Lady—who had been popping tranquilizers in the ladies' room during film breaks—stumbling her way through the words, giving what one journalist called a "sloe-eyed [sic] sleepy-tongued performance."[36]

But it wasn't until she retired from public life that Ford's drug problem prodded her family to act. In Palm Springs, family members staged not one but two interventions, confronting the surprised Ford and demanding that she trade her pharmaceutical aids for professional help. Ford finally relented. The nearby Long Beach Naval Hospital had set up a covert rehabilitation center in 1965 in a condemned Quonset hut because, in a revealing sign of the taboo surrounding addiction, the armed forces refused to admit the existence of drug or alcohol problems among active duty naval personnel. In 1974, when the navy went public with the problem, the program was relocated to the hospital's fourth floor. There Ford attended group therapy sessions, modeled after the twelve steps program of Alcoholics Anonymous, and slept in a shared room with other addicts. During those difficult weeks, she received flowers and bags of mail from well-wishers around the country. Newspapers and magazines applauded her humility and courage. As addiction specialist Muriel Nellis proclaimed in *Harper's Bazaar,* the former First Lady had again performed an invaluable public service by admitting her dependence on Valium and alcohol, creating "a public awareness which will affect the lives of millions of women." Ford went on to cofound, with Ambassador Leonard Firestone, the now famous Betty Ford Center in Rancho Mirage, California, a nonprofit facility devoted to treating patients and their families suffering from chemical dependency.[37]

Similar accolades were bestowed on renowned television writer and documentary filmmaker Barbara Gordon, whose harrowing story of Valium addiction and unsupervised withdrawal was captured in gripping prose in her memoir, *I'm Dancing As Fast As I Can*. Born in Miami to an upper-middle-class family, she graduated from Barnard with a "head full of philosophy, economics, history, psychology [and] English literature." At age twenty-one, she began work as a secretary at NBC, and through grim determination, sheer talent, and some luck navigated her way through the largely male television labyrinth, filming controversial documentaries on Vietnam veterans, slum landlords, and the FBI's use of *agents provocateurs* to infiltrate and subdue New Left organizations. After her marriage ended, she began seeing a psychiatrist every week. It was a "routine, like brushing my teeth, a normal part of my life," she wrote. She had previously taken Valium for two herniated disks in her back. When her psychiatrist prescribed Valium for occasional anxiety attacks, she felt secure: "It was like returning to an old friend." But neither the drug nor weekly therapy sessions stemmed the tide of panic attacks. Instead, after ten years of psychiatric and pharmaceutical care, her anxiety had soared to new, terrifying heights. Successful, respected, and with three Emmys to her credit, the once "aggressive and outgoing" woman now feared leaving her office for lunch. "Just thinking about crowded streets and noisy restaurants and a gnawing panic would begin, a panic that had become all too familiar, filling my mind, my body, almost immobilizing me." As the anxiety worsened, her psychiatrist increased her dose. On the outside, life looked perfect. There was just one problem. "I couldn't cross the street or go near a department store or ride a bus without those bloody pills in my pocket."[38]

Gordon told her psychiatrist she wanted to stop taking pills. They weren't helping, and yet she had become completely "dependent on something other than myself to function." He reassured her that Valium was not addictive and couldn't hurt. In lieu of a higher dose, he offered her Thorazine. Gordon refused. The psychiatrist acquiesced to Gordon's request but insisted that there was only one right way to stop Valium: "don't take one, not one. Do it absolutely cold." She heeded his advice. "It didn't occur to me to do it any other way," she remembered. "Besides, my doctor [was] not an ordinary doctor, but a friend, a man, a psychiatrist, who had known me for ten years. He wouldn't tell me to do the wrong thing."[39]

In fact he had. By the late 1970s, studies had demonstrated the therapeutic benefits of a tapered withdrawal, in which patients are weaned from progressively lower doses of benzodiazepines over weeks and even months. Deferring to her doctor, Gordon suffered the ghastly side effects of a sudden cessation: insomnia, agitation, paranoia, weight loss, tremors, even difficulty concentrating. "I couldn't think anymore, reason anymore. I didn't know right from wrong." Some days it felt like her scalp was on fire and her body was nothing but "a skeleton with flesh." After seventeen days of hospital care for withdrawal-induced problems, the symptoms continued, and she entered a second psychiatric hospital where, over a period of five months, she began the slow and grueling process of recovery. With the help of a psychologist, she realized that she had "made the mistake of thinking of [Valium] as a medicine, not as a drug which should be handled with care." She was not alone; millions of other women had made the same mistake. Gordon wrote of the haunting specter of "thousands of women all across the country being given pills by male doctors."[40]

After her hospital discharge, the stigma of mental illness, addiction, and institutionalization trailed Gordon into the workplace, where colleagues who had previously lauded her acuity and drive now gave her frosty snubs and stares but no job offer. Demoralized, unemployed, and struggling to make ends meet, she revisited a lifelong passion: writing. As a child, "I always wrote," she told me. Her desk and typewriter had long served as a personal sanctuary, a "safe and favorite place." Hoping to make sense of her dramatic journey from CBS superstar to institutionalized addict, she began writing her groundbreaking book, which wasn't meant for publication. It was, at its inception, a private quest to explain her lost year: "I wrote it to make order out of [the] disorder," she explained. Friends asked to read her memoir, and one passed it to an agent. The first editor rejected it, and then Gordon got lucky. An editor at Harper & Row liked it, took a chance, and offered Gordon a book contract.[41]

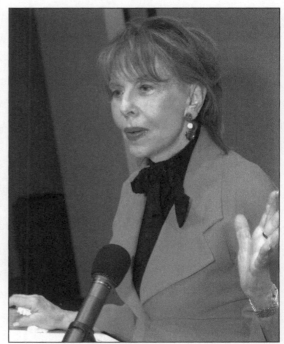

Barbara Gordon. An award-winning television producer and writer, Barbara Gordon is also author of the bestselling *I'm Dancing As Fast As I Can.* Published in 1979, the book helped Americans understand the hazards of an untapered withdrawal from a drug that, at the time Gordon's book was published, was the world's most widely prescribed. Copyright © Kathy Gurfein.

Published in the summer of 1979, *I'm Dancing As Fast As I Can* became an overnight sensation and a cultural phenomenon. It quickly made its way onto the *New York Times* bestseller list, launched women's book clubs, inspired a 1982 Paramount film (in which Jill Clayburgh played Gordon), and landed Gordon coveted appearances on *Donahue, The Today Show, Good Morning America,* and other prime-time programs. It also put her into the uncomfortable role of medical adviser. She began receiving phone calls at home from panicked women: "I take two, I take four, I take six. . . . Do you think I'm addicted?" According to an interview with *People,* Gordon would reply: "I'm not an expert. Go doctor hunting." Boxes of fan mail from all over the world would await when she returned from speaking tours.[42]

No one was more surprised by the public response than Gordon. "I thought I had written a book about the screwed-up year of one woman's life," she remembered. "I wasn't trying to 'tap into' anything else. I wasn't trying to write a cosmic book that applied to many people. I didn't even see it as a powerful, cautionary tale." But Gordon's story struck a resonant chord with thousands of readers who found in her memoir a way to make better sense of their own anguish and struggles. "You describe my life. My aunt's life. My cousin's life," grateful readers wrote. "My sister is like you. She won't go out of the house or go to sleep without that pill." There were too many letters to answer, but Gordon did her best. Decades later, there is one she still remembers vividly. A woman wrote to say *Dancing* had saved her vision. The woman had experienced difficulties seeing, which her doctor attributed to hysterical menopausal blindness. He prescribed Valium to placate her. Not surprisingly, her vision problems continued. Then the woman learned about *Dancing*. It made her realize the danger of trusting doctors on faith and the importance of taking health matters into one's one hands. She and her husband consulted a second physician who ordered diagnostic tests that revealed an operable tumor. Gordon met the grateful couple for dinner at the Four Seasons. She remembers that the woman "put her arms around me and we were both crying."[43]

Gordon refused to condemn Valium or other tranquilizers. Valium "is a superb anti-anxiety agent as well as a muscle relaxant," she insisted. Nor did she criticize its use to help people cope with a genuine crisis: "death in the family, a divorce, a sick child or major surgery." But patients should be informed of its risks and instructed how to withdraw safely. Gordon also defended the psychiatric profession (at a time when the antipsychiatry movement was vehemently attacking it); after her second hospital discharge, she sought the care of a therapist she considered a great psychiatrist. However, as she told *People* in 1979, "the profession needs a Ralph Nader. We give much more thought to buying a car or winter coat than shopping for the right doctor."[44]

Valium's Victims

What united these disparate tranquilizer tales was their characterization of women as victims of a health care system that increasingly resorted to chemical answers to human problems and devalued the expression of normal human emotions and frailties. They were victims of physician ignorance about the side effects of powerful drugs and their own willingness to place their trust in a medical system they had been encouraged to not question. Although researchers disagreed about why women consumed more tranquilizers than men, they stood united in their depiction of women as "accidental accidents," hooked on prescription pills through no fault of their own.[45]

Some people blamed the alleged epidemic on women's greater tendency to consult doctors. Shorn of cultural explanations, the problem could be distilled to medical exposure. Women saw doctors on average twice as often as men in the 1970s. It only stood to reason that they represented two-thirds of tranquilizer users.[46]

Others argued that it was the gender-specific reasons for medical consultations that increased the likelihood that women would leave a doctor's office with a script. "When men go to the doctor," explained activist Belita Cowan, "it is usually because they are ill." Women, on the other hand, were more likely to seek medical care when they were healthy—to check in with their or their children's doctors for regular visits and the like. Such checkups readily lent themselves to discussions of how women were faring overall, discussions of everyday health that encouraged prescriptions for a drug meant to relieve everyday problems.[47]

Others noted that the stereotype of the emotive woman, while thwarting opportunities for professional mobility, also enabled women to discuss psychological problems with doctors more freely than men did. The doctor's office functioned as a safe space where women could vent with impunity. High prescription rates reflected medical responsiveness to women's expressions of distress but also a willingness among doctors, more than 90 percent of whom were male in 1970, to code nervousness, stress, and insomnia as distinctly "female" problems. Men were no less psychologically conflicted, researchers averred, but they resisted sharing their problems with doctors. "If a man is tense or nervous, he can go into a bar," observed one contemporary. "A woman, because of social pressures, doesn't have that outlet . . . [so] she goes to the doctor for a tranquilizer." Men's miseries were temporarily rectified with liquor and male sociability at bars, business functions, and sporting events, coping mechanisms that reinforced symbols of masculine fortitude and self-help. Isolated at home, women's woes got managed by experts and prescription drugs.[48]

Significantly, this characterization of Valium's victims ignored contemporary and historical realities. It overlooked the thousands of women like Betty Ford or Barbara Gordon who had gotten hooked as career women or public figures. In addition, the stereotype of the tranquilizer-averse man glossed over a long history of male use and discounted the fact that millions of men—not just soldiers and veterans but also businessmen, athletes, teachers, and politicians—had used, praised, and even demanded tranquilizers. That is not to say that men had consistently and uniformly sought medical or pharmaceutical help. Even in the 1950s and 1960s, which likely witnessed the height of male tranquilizer consumption, many men, like many women, had resisted taking a pill for everyday nerves.

Sometimes the shame attached to seeking help sparked tragedy. In one case, an anguished woman wrote the FDA to detail the circumstances surrounding her husband's death. Her husband had been "the perfect husband and father, well known and very well thought of in the community, a professional man with the usual pressures of his position." He was also an exercise and healthy diet enthusiast. Unfortunately, healthy living alone could not lower his high blood pressure. His doctor prescribed Librium, which he took three times a day. Mindful of the stigma associated with tranquilizers, the doctor told him they were blood pressure pills: a little white lie intended to protect his male pride. "My husband was very strong in every way and considered it an expression of weakness to take even one tranquilizer," the devastated woman explained. "I know, because I had some for myself that he chided me about on the rare occasion when I would resort to them." All went well for five months. Then the man learned the truth about his drugs and stopped taking them immediately. What followed was a cascade of psychological and physiological symptoms that, in the wife's estimation, triggered his suicide days later.[49]

The stigma associated with mother's little helpers functioned as a double-edged sword. Discrediting tranquilizers as crutches for emotionally needy women made it more difficult for men to regard them as something they might benefit from. Attributing women's penchant for pill taking to social roles that allowed them to be more emotionally expressive, the stigma typecast men as withdrawn and emotionally stunted. Both were unflattering and exaggerated stereotypes that, with enough cultural currency, legitimized the very behaviors their invocation sought to explain. Although impossible to quantify with precision, it is likely that the conjoined stigmatization and feminization of tranquilizers in the 1970s further tainted antianxiety drugs as something "real" men should avoid.

People also blamed physicians for, in the words of one journalist, prescribing tranquilizers promiscuously. Instead of taking time to discuss patients' problems, doctors hurried them out the door with a quick fix, applying a band-aid to a bullet wound. Betty Ford recalled: "It was easier to give a woman tranquilizers and get rid of her than to sit and listen to her." One disgruntled man implored the FDA to stem the tide of tranquilizer use by monitoring physicians who "prescribe [Valium] as liberally as if they were handing out candy." Others explained doctors' prescription behavior in the context of the political economy of the American health care system. As general practitioners and internists increased their patient load, as health maintenance organizations sought to thwart spiraling health care costs by compressing doctors' schedules, doctors had less time to devote to each patient. By the late 1970s, it was common for a routine doctor's visit to last ten minutes or less. This structure impeded lengthy consultations and encouraged pill prescribing. As one physician said bluntly, "It takes thirty seconds to write a prescription for Valium but thirty minutes to explain why a patient shouldn't have it." "What might well be the best prescription," avowed psychiatrist Nathan Kline, "is something that the doctor usually cannot give: an hour of his time, listening to ill-defined complaints and offering understanding reassurance." Charged one less forgiving critic, "Get the hysterical female tranquilized and get her out of here."[50]

A handful of researchers linked the Valium phenomenon to a broader feminist critique of society's mistreatment of women. Harking back to Betty Friedan's analysis, they insisted that the real problem was the circumstances that encouraged women to seek escape. Why should a woman feel calm minding five children alone? How fulfilled could any person be cleaning dirty floors and toddler spit-up? Why did society expect women to look and act a certain way? Tranquilizer use was a logical result of an unhealthy ordering of gender roles. According to a study by feminist sociologist Ruth Cooperstock, wage-earning women were significantly less likely to take tranquilizers than women who stayed at home. Indeed, employment had a salutary effect on women's well-being. Women often got locked into roles that made them feel atomized and anxious, powerless to change their situation.[51]

Testifying before a congressional hearing on women's use of prescription drugs, Barbara Gibson, an addiction expert, suggested that the Equal Rights Amendment might better remedy women's drug abuse than simplistic denunciations of doctors, drugs, and pharmaceutical firms. With so many roadblocks—sexist attitudes, discriminatory policies, unequal pay—in women's way, it was no wonder so many "take something to survive." Gibson feared that media interest in women's drug use would encourage political quick fixes rather than a necessary reevaluation of systemic and cultural discrimination that would best effect permanent change: "What is it that prevents congressional persons from looking at the ERA, not in terms of a threat, but in terms of a minute facilitator for some easier processes for going from day to day for women? . . . I just don't think that we can afford to be so [narrowly focused] in terms of our concerns."[52]

In a different time and place, such appeals might have facilitated a political discussion of the mistreatment of women and created a political road map to help them experience their full potential as humans. But America's antidrug fervor favored simplistic solutions over more complicated explanations that shared the blame, explanations that would have acknowledged the myriad cultural, political, medical, and economic factors underlying the tranquilizer problem. Politicians and the mainstream media projected a simplistic and reassuring message that discounted broader grievances and gave people someone to blame. Doctors and drug companies were portrayed as "pushing" dangerous drugs onto hapless victims. "Drug Abuse—Just What the Doctor Ordered" and similar headlines depicted physicians as puppets of the avaricious drug establishment. "Millions of women have become victims of their physicians who, in turn, have been brainwashed by drug manufacturers," claimed one article. Pharmaceutical firms were blamed for promoting drugs in excessive and sexist ways and marketing tranquilizers for everyday problems. At the 1979 hearings on benzodi-azepines, Senator Edward Kennedy told the audience that "the whole pitch appears to be to sell and market, to sell and market."[53]

At the same time, regulators' critiques stopped short of calling for a radical overhaul of the medical system: politicians lobbied for reform, not revolution. Indeed, the public trials of tranquilizers and the attendant fin-ger pointing and rapping of corporate knuckles can be regarded as another chapter in a long history of American political reform. Hearings, rhetori-cal mud slinging, and the adoption of new regulations ultimately served to *preserve* the existing political order. It was important for politicians and liberal journalists to present themselves publicly as virtuous defenders of victimized mothers, but there was a telling gap between the rhetoric of blame and the politics of radical change. No one advocated the banning of benzodiazepines, the dismantling of private health care, or a restructuring of the pharmaceutical industry, never mind the adoption of the ERA or universal day care. Politicians knew who buttered their bread. In fact, the American Medical Association's political action committee dispersed over $1.5 million in campaign contributions (making it one of the most gener-ous contributors) to help elect the Ninety-sixth Congress in session during the Kennedy hearings. Denouncing the excesses of industry and American doctors, politicians continued to rely on both groups for financial and po-litical support.[54]

Americans emboldened by the Kennedy hearings, Betty Ford's disclo-sure, and Barbara Gordon's tell-all memoir blamed drug companies and doctors for their own misfortunes. Others did more than vent. They sought financial compensation for their suffering. In one case a family physician prescribed Valium for a woman he diagnosed with free-floating anxiety. Years later, the patient read *I'm Dancing As Fast As I Can*. Suffi-ciently alarmed by her decade-long use of Valium, she confronted her doc-tor about the drug's side effects. The doctor reassured her that she was taking a very low dosage and that addiction would not be a problem. Later the woman read Betty Ford's autobiography. Once more, she confronted her physician. Again he reassured her. When the woman insisted that she wanted to stop taking Valium under medical supervision, he referred her to an alcohol and drug treatment center. The detoxification program caused acute "insomnia, contractions, headaches, and sensations of burning." The patient sued both her physician and the rehab facility for medical malpractice. Court cases such as these became increasingly common in the 1980s as patients' concerns about the side effects of tranquilizers—which had in the 1950s and 1960s prompted a steady stream of private letters to the FDA—were rechanneled in an era of congressional hearings, activism, and published memoirs into political and legal demands. In another case, a plaintiff addicted to Valium filed suit against Hoffman-La Roche and Medical Economics, the publisher of the *Physicians' Desk Reference*, for "gross negligence" in failing to disclose to doctors and consumers the addictive character of Valium.[55]

Explanations that blamed doctors and drug companies for the nation's tranquilizer epidemic resonated with Americans in part because they were true. Doctors had prescribed tranquilizers carelessly; companies had promoted them excessively. Companies had downplayed the risk of dependence and the discomfort and medical hazards of sudden benzodiazepine withdrawal. At the same time, media reports neglected the nuances of the complicated history of the development and use of minor tranquilizers. Nowhere did they detail the commercial restraint that had characterized Miltown's release in the 1950s. Nor did they discuss patient demand and the ebullient cultural enthusiasm for minor tranquilizers that had transformed benzodiazepines like Valium into the world's leading pharmaceutical moneymakers. Rarely did they mention that evidence of the drug's dependence liability had been documented since 1961, or that by the time the American media and government officials "discovered" the extent of Valium's use, new prescriptions for the drug were beginning to wane. Nor did they try to sort out the vexing question of what made Americans so receptive to tranquilizers in the first place. In the years ahead, Americans would continue to wrestle with the many meanings of tranquilizers in a society whose pace and politics often seemed no less frantic than they had to millions during Miltown's halcyon years.

(9)

Tranquilizers on Trial

Addiction narratives have been told and retold in the news, in published memoirs, before expert committees and government task forces, in courtrooms and legislatures, and in the privacy of doctor's offices and patients' homes. For disturbed listeners, these stories became a rallying cry for reform. Bad publicity put tranquilizers on trial and elicited legislative and legal reforms to curb their use.

The benzo backlash played itself out at both federal and state levels. In 1975 the Justice Department designated Valium and Librium Schedule IV drugs, a classification that curtailed the number of times a patient could refill an original prescription. Stiff criminal sanctions were also adopted; the illegal sale of benzos became punishable by a fine of up to $10,000 or a prison sentence of up to three years. The FDA also got involved, brokering a widely publicized agreement with tranquilizer manufacturers. The new information package manufacturers sent to doctors was expanded to include the solemn edict: "Anxiety or tension associated with the stress of everyday life usually does not require treatment with an anxiolytic (antianxiety) drug."[1]

Federal action was paralleled by state initiatives to reduce government spending and control excessive or illicit benzo use. Convinced that expenditures on tranquilizers—newly recast as overprescribed rather than essential medications—were inappropriate, Medicaid programs in Georgia,

Pennsylvania, South Carolina, and Washington, D.C., eliminated benzo-diazepines from their list of covered drugs in the 1970s or severely re-stricted how many scripts or pills would be paid for by the state. The poor were now effectively denied access to drugs whose legitimacy was openly questioned. In 1989 New York State enacted a pioneering and controver-sial measure to reduce benzodiazepine prescriptions. Proponents justified the plan by pointing to a whopping 8 million prescriptions (about 4 per-cent of *all* prescriptions dispensed in the state) that had been filled the year before. Lauded by supporters as a progressive public health measure, the initiative limited each prescription of benzodiazepines to a one-month supply without a refill in the absence of compelling circumstances, which had to be carefully documented by physicians. Patients requiring more than a thirty-day supply were obligated to schedule a follow-up appoint-ment. Dispensing pharmacists now had to register prescriptions, along with the names of doctors and patients, with Health Department author-ities in Albany. The information was entered into a computer database and analyzed. Physicians identified as "permissive prescribers" could be investi-gated, sanctioned, and fined. Six months after the program began, about three hundred practitioners had been placed under investigation for pre-scribing too many tranks.[2]

State legislatures also made the illegal possession or sale of benzos felony offenses. Consistent with the reigning punitive mind-set, courts and juries strictly enforced them. In 1978 a guard at an Illinois peniten-tiary discovered seven Valium pills in a woman visitor's jacket. Confronted with the evidence—an unauthorized substance inside a prison—the woman apologized and appealed for leniency. Her contrite confession was deemed irrelevant, and the circuit court sentenced her to two to six years of imprisonment. The defendant appealed, arguing that the sentence was excessive, only to have an Illinois appellate court uphold it. In Alabama, a man who accidentally dropped a matchbox containing "nine yellow med-icine tablets" in the presence of a police offer met an equally grim fate. The man admitted that the drugs, acquired from his roommate, were Val-ium. The yellow pills were sent to the Alabama Department of Forensic Sciences, which confirmed their chemical properties. The man was charged, tried, and sentenced to four years in prison for "unlawfully, willfully, and feloniously possess[ing] Diazepam." Fifteen years earlier, the policeman might have looked the other way. Sharing tranquilizers with friends and relatives was commonplace. But this was 1979, and times had changed.[3]

Not surprisingly, in an era when tranquilizers were discredited, doctors scrutinized, and users stigmatized, sales of benzos declined. In the United States, prescriptions for Valium plunged from 61.3 million in 1975 to 33.6 million in 1980. A similar trend occurred in the United Kingdom. After the BBC program *That's Life!* profiled three people battling to get off benzos, thousands of viewers responded to share similar struggles. The BBC teamed up with MIND, the leading mental health charity in England and Wales, to survey the extent of tranquilizer use and dependency. The results, published in a pioneering handbook by the BBC, kept tranquilizers in the public spotlight and fueled a comparable backlash that included the adoption of stricter dispensing regulations. Sales were roughly halved between 1981 and 1989. Judging by the numbers at least, the tranquilizer "epidemic" had apparently been contained.[4]

But this was not the full story. Indeed, far from settling the tranquilizer debate, the benzo backlash opened up a Pandora's box. Across the United States, outraged Americans assailed the new restrictions, insisting that their medical needs were being shortchanged as a result of pundits' smug platitudes and policies. Sanctimonious schemes, they charged, might make for good sound bites in an era of pharmacological Calvinism, but in fact tranquilizers counted numerous success stories, people who credited their well-being to the maligned drugs. Mental health lobbyists and legions of psychiatrists decried the medical and social costs of underutilization and called for flexible guidelines—not one-dose-fits-all policies—that would accommodate the range of patients' predicaments and pharmacological needs. Faced with a mountain of bad press and formidable restrictions, Hoffman-La Roche implored doctors and an increasingly skeptical public to remember Valium's clinical upside. Millions of Americans had benefited from it, company spokespersons insisted. Valium-related problems, while real and devastating, were relatively uncommon. (Not unexpectedly, the company downplayed its own culpability in failing to reveal the full extent of Valium's risks.)[5] In response to the FDA press release regarding the revised 1980 advisory, Roche published a series of provocative ads to court medical support. Entitled "Examine Me" and "Feelings vs. Facts," the ads exploited the rhetorical power of subjective experience. They asserted competing narratives and implored doctors to let their own experiences, rather than media headlines, be the final arbiters of Valium's worth. "Examine Me" urged doctors to look anew at the controversy from the drug's perspective:

During the past several years, I have heard my name mentioned in movies, on television and radio talk shows, and even at Senate subcommittee sessions. And I have seen it repeatedly in newspapers, magazines, and yes, bestsellers. Lately, whenever I see or hear the phrases "overmedicated society," "overuse," "misuse," and "abuse," my name is one of the reference points. Sometimes even the reference point.

These current issues, involving patient compliance or dependency-proneness, should be given careful scrutiny, for they may impede my overall therapeutic usefulness. As you know, a problem almost always involves improper usage. When I am prescribed and taken correctly, I can produce the effective relief for which I am intended.

Amid all this controversy, I ask you to reflect on and re-examine my merits. Think back on the patients in your practice who have been helped with your clinical counseling and prudent prescriptions for me. . . . Recall how often you've heard, as a result, "Doctor, I don't know what I would have done without your help."

You and I can feel proud of what we've done together. . . . If you examine and evaluate me in the light of your own experience, you'll come away with a confirmation of your knowledge that I *am* a safe and effective drug when prescribed judiciously and used wisely.[6]

Roche also referenced escalating and (socially noncatastrophic) use of benzodiazepines in other countries as evidence of how capricious politics, rather than objective science, were driving the tranquilizer wars. Meanwhile, rival pharmaceutical firms capitalized on the commercial vacuum created by the benzo backlash and America's affinity for psychiatric pill popping to help make Prozac and other SSRIs, a new generation of antidepressants, the biggest psychiatric blockbusters since Miltown and Valium. By the 1990s, manufacturers were repositioning SSRIs as antianxiety agents. In the end, the failure of SSRIs to capture the anxiety market, expanded and politicized after 9/11, revealed much about America's long-standing fascination with tranquilizers, a class of drugs whose arrival had initiated the age of mass-prescribed psychiatric panaceas.

Voices of Protest

Tranquilizer users were among the first to denounce new restrictions. The tone of their complaints indicated a new strand of patient activism as trust in regulators, so pronounced after Frances Kelsey's thalidomide triumph, had yielded to entrenched skepticism of government authority. Some of this mistrust was stoked by health activists' wariness of medical institutions in general. Revelations regarding the Tuskegee trial, a multidecade clinical study sponsored by the U.S. Public Health Service in which African American men were denied treatment for syphilis, compounded the climate of doubt. So too did the federal government's apparent indifference to the HIV/AIDS crisis. The protests also reflected the medical libertarianism enshrined in the Supreme Court's decisions in *Griswold v. Connecticut* (1965), in which a right to privacy—including the privacy to use contraceptives without state interference—was acknowledged to exist within the penumbra of the Bill of Rights, and *Roe v. Wade* (1973). Women had the legal right to use contraceptives or obtain an early abortion on the grounds that these were private medical matters that required shielding from state interference. Car bumper stickers that appeared after *Roe* brandished the well-known message, "keep your laws off my body," to warn regulation-happy legislators that they would not tolerate further state intrusions.[7]

A determination to curtail legislators' prerogatives to interfere with existing prescription practices informed the protests of angry tranquilizer

users. Irate patients portrayed themselves as seasoned experts whose experience allowed them to discern the risks of medication. Repeatedly, they
beseeched regulators to butt out. "Bureaucrats have again scored a victory,"
seethed one Wisconsin man in a letter to Senator Gaylord Nelson, upon
learning that refills would be limited to a six-month supply:

> How can you judge if I need the drug for a week or [for] the rest of my
> life? I didn't know that the Senators and Congressman are becoming
> M.D.s . . . which way do we go Senator? Are we to be a free society and
> live according to the Bill of Rights and our Constitution? You're taking
> away my right to the pursuit of Health and Happiness. You have a lot of
> good ideas but please don't be my doctor.[8]

Similarly, a Librium user wrote both her senator and congressman to
criticize the new restrictions. "Millions of us have used these products for
many years in a quite normal manner, in order that we function better," she
noted. Now, bureaucrats were impeding their efforts to have full and pur-
poseful lives.

> Government has loaded us down with far too many restrictions, rules,
> regulations as it is—it seems bent on interfering in the private business of
> the normal people rather than winnowing out of society the abnormal
> drug traffic with its terrible human specimens of disaster—it cries of the
> plight of abnormal humans "downtrodden" by society but does nothing
> which will help those who are the victims of abnormal specimens. . . .
> We are not a variety of sheep to be fed, led, herded, and told what to
> think—what to eat—what to wear—we are decision-making, responsible
> people. . . . We don't need to be regulated to death.[9]

Patients went to great lengths to distinguish themselves from junkies.
Rejecting the implicit conflation of illicit drugs such as marijuana or cocaine with prescription medications, they demanded to be recognized as
law-abiding citizens. "We have a tremendous drug problem in our country," one woman raged. "Why can't government enforce the laws we have

and try to stop the law-breaking drug pushers and users?" A Librium user suggested that Congress ban the sale of alcohol, "the real demon in our midst." Ill-advised restrictions on prescription drugs diverted government attention from real problems, penalizing millions of "conscientious users." Another frustrated user urged politicians to review their own medicinal habits before passing judgment on patients and doctors: "Does the DEA ever count the number of cocktails sold in Washington, D.C.?" she fumed. "Do they propose a limit on the amount of alcoholic beverages a government worker may consume in 6 months?" Another demanded, "What about alcoholic drinks and marijuana and heroin and the like, why don't you do something about those things?" She likened tranquilizers to antibiotics, which had retained their mystique as the emblem of "good" medicine. She taunted zealous regulators to take antibiotics off the market as well: "[Maybe] you will be satisfied then, when all of us will either die of disease or become mental patients."[10]

These complaints mirrored several undulating currents: mistrust of government, contempt for misplaced and excessive regulation, and a rejection of the assumption that tranquilizer users shared the same social address as other addicts. Also resonant in patients' criticisms were the economic hardships endured by low-income Americans already struggling with rising food and energy costs in an era of galloping inflation and economic recession, the first since the Eisenhower years. Limiting prescription refills forced patients to consult doctors more often. Although keeping patients better monitored was the putative objective of the revamped system, this meant time-consuming and costly visits to the doctor's office. An eighty-nine-year-old man, a self-identified church member uninterested in taking drugs to get high, denigrated the new financial strain: "A new prescription, at $10.00 every three months [the cost of a doctor's visit], plus the $8.00 for a hundred pills is a considerable hardship to a man with no income but Social Security." There was no question that "youngsters need to be restricted," another user sniped, "but why punish the elderly who are on small Social Security checks?" Another patient wondered if the new regulations didn't suggest an unholy alliance between politicians and physicians, a collusion meant to fatten the wallets of doctors, who could charge top dollar for extra consultations. The law was particularly "unfair to the people [who] have taken [tranquilizers] for years and not abused them," he complained to his congressman, Tennessee Republican Robin Leo Beard. Perhaps it was time to change political leadership rather than limit prescription refills. "Me and my family supported you in the last election and intend to this time, but we are beginning to see why the Republicans get the name of being for the fat cats instead of the average working-class people," he complained.[11]

Others focused on the undertreatment of anxiety and the anguish resulting from the drug controversies. A barrage of bad publicity had created a cultural and medical milieu where stigma, shame, and the specter of addiction discouraged people from seeking help. Virginia Ironside, the "agony aunt" for the *Independent* (London), feared that the backlash had exacerbated a grin-and-bear-it mentality that left many people feeling needlessly frantic and tired. Ironside had used Valium on and off for years and still kept some in her handbag for emergencies and periodic insomnia. "It saves an enormous amount of grief," she explained. "I meet people looking haggard and they say they have been so worried and can't sleep, and I think, you stupid wallies—take a Valium and it'll all look different in the morning." One reporter she spoke with speculated that millions of Britons had similar stories but didn't share them because of the stigma attached to Valium. "No one would wish to downplay the suffering of people . . . whose lives have been ravaged by an unwitting benzodiazepine addiction," conceded Ironside. "But the truth is that their numbers are small in comparison to those who have been quietly helped along their way by these drugs."[12]

Doctors who had followed the evolving perceptions of tranquilizers also wondered if their stigmatization had done more harm than good. The eminent psychiatrist Heinz Lehmann, known for his earlier clinical studies of Thorazine, was among them. In 1960, Lehmann had warned a U.S. Senate subcommittee that the popularization of minor tranquilizers such as Miltown and Equanil had led to tremendous abuse. Doctors were prescribing beyond normal ranges and patients were becoming dependent. Decades later, Lehmann worried that the pendulum of political opinion had swung too far in the opposite direction. In the 1980s, Lehmann told reporters that patients had been hoodwinked by "sensational horror stories." As a result, thousands of unmedicated patients were "suffering needlessly."[13]

Other physicians feared that restrictions were encouraging doctors to prescribe older and more dangerous compounds. This was one unexpected result of New York's 1989 measure to curb benzodiazepine use. While many clinicians, civil libertarians, and advocates of the poor decried New York's pilot program, no one disputed that the prohibition had worked in a narrow sense. A year after the measure went into effect, benzo prescriptions had decreased by 44 percent in New York, compared with a national decrease of 11 percent. But the drop was accompanied by a simultaneous rise in prescriptions for riskier sedatives such as barbiturates and chloral hydrate. One psychiatrist attributed the shift to the fact that cautious physicians were running scared. "It's a horrible, horrible direction to go," complained Dr. Fritz Henn, director of the Department of Psychiatry at the State University of New York at Stony Brook. "It means that people are so afraid of the regulation that they're prescribing what are really relatively dangerous and very addictive drugs for the same thing they would have prescribed somewhat addictive, rather safe drugs for. It's really sad." The law was particularly burdensome for low-income patients, many of whom were on Medicaid, because the number of medical consultations was capped. As one physician in Queens put it, for public health officials "to proudly point to the reduction of the number of written prescriptions as an indicator of some kind of success against alleged prescribing abuse is scientific naiveté."[14]

Restricted access also nurtured a bootleg benzo market. Polydrug users and opiate and cocaine addicts who took benzos to enhance a high or ease a crash obtained them illicitly from street dealers, Internet vendors, or unscrupulous physicians or pharmacists. Some forged prescriptions; others stole pills from family, friends, health centers, drugstores, and even pharmaceutical warehouses. Tranquilizers had been bootlegged in the 1950s too, but restrictions limiting patient access to these drugs caused the black market to grow, especially among the addicted. In 2000, a Nashville man hooked on Xanax, a newer benzodiazepine, walked into a neighborhood

Walgreen's and threatened a pharmacist with a barbecue fork. After receiving the tablets, the belligerent man swallowed them and waited calmly in the pharmacy chair for the police to apprehend him and escort him to jail. The problem transcended class and social divisions. In January 2002, Noelle Bush, daughter of then Florida governor Jeb Bush, made national headlines when she was arrested after being accused of trying to procure Xanax with a forged prescription.[15]

The popularity of Xanax was a curious by-product of the Valium backlash. A recurring concern about Valium in the 1970s was its long half-life—the time it takes for a drug to be metabolized and eliminated from the body (literally, the time required for the concentration of the drug to fall to half its initial value in the bloodstream). Valium's half-life is twenty to one hundred hours, longer than most benzodiazepines.[16] Critics worried that Valium's half-life left habitual users, who in the late 1970s numbered in the millions, permanently drowsy and impaired. The image of a drugged-around-the-clock nation figured prominently in the 1979 Kennedy hearings on the hazards of benzo use and in the media maelstrom it unfurled.

Enter Xanax, a shorter-acting tranquilizer. Introduced by Upjohn in 1981, Xanax had a half-life of only six to twelve hours, and thus seemed tailor-made for the problem of long-term sluggishness. Indeed, one of the cultural and medical appeals of Xanax was that it tranquilized users for a shorter period of time. Upjohn promoted Xanax as a new type of benzodiazepine that was safer than Valium: no hangover, no physical dysfunction. Upjohn also reaped the benefits of two important events. One was the expiration of Valium's patent in 1985, which allowed other companies to manufacture it as an inexpensive generic (diazepam). Once Valium went off patent, there was no financial incentive to promote it, creating a commercial space for a new, presumably better, and certainly more costly brand-name benzo. Pushed as a technologically upgraded successor to Valium, Xanax had already overtaken Valium as the country's leading benzodiazepine by 1986.[17]

Upjohn's other marketing coup, delivered a few years later but set in motion in the early 1980s, was Xanax's therapeutic monopoly as the first

FDA-approved drug for the treatment of panic disorder, recognized as a separate and distinct condition for the first time in the DSM-III (1980). As researcher David Sheehan remembered, there was nothing unique about Xanax's antipanic properties. Other benzodiazepines such as Ativan (lorazepam) and the antidepressant Tofranil (imipramine) also treated panic effectively. What distinguished Xanax was a shorter half-life (imipramine's was roughly double) and Upjohn's shrewd marketing acumen which, according to Sheehan, seized on the "confusion that existed in the classification system for anxiety disorders in DSM-III to create a perception that a drug had special and unique properties that would help it capture market share and displace [Valium] from the top position."[18]

The arrival of panic disorder on the diagnostic scene enabled Upjohn to launch one of the first multinational clinical drug trials in the annals of psychiatry. The Cross-National Collaborative Panic Study recruited almost two thousand patients in fourteen countries and four continents from 1982 to 1987. Because Ativan and Tofranil were no longer protected by patent, they lacked Xanax's commercial potential. Understandably, no other company was willing to run trials of comparable scale to assess whether a low-cost generic might work just as well. Armed with expensively procured trial results demonstrating Xanax's safety and efficacy for treating panic, Upjohn got FDA approval—and a green light to create a new marketing niche. The FDA's decision was trumpeted in multipage color advertisements:

XANAX:
THE FIRST AND ONLY MEDICATION
INDICATED FOR PANIC DISORDER[19]

With verve and money, Upjohn promoted Xanax aggressively, charging consumers more than twenty times what Wyeth charged for Ativan (on the market since 1971). By 1991 Xanax was a top-selling drug, accounting for almost one-fourth of Upjohn's global sales.[20]

But there was serious downside to the drug's advertised virtues. Xanax's rapid elimination, a benefit for those concerned with long-term accumulation, precipitated more severe and rapid withdrawal symptoms in users than the longer-acting benzos. As one addiction specialist put it, the drug was *so* short-acting "that you eventually need to be dosed rapidly throughout the day." For someone "predisposed to addiction, it is a very addicting drug. It's the crack [cocaine] of the benzodiazepines." In fact, 73 percent of patients in one study were able to taper off Valium successfully; only 43 percent were able to stop Xanax. Ironically, in cases of Xanax or Ativan addiction today, doctors often prescribe longer-acting benzodiazepines such as Valium or Klonopin to help patients ride out withdrawal symptoms. The history of Xanax (like that of other tranquilizers) illustrates the social concerns that frame evaluations of a drug's therapeutic value. How doctors, patients, legislators, activists, and other groups have perceived Xanax—as an antidote to sluggishness, a panic-fighting panacea, or a recipe for addiction— reflects cultural and political preoccupations.[21]

Doctors' responses to the benzo backlash, which included an ongoing willingness to prescribe Xanax, were also informed by concerns that anxiety disorders were underdiagnosed and undertreated, particularly in the United States. Despite long-standing efforts to classify and standardize anxiety, estimating its incidence remains a contested issue, enmeshed in a broader, high-stakes debate about the diagnostic reliability of DSM, the power of pharmaceutical promotion to pathologize what some consider nonmedical problems, the subjective character of doctor-patient encounters, and the idiosyncrasies of anxiety. Still, many doctors and mental health organizations contend that, on balance, anxiety disorders are both prevalent *and* underdiagnosed. In 2006, the National Institute of Mental Health estimated that as many as 40 million adult Americans suffer from an anxiety disorder in any given year: more than double the number thought to have such a disorder in 2001. The Anxiety Disorders Association of America (ADAA) also puts the figure at about 40 million, characterizing anxiety as "the most common mental illness in the United States." A study commissioned by the ADAA estimated that anxiety cost taxpayers $42.3 billion a year—about a third of the nation's $148 billion mental health bill. Workplace absenteeism and low productivity were other hidden costs, to the tune of $256 per year per anxious worker. Resurrecting arguments made in the 1950s by Mike Gorman and other mental health activists about the social and economic burdens of psychological illness, modern proponents of psychiatric intervention have depicted anxiety as too costly to ignore.[22]

What role should drugs play in alleviating it? Various studies suggest that despite alarm about the country's psychiatric overmedication, a concern amplified by the Xanax controversy, only a minority of patients meeting DSM criteria for anxiety disorders are prescribed medication or receive therapy. In one study, 73 percent of persons suffering from generalized anxiety eschewed medical treatment. Many doctors worry that media sensationalism in the 1970s and 1980s has exaggerated the abuse potential of benzodiazepines, depriving legitimate sufferers of useful treatment. The burning question, one medical study somberly concluded, was "whether attitudes strongly biased against the use of these drugs work to deprive the majority of severely anxious patients of appropriate treatment."[23]

The possibility that media hype had distorted reality was echoed in various milieus in the 1980s and 1990s. "Where are all the tranquilizer junkies?" inquired a 1983 editorial in the *Journal of the American Medical Association*, which suggested that accounts of widespread benzodiazepine addiction were the stuff of legend. Irresponsible, overprescribing physicians were the exception, not the norm. A 1990 report by the American Psychiatric Association task force found that most Americans took benzodiazepines intermittently, largely for punctual symptom relief. When recreational abuse did occur, they noted, it was "almost always among persons who [were] also actively abusing alcohol, opiates, or other sedative hypnotics." The report discussed benzo-related risks, including memory impairment, psychomotor dysfunction, and discontinuance symptoms when the drug was abruptly stopped. Yet it also advised clinicians not to be discouraged from prescribing a benzodiazepine when necessary, and to recognize that "at least on [a] short-term basis, for most patients the benefits outweigh the risks." A task force established by the World Psychiatric Association reached a similar conclusion, suggesting that use rates were low "relative to the proportion of the population with defined clinical needs." The tone of these recommendations, urging doctors to prioritize patients' individual needs over generic clinical guidelines (much as many tranquilizer users had done) was further supported by studies showing that benzodiazepines not only retained their efficacy over long periods but did not lead to abuse, even in high doses.[24]

As patients and doctors appealed for personalized evaluation at a time when policy makers were swayed by the notion of collective hazards, some wondered if semantics weren't impeding a peaceful resolution to the tranquilizer wars. Patients, doctors, activists, politicians, and journalists were talking about the same drugs, but the divergent vocabulary they used made a bewildering matter even more baffling. Each group effectively talked past the others, ensuring that conversations failed to converge in a constructive way. One study insightfully suggested that a consensus on the risks and benefits of benzodiazepines was unlikely to emerge because the words most salient to the discussion—dependence, addiction, abuse, withdrawal, craving, euphoria, tolerance, and rebound—had historically been defined differently by different groups and individuals, even within the psychiatric community. While some people used terms like "addiction" and "dependence" interchangeably, others disaggregated them, linking addiction with recreational abuse and pleasure seeking. Dependence, on the other hand, was a "normal consequence of long-term pharmacological receptor-site activity," affected by dosage and duration of treatment. In a world where the vocabulary used to discuss tranquilizers was so nebulous and unstable, could social or scientific consensus ever prevail?[25]

The SSRI Encroachment

As the tranquilizer wars were being fought on various fronts, SSRIs made their way into the clinic. The blockbuster Prozac came first (in 1987), followed by Paxil, Zoloft, and countless others. Although the DSM-III had divided anxiety and depressive disorders into distinct clinical entities, the term "anxious depression" denoted the presence of symptoms of both disorders in a single person. Today, mental health experts discuss "comorbidity rates" to acknowledge the simultaneous but independent existence of a depressive or anxiety disorder; someone who primarily suffers from depression may also have symptoms of anxiety. Capitalizing on heightened medical interest in associations between the two disorders and hoping to grab some of tranquilizers' market share, pharmaceutical manufacturers sponsored clinical trials that demonstrated that serotonergic agents (mainly SSRIs and SNRIs, serotonin-norepinephrine reuptake inhibitors, such as Effexor, which acts on two neurotransmitters) improved the symptoms of anxiety disorders. By the 1990s, most SSRIs had acquired a broader, FDA-sanctioned treatment profile that included both depression and certain forms of anxiety: obsessive compulsive disorder, panic, social phobia, and generalized anxiety disorder. New clinical guidelines, incorporating wariness of the habit-forming potential of benzos and the availability of antidepressant alternatives, recommended that SSRIs and SNRIs be considered first-choice drugs for anxious patients.[26]

Manufacturers also worked hard to reposition antidepressants as effective antianxiety agents. The campaign surrounding social anxiety disorder or SAD (originally called social phobia) was a case in point. Characterized by debilitating shyness, anxiety in the face of observation or scrutiny, and a persistent fear of humiliation, SAD was once considered a rare malady in North America and Europe. When discussed in psychiatric circles, it was generally seen as an "Asian disorder." In 1997 and 1998, it was mentioned a mere fifty times in the American press, but by 1999 it had been referenced over a billion times, giving it a visibility one might expect to see reserved for a global pandemic.[27]

This change was driven by a well-funded educational and advertising campaign to publicize anxiety disorders and to associate their amenability to treatment with antidepressants. The most successful of these was coordinated by Cohn Wolfe, a PR firm retained by GlaxoSmithKline (GSK) to cultivate awareness of SAD. GSK launched Paxil in the United Kingdom in 1991 and in the United States a year later. Sporting the catchy slogan "Imagine Being Allergic to People," the SAD campaign began just before the company won FDA approval in 1999 to market the antidepressant as the first and only FDA-approved treatment for SAD. As Paxil's product director boasted, "Every marketer's dream is to find an unidentified or unknown market and develop it. That's what we were able to do with social anxiety disorder." The campaign cost GSK more than $92 million in a single year (millions more than Pfizer spent promoting Viagra). It characterized SAD as America's third largest mental health problem after alcoholism and depression, affecting more than 10 million people (although the National Institute of Mental Health and the American Psychiatric Association estimated that the number of true sufferers was much lower). "You blush, sweat, shake—even find it hard to breathe. That's what social anxiety disorder feels like," explained one poster. No mention of GSK appeared in the hundreds of newspaper and magazine articles, and radio and television segments, profiling SAD. Instead, concerned parties were directed to the industry-funded Social Anxiety Disorder Coalition for more information. GSK was a more ubiquitous presence in Cohn Wolfe's direct-to-consumer advertising (DTCA) blitz, made possible by an FDA decision that relaxed restrictions on pharmaceutical marketing. By 1995, expenditures on DTCA for prescription drugs had reached $380 million; a decade later they exceeded $4 billion. Ads for Paxil and SAD were part of this whirlwind campaign. The company filled women's magazines and prime-time commercials with images of distraught social phobics—male businessmen (the modern incarnation of Miltown's frazzled executives), housewives, and career women—afflicted with chemical imbalances that Paxil, the "anxiolytic antidepressant," could correct. One print ad featured a thirty-something, suited businessman, face against the wall, eyes shut, devastated by his dismal work performance. The captions running down the left margin narrated the failures that besieged him. "I should have joined in more often, I could have taken the promotion, I would have found someone special. . . . only I can't. I just can't." To the right: "Show them you can," in bold letters tinged with a beckoning orange hue. The man could be saved by chemical enlightenment: "Paxil. Relieve the anxiety. Reveal the person." Another Paxil ad updated the stock female antiheroes of 1970s Valium ads (Jan, the psychoneurotic single, Mrs. Raymond, the menopausal misfit) with a feminist veneer. It showcased a determined woman, clad in bold red, once overpowered by anxiety, newly "empowered by Paxil."[28]

The media sweep also included strategically placed television testimonials from physicians, advocates, and patients highlighting the deleterious consequences of untreated social anxiety disorder. In the new DTCA era,

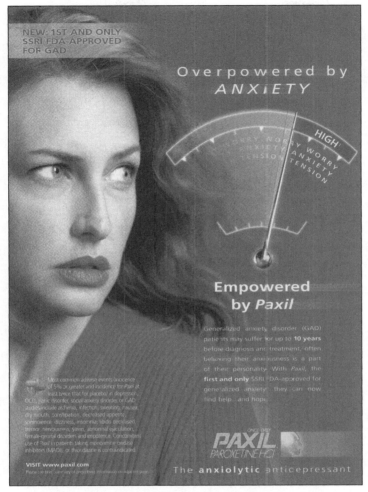

Empowered by Paxil. In the 1990s, manufacturers of SSRIs repositioned them as antianxiety agents, successfully securing FDA approval to have them prescribed for a range of anxiety disorders, including GAD and SAD. Direct-to-consumer ads updated time-worn themes in tranquilizer marketing, such as executive anxiety and female timidity, by associating pill popping with personal liberation and professional advancement. *American Journal of Psychiatry,* July 2001.

pharmaceutical companies often select well-known individuals to promote specific products. In some of the first Viagra ads, Republican Bob Dole openly discussed his erectile dysfunction. Similarly, Cohn Wolfe hand-picked public figures to discuss their pharmaceutical experiences with the masses. In the days of Miltown, compensated endorsements were illegal, although many Miltown devotees shared their trank tales with unbridled enthusiasm. But the mood had changed since the 1950s; anxiety was a mental health disorder and taking tranquilizers was no longer a playful rite of personhood. Americans were understandably more circumspect discussing the problem. In the meantime, pharmaceutical promotion had become more sophisticated, expensive, and slick. Because the use of antianxiety agents, especially by men, had been increasingly veiled by social secrecy and medical stigma, marketing firms in the late 1990s jockeyed to draw attention to men's emotional suffering and pharmacological relief.

Miami Dolphins running back Ricky Williams was among those hand-picked for the cause. On *Oprah* and other outlets, he told viewers about how his fear of people had once made him dodge approaching fans and wear his helmet, equipped with a visor, to shield him during interviews. The former Heisman Trophy winner had always been shy, but when his avoidance behavior escalated—prompting journalists to depict him as aloof and eccentric—he sought help. Diagnosed with SAD, Williams started Paxil and began seeing a therapist. "The moment I started treating my social anxiety disorder, I started feeling better," he told an online chat group. He now welcomed interviews. Unfortunately for GSK, Paxil and therapy were not enough for the sports superstar. In 2004 Williams was fined and suspended for testing positive for marijuana use. Williams told the *Miami Herald* that marijuana had fewer side effects "and worked 10 times better for me than Paxil." Besides, unlike synthetic pills manufactured by corporations, "it's just a plant."[29]

If Williams had become a public relations liability for GSK, this was not reflected in Paxil sales. Between 1999 and 2000, prescriptions for Paxil rose by 18 percent. Paxil had become GSK's most profitable drug as well as the most popular SSRI in the United States. Racking up $2.1 billion worth of sales, it outdid two other profit-making workhorses, Zoloft and Prozac. Paxil's success was enhanced by the FDA's decision to approve it for generalized anxiety disorder, panic disorder, obsessive compulsive disorder, and posttraumatic stress disorder, testimony to the antidepressant's attempted takeover of the anxiety market. To encourage the use of Paxil as an antianxiety drug, GSK financed an *Anxious Moments* film series for distribution to physicians, with separate films profiling each disorder, its associated symptoms, and treatments.[30]

The hype surrounding social anxiety disorder and the push for Paxil have raised concerns that echo those voiced by Americans in the past. One is the extent to which pharmaceutical companies have pathologized problems that are simply part of the normal vagaries of life. How many Americans would identify social anxiety as a disorder requiring medical consultation or pharmacotherapy in the absence of well-placed ads or awareness campaigns? Where does the boundary separating extreme shyness and social phobia begin? When does normal anxiety bleed into something more closely approximating pathological illness? Physicians and social commentators debated this issue in the 1950s and 1960s too, but the present-day multimillion dollar campaigns—replete with educational initiatives, websites, self-diagnostic Internet and magazine tests, and a flotilla of slick ads and jingles—have sought to reframe how we perceive mental wellness and illness in a way that is culturally resonant yet equally controversial.

Critics worried about corporate-sponsored medicalization contend that the pharmaceutical industry has artificially inflated the prevalence and severity of psychiatric disorders more to increase profits than to protect the public's health. As Marcia Angell, the former editor of the *New England Journal of Medicine* avers, the chief objective of pharmaceutical campaigns is to push products: "They are no more in the business of educating the people [about health] than a beer company is in the business of educating people about alcoholism." A short film spoof entitled *A New Epidemic,* cleverly placed on www.youtube.com, profiles, with seeming sincerity, a fictitious psychiatric illness—motivational deficiency disorder—alleged to be underdiagnosed but rampant. Its symptoms range from the mild (a reluctance to get out of bed on Monday morning) to serious (a potentially life-threatening lack of motivation to breathe). One disheveled patient is pictured asleep in front of his television, surrounded by stacks of papers and unwashed dishes. He plaintively admits: "All my life people have called me lazy, but now I know I was sick." One wife weeps with gratitude that her afflicted husband has finally gotten help. On meds, he has mowed their lawn, repaired their gutters, and paid the electricity bill: all in one week! In my experience, most medical and history students find the clip entertaining. It sardonically captures what Peter Kramer, author of *Listening to Prozac,* terms "diagnostic bracket creep": the relentless expansion of illnesses to accommodate new medications that purport to treat them.[31]

Many physicians and mental health lobbyists counter that nonpartisan awareness campaigns serve a vital public function. In publicizing anxiety disorders, they demistify the stigma that has long plagued mental illnesses without trivializing tranquilizers as the earlier media frenzy surrounding Miltown may have done. "I believe the industry has done a very good job at raising awareness and getting a lot of people help [who] otherwise wouldn't have got it," asserts one psychiatrist. Undertreatment is the norm. "I know there's lots of concern about 'Are we medicalizing normative things?'" admitted another consultant. But "the people I see talking about that have not seen these patients. These patients are genuinely distraught." He urged others to respect patients' suffering and the meaning behind their help-seeking behavior. Medications have benefited and continued to benefit countless Americans whose anguish, while hard to measure objectively, shouldn't be blithely dismissed as a commercial fabrication.[32]

Even among those favoring greater intervention, there are important overlapping and contradictory differences in orientation and approach. Some groups have expressed alarm that emphasizing the prevalence of anxiety disorders such as SAD detracts attention from rarer and more life-threatening psychiatric illnesses. Does the (disputed) assertion that as many as 10 million people have treatable SAD trivialize the gravity of other mental illnesses? If Americans come to regard SAD as commonplace, will their compassion for schizophrenics or the suicidal diminish? Although some critics charge that company-sponsored awareness campaigns are tantamount to drug promotion, nonprofit advocacy groups such as the ADAA or Freedom from Fear support such awareness initiatives, but their goal, they insist, has been to educate people about treatment options, not push pills. "We have never, ever promoted any drug," maintains Jerilyn Ross, the founder of the ADAA. And indeed, the organization's website lists medication options without endorsing any particular drug and emphasizes the efficacy of cognitive and behavioral therapy. It even provides browsers with a link to help them find an accredited therapist. These and other examples illustrate the plurality of views within the advocacy community.[33]

If the SSRI campaign has drawn attention to anxiety and the benefits of drug therapy, it hasn't persuaded all physicians that antidepressants are necessarily better than benzodiazepines. Tranquilizers and SSRIs work differently, and those differences help explain their enduring appeal to doctors and patients. At issue are their relative tolerability, efficacy, and cost. SSRIs typically achieve maximum potency after weeks of use and can cause side effects (dry mouth, fatigue, sexual dysfunction, and heightened feelings of anxiety in the first weeks of use) intolerable to some patients. Even when they work, SSRIs typically reduce (often by only 50 or 60 percent) rather than eliminate anxiety symptoms outright. Growing evidence suggests that some SSRIs may be no less habit-forming than the benzodiazepines they sought to replace. This is an important finding: one of the rationales behind the repositioning of SSRIs as anxiolytics was manufacturers' claims that they lacked benzodiazepines' habit-forming potential. Benzodiazepines also have a different therapeutic profile. They work rapidly and generally eliminate most symptoms promptly. As a result, they can be used as needed, making them preferable to SSRIs for situational anxiety. As Dr. Carl Salzman, a psychiatrist affiliated with the Massachusetts Mental Health Center and the former chair of the APA's task force on benzodiazepines, recently observed, benzodiazepines have a compelling safety, compliance, and efficacy record. This may yet lead to their reinstatement as primary antianxiety agents in treatment guidelines being adopted by medical groups, insurance companies, and health departments to standardize clinical practice.[34]

Critics of the benzo backlash also insist that international patterns should be taken into account when Americans evaluate the medicinal merits of tranks. In 1979, when the Kennedy hearings and media reports decried the overmedication of America, a study published in the *New England Journal of Medicine* reached a somewhat different conclusion. It showed that adults in some Western European nations, including Belgium, Denmark,

France, Germany, and the Netherlands, used more antianxiety agents, particularly benzodiazepines, than Americans did. In fact, compared to nine European countries, the United States ranked an unimpressive sixth; neither unique nor atypical, the frequency and duration of tranquilizer use in the United States made Americans altogether average. Robert B. Clark, the president of Hoffman-La Roche in 1979, tried to marshal this data to strategic advantage—attempting to disentangle the drug's clinical record from its social and political baggage—but his entreaties fell on deaf ears. Politicians and pundits held fast to the idea of America as an excessively tranquilized nation.[35]

As sales of benzodiazepines fell in the United States and the United Kingdom in the 1980s, they increased globally by as much as 18 percent, according to one estimate. France and Japan are two interesting examples. In the 1970s, cross-national studies revealed that per capita tranquilizer consumption was slightly higher in France (where 17 percent of the public took benzodiazepines in a single year) than in the United States (where only 15 percent did). As benzodiazepine use dropped in the United States, it increased in France, widening the disparity in drug use between the two countries. Studies undertaken in the late 1990s and early 2000s confirm the prevalence of benzodiazepine use in France. One study found that more than 75 percent of French benzodiazepine users had taken pills regularly for over six months. Indeed, France appears to have realized the greatest fear of American journalists and policy makers: millions of people for whom long-term benzo use is the norm.[36]

Some public health officials have encouraged French general practitioners, who write more than 80 percent of benzodiazepine prescriptions, to modify their practices. However, as far as the French are concerned, there is no crisis. This may reflect a principled rejection of the parochial idea that what holds true in the United States or the United Kingdom should hold sway in France. As a growing number of scholars have demonstrated, the history of Western medicine is replete with variations in clinical practices, despite efforts to standardize them. But the French attitude toward benzodiazepines may also reflect a suspicion that the urgency behind the U.S. campaign says more about American cultural values than about the social and medical liabilities of benzodiazepines. "I think Americans are basically puritans," admitted the eminent psychopharmacologist Karl Rickels. "Maybe Great Britain too. . . . Certainly France is more relaxed and they're prescribing it more." Nor have any catastrophes befallen the country as a result. "I don't see that [French] people are dying more on the roads in car accidents. I don't see that in any way their society is more affected."[37]

A parallel story developed in Japan, where the market for benzodiazepines grew even as other countries moved away from them in favor of antidepressants to treat depression or anxiety. An important reason for the Japanese difference is that the diagnosis and treatment of depression has only recently become medically and cultural respectable. While the United States and the United Kingdom began to experience depression "epidemics" in the late 1980s, Japan, for all appearances, remained anxious. Unlike depression, anxiety was sanctioned by Japanese culture and tradition. Indeed, until recently, Japan did not have a cultural idiom for what in the West would be termed depression. Sadness and suffering in Japan have long been intertwined with spiritual values that link an individual's experience of grief to a shared and valued identity. Rather than being a problem to be muted with medication, a person's capacity to suffer loss was culturally accepted as essential to the individual but also to the community's moral and spiritual growth. The medical model of mild depression, which attributes emotional suffering to a chemical disorder of the individual, was at odds with traditional ways of interpreting and responding to pain. "Melancholia, sensitivity, fragility—these are not negative things in a Japanese context," explains Japanese psychiatrist Tooru Takahashi. Japanese physicians' willingness to prescribe benzos was aligned with the country's tradition of psychosomatic medicine and a culture that encouraged patients' reportage of anxiety symptoms.[38]

In Japan, where the predominant culture sanctions cohesion, deference, and calm, the pharmaceutical containment of anxiety continues to have political and social import. The value of a functioning, "tranquilized" state has allowed the benzodiazepine market to expand with social impunity. Japanese psychopharmacologist Toshi-Hiro Kobayakawa explains how cultural and political variables converged to legitimize benzodiazepine prescribing practices there:

> People have very few problems with addiction over here. There is a strict control of prescribing. . . . In the West, people are always preoccupied with themselves, whereas the Japanese system is much more modest and co-operative—people work together much more. Against this background, amphetamines are much more of a problem than are the benzodiazepines; we are much more sensitive to the changes, the exaggerations of behavior, produced by the amphetamines. . . . Sedative agents are seen as much less of a problem in Japan. . . . There is something of a preference for an agent that will be sedative rather than arousing, like perhaps, Prozac.[39]

The future of benzos in France and Japan remains uncertain. Antidepressant consumption has risen in both countries, where the diagnosis of depression and the benefits of SSRIs for treating both depression and anxiety, bolstered by pharmaceutical awareness campaigns, have gained traction among physicians and patients. In the five years since the Japanese government authorized the prescription of SSRIs, antidepressant sales have quintupled. As Harvard anthropologist Arthur Kleinman has noted, the expansion of American psychopharmacology reflects "one of the most powerful aspects of globalization."[40]

Back to Benzos: Tranquilizers and Anxiety After 9/11

At the apex of the benzo backlash and before the tragic events of September 11, American military officials were stealthily evaluating tranquilizers as potent weapons to subdue terrorists. In 1986, the U.S. Army Chemical and Research Development Center sponsored a workshop on incapacitating agents to "assess the feasibility of using central nervous system drugs as incapacitating agents against terrorists." At the Aberdeen proving ground in Maryland, the U.S. Army's multiacre site for weapons development and chemical engineering, the government gathered some of the nation's top clinical pharmacologists, anesthesiologists, and psychiatrists to help strategists identify pharmaceutical compounds that would "rapidly incapacitate a terrorist in order to render him incapable of reprisals." Tranquilizers, used orally or as an aerosol, were voted ideal in a "protracted scenario where immediate assault is not required."[41]

Tranquilizers continue to receive top marks for their potential as tools in America's struggle to maintain a strategic military edge. In 2000, the Pentagon commissioned scientists at Pennsylvania State University's applied research laboratory to investigate how Valium and dexmedetomidine (a sedative with analgesic properties approved by the FDA in 1999) could be employed to pacify enemy forces and subdue hostile populations. According to scientists, the tranquilizers had military promise as nonlethal chemical weapons that "produce a less anxious, less aggressive, more tranquil-like behavior" in targeted populations such as unruly crowds. As it had during the cold war, when psychopharmacology stoked fear of a communist takeover (powered by pills invented by Russians to enable them to operate at full capacity without sleep) and faith in America's scientific supremacy, the U.S. government was again searching for the right chemical cocktail to strengthen its position as a superpower.[42]

Critics charge that the use of Valium and other calmatives as weapons violates the terms of the 1997 Chemical Weapons Convention, but this hasn't stymied the resolve of U.S. government agencies to accelerate the pace of research. In November 2002, the Naval Studies Board of the National Research Council issued a report urging military strategists to increase research on using tranquilizers to control and contain hostile groups. The board's request couldn't have been more timely; terrorist attacks, past and future, were on many people's minds. The report was issued days after Russian troops had deployed a gas to pacify Chechen rebels who, in late October, had taken seven hundred hostages at a Moscow theater. Although the gas (a nebulized aerosol alleged to contain the opiate fentanyl) killed more than one hundred hostages, it highlighted the importance of military preparedness and positioned tranquilizers front and center in the politics of containment once again.[43]

The use of antianxiety agents by ordinary Americans has found new currency in the current administration's "war against terror." As in the

1950s, when the political rhetoric urged Americans to adopt readiness rituals to prepare for a nuclear attack with steadfast calm, the Department of
Homeland Security actively promotes citizen preparedness. The department's website provides links to inform citizens from all walks of life (including pet owners and seniors and other groups with special needs) on
how to prepare for a "terrorist attack, natural disaster, or other large-scale
emergency." Valium is mentioned as one of some thirty pharmaceutical
agents (others include antibiotics, analgesics, steroids, and anesthetics) authorized for transport in vehicles designated to respond to chemical, biological, radiological, or nuclear emergencies.[44]

Although duct tape and Cipro (an antibiotic approved for use after exposure to inhalational anthrax) rather than duck-and-cover drills and fallout shelters are the watchwords of today's containment campaign, mental
health experts have made anxiety management an integral part of our present political landscape. Backed by a slew of survey data, doctors and researchers warn that the events of 9/11 and their aftermath—anthrax
attacks, airport closures, the federal government's color-coded alert system, and a barrage of new security precautions—have triggered a new anxiety epidemic.

Across the board, the news is grim. A study of schoolchildren commissioned by New York City's board of education concluded that months
after the World Trade Center attack, 75,000 children in grades 4–12 were
suffering from posttraumatic stress disorder (PTSD) and that even more
had developed agoraphobia. Schools chancellor Harold O. Levy believed
that the study's results cried out for intervention: "This is powerful information to help teachers, guidance counselors and others identify kids who
are experiencing these symptoms and do what we can to reduce the severity of it," he told the *New York Times*. Adults in the city were also experiencing similar symptoms: rates of PTSD among a representative sample
assessed weeks after 9/11 were estimated at 7.5 percent for persons living
south of 110th Street and 20 percent for those residing south of Canal
Street (closer to the Twin Towers).[45]

Anxiety levels are reportedly higher among Americans who did *not* live
in Manhattan but experienced the catastrophe through "immediate,

graphic, and pervasive" television coverage. A study published in the *New England Journal of Medicine* in November 2001 reported that graphic video footage of the plane attacks, the collapsing towers, and the desperate and often futile efforts to evade death had unexpectedly rattled a large part of the population. In a technologically sophisticated world where media technologies have blurred geographic boundaries, television, radio, and the Internet may have redefined what it means to experience trauma. The authors concluded that the psychological effects of the acts of terrorism on 9/11 are unlikely to disappear soon. "Ongoing media coverage may serve as a traumatic reminder, resulting in persistent symptoms."[46]

Eventually *Newsweek* and *Time* published cover stories on the prevalence and treatment of American anxiety. Lest there be any doubt as to what Americans should be anxious about, *Newsweek* depicted a man's brain clouded with images of Osama bin Laden and Saddam Hussein, bridged by a rendition of the government's alert index coded orange and red. Although the immediate shock of September 11 had faded, *Time* warned its readers that millions of Americans continue to share a collective anxiety: "We live in a particularly anxious age," the reporter concluded, reiterating an adage that has been asserted countless times in modern American political history.[47]

The existence and exact dimensions of a post–9/11 mental health fallout among Americans is unclear. What *is* clear is that after 9/11 anxiety and its medical treatment commanded greater attention from health practitioners and patients. The number of patients who seek medical advice for anxiety has risen, from 13.4 million in 2002 to 16.2 million in 2006. Anxiety is currently the fifteenth most common reason for visiting a doctor—eclipsing consultations for back or joint pain or migraine headaches.[48]

An intriguing twist is that the drug Americans are most likely to take for anxiety is not an antidepressant like Paxil or Zoloft but a tranquilizer: typically generic Xanax, Ativan, or Klonopin. In the two weeks after September 11, prescriptions for generic Xanax (alpraxolam) spiked 22 percent in New York and 9 percent nationally. Between 2002 and 2005, the number of prescriptions for alpraxolam rose from 29.9 to 35 million. Despite political and cultural opposition, restrictive policies and practice guidelines, and an

expensive advertising campaign to reposition SSRIs as safer antianxiety
agents, the American tranquilizer market is quietly expanding. While antidepressant sales have grown astronomically in recent years and have made
significant headway into the anxiety market, they have failed to displace
benzodiazepines as America's antianxiety agent of choice. In 2006 the three
most frequently prescribed drugs in the United States for anxiety states were
benzodiazepines. And of the 71.4 million prescriptions written for anxiety
disorders in 2006, most—more than 40 million—were for benzos.[49]

How do we explain the disjunction between widespread condemnation
of benzodiazepines on the one hand and their increased use on the other?
Perhaps Americans who feel well served by benzos or (more unsettlingly)
think they are too difficult to withdraw from have created a steady market
of users. This doesn't account for the drug's increased use, however, a trend
that has augmented this preexisting market. Contributing to the resurgence of tranquilizers is the visibility of anxiety education campaigns, from
those trumpeting SAD to those promoting anxiety management in a
post–9/11 world. Once aptly characterized as the stepchild of the country's psychiatric health care system, anxiety disorders are now identified as
a growth industry. One suburban mall actually offers customers an anxiety
screening kiosk, where shoppers can break from buying clothes at Guess or
Tommy Hilfiger to get screened for social phobia, panic attacks, generalized anxiety disorder, and more.[50]

Another contributing variable is the therapeutic track record of benzos: the immediate, robust efficacy and tolerability that psychiatrists and
patients have known about for decades. Awareness campaigns have helped
expand the market for tried-and-true (but sometimes risky) tranquilizing
drugs. Here the physiological differences between antidepressants and
benzodiazepines—rather than the social and political commonalities the
drugs share—help account for the popularity of tranquilizers. The fact
that benzos are well tolerated and relatively safe when used intermittently
makes them, in the eyes of many clinicians and patients, superior anxiolytics. And they're cheaper. A thirty-day supply of generic Paxil currently
costs about four times as much as generic Valium, and name-brand Paxil
costs much more. Given the choice between antidepressants and benzodi-

azepines, many physicians and patients have put pragmatism ahead of addiction concerns.[51]

The mainstreaming of tranquilizers also reflects the agility and financial capacity of American corporations to invent new benzos that purportedly rectify older variants' failings, without depicting them as the playful pharmaceutical accessories of yesteryear. (Leaked stories and chilling autopsy reports have revealed that modern celebrities such as Paris Hilton, Heath Ledger, and Anna Nicole Smith used benzodiazepines as part of a celebrity culture of dangerous polydrug use.) Drug firms have tinkered with their tranquilizers, providing anxious Americans with new twists on old drugs. In 2003, Pfizer introduced Xanax-XR, a patented extended-release once a day formula that redresses the problem of the previous version's short half-life and concomitant rebound symptoms. Company advertising reassured patients that they would no longer have to "watch the clock" or worry about where they would be when they would have to take their next dose. "And that can help you relax."[52]

In 2003, Hoffman-La Roche, in partnership with Solvay Pharmaceuticals and Cardinal Health, introduced Klonopin Wafers, a new drug delivery system that addresses patient convenience and privacy. Because the tablets disintegrate on contact with saliva, they can be taken discreetly anytime, anywhere. The marketing campaign deftly merged the drug's established clinical history—"the confidence that comes from years of experience"—with the modern emphasis on consumer empowerment, convenience, and social camouflaging. With Wafers, there is no telltale glass of water or vial to signal that a patient needs a benzo to get by. The delivery system acknowledges the embarrassment that may come with openly taking a trank. Promoted as "therapy designed with patients in mind," company marketing emphasized that patients would "have the confidence of knowing that they can conveniently and discreetly take their prescribed therapy anywhere . . . at least 70% [of patients] preferred quick-dissolve delivery systems over conventional tablets." Promotional packets left in doctors' offices pictured iconic pills with anxiety-free women and men functioning at full capacity: before a podium, at a meeting, about to board a plane. Implicitly tackling the troubling half-life issue, which

Xanax-XR also addressed, the packet referenced the range of available low-dose strengths that would enhance a clinician's flexibility for "initiation, optimization, and gradual discontinuation." The punch line? Klonopin Wafers: easy to take, easy to titrate. An old drug repackaged in a new way promised to conquer myriad social and medical ills.[53]

Today, pharmaceutical firms adroitly promote the scientific laurels of a class of drugs whose tumultuous political history has neither eclipsed their chemical efficacy nor discouraged legions of loyal users. Promoting the virtues of a speedy calm, the newest batch of tranquilizers appeals to a frenzied culture of consumer gratification that took root in the 1950s and has intensified over time. Our need to calm down fast is bound up in our harried race to do it all as effortlessly and as quickly as possible, with minimal stops (who has time for therapy or a vacation?) on our way to the finish line. Our modern tranquilizer culture is constructed around a muscular competition between pills freighted with different social meanings: tranquilizers that slow us down faster, quell our fears discreetly, keep us functioning for longer *or* shorter periods of time—our choice.[54]

Of course, pharmaceutical firms also supply medications that enable untold numbers of Americans to survive a world associated with psychological pain. Betwixt and between these multiple meanings—the cultural power of tranquilizers as tools of gratification, the therapeutic benefits of tranquilizers as chemical agents of calm—the medical and the social overlap and converge, as they have since Miltown inaugurated our tranquilizer age. Our abiding attachment to tranks speaks volumes about America's long and turbulent affair with a class of drugs whose unique history illuminates the ways in which millions of Americans today choose to confront the struggles and strife of twenty-first-century life.

ACKNOWLEDGMENTS

This book grew out of one historian's rendering of the past but, like every work of history, it is the by-product of collective discussions and effort. It is with pleasure and gratitude that I thank the many individuals and institutions who helped make its research and writing possible.

Much of this book draws from research at archives whose use benefited from the expertise of a wealth of talented archivists and curators. I'd particularly like to thank Suzanne White Junod and John P. Swann at the Food and Drug Administration's History Office for accommodating my multiple visits; without their generosity, this book would not have been possible. Thanks also to Christopher Lyons at McGill's Osler Library, Jeremy Nordmoe at the International Archives of Neuro-Psychopharmacology at Vanderbilt University, Stephen Greenberg and Michael Sappol at the National Library of Medicine, Linda Leahy at Harvard's Schlesinger Library, Patricia Gossel at the Division of Science, Medicine, and Society at the Smithsonian, Chris Warren and Arlene Shaner at the New York Academy of Medicine, Amy Crumpton at the American Association for the Advancement of Science, Isaac Gewirtz of the Berg Collection at the New York Public Library, RoseMary Russo at the Drug Enforcement Administration Agency Library of the Department of Justice, Darcy Taube at the Special Collections Division of the University of Southern California, Ned Comstock at the USC Cinema-Television Archives, Julie Snelling at the BBC Written Archive Centre in Reading, and Shelley Jofre and Andy Bell at the BBC London Office. I'd also like to thank the staff at the Jimmy Carter Library and Archives in Atlanta, the Chemical Heritage Foundation, the libraries at Emory University, the Georgia Institute of Technology, and McGill University, the Library of Congress, and the Special Collections Manuscripts Division of UCLA. Thanks, also, to Christine D. Albino at IMS Health Canada and especially Gary Endlein at IMS United States for their help amassing prescription data.

Portions of this book were first presented to the American Association for the History of Medicine, the New York Academy of Medicine's History of Psychiatry Lecture Series, the Canadian Psychiatric Association, UBC's Department of English and Peter Wall Institute for Advanced Studies, the American College of Neuropsychopharmacology, the University of Pennsylvania's Department of History and Sociology of Science, Emory University's Center for Health, Culture, and Society, the University of Toronto's Symposium on the Social Origins of Psychopharmacology, Yale University's History of Medicine and Science Lecture Series, UCSF's Department of Anthropology, History, and Social Medicine, McGill's Epidemiology and Biostatistics research seminar series and its Department of Psychiatry's Division of Social and Transcultural Psychiatry Advanced Study Institute, Case Western Reserve University's workshop on Biological Psychiatry in History and Culture, and the Danish Institute for Psychosocial Medicine in Copenhagen. I benefited immeasurably from the excellent feedback I received on each of those occasions.

Countless friends and colleagues in the field nurtured this book with research leads and fruitful suggestions, including Joel Braslow, Charles Cahn, Alberto Cambrosio, David Courtwright, Ruth Schwartz Cowan, Joe Dumit, Erika Dyck, Max Fink, Kathy Glass, Patricia Gossel, Stephen Greenberg, Wendy Klein, William Hefland, Howard Kushner, Dan Horowitz, Jonathan Kimmelman, Laurence Kirmayer, Stephanie Lloyd, Liz Lunbeck, Christopher Lyons, Erin McClure, Charles Medawar, Jonathan Metzl, Nathan Moon, Hans Pol, Kathy Peiss, Oakley Ray, Karl Rickels, Naomi Rogers, Charles Rosenberg, Jonathan Sadowsky, Jamie Saris, Edward Shorter, William Siedelman, Mickey Smith, Sarah Starks, Leonore Tiefer, Nancy Tomes, Liz Watkins, George Weisz, Dennis Worthen, and Allan Young. David Healy took a pivotal interest in this project from the very beginning. For the countless hours (I suspect days is more accurate) he spent nudging it and me along, answering questions, posing challenges, and connecting me with people in the field, I owe him a great debt.

Frank Berger allowed me to interview him on several trips to New York and then, almost as an afterthought, muttered words every historian longs to hear: "My sons assembled scrapbooks chronicling my career. . . . Would you like to see them?" For granting me unimpeded access to his life and his work, and for the interest of his family, especially his wife Christine and son Franklin, I offer my heartfelt thanks. I am indeed sorry that his death prevented him from seeing this book in print. I am also grateful to Leo Sternbach and his family for permitting me to conduct a full-day interview with him shortly before his passing.

Research for this project was funded by the Canadian Institutes of Health Research, McGill's Faculty of Medicine, and the Georgia Tech Foundation. My thanks to each of these organizations for their generous support. I was particularly fortunate to have a succession of superlatively efficient and caring department chairs to help me navigate the inevitable challenges of holding a joint appointment in two departments and faculties; I especially want to thank Alberto Cambrosio of the Department of Social Studies of Medicine and Brian Lewis of the Department of History for their friendship, humor, and help. Thanks to Adele Tarantino, Colleen Parish, Georgii Mikula, and especially Heike Faerber for administrative support. I benefited enormously from the skills and dedication of several research assistants: Brian Pierce, Nathan Flis, Eric Hardy, Theresa Howard, Kristen Keerma, and especially Lana Povitz, who embraced this assignment with a professionalism and enthusiasm that has made it an altogether better book. Students in my history of psychiatry, social history of medicine, and gender and medicine seminars, as well as graduate students at Georgia Tech and McGill, were excellent sounding boards as I gingerly offered up new thoughts and inchoate arguments.

Numerous physicians answered questions, granted interviews, and practiced good medicine; thanks especially to Michael Aube, Samuel Barondes, Dennis Doherty, Max Fink, David Hewitt, Laurence Kirmayer, Anne-Louise Lafontaine, Herb Meltzer, Maggie Mermin, Greg Meterissian, Jonathan Simonds, Stephen Stahl, Sophia Tchervenkov, Ronald Ucha Udabe, Izabella Verbitsky, and Mark Ware.

Countless colleagues, family members, neighbors, and friends helped in too many ways to catalog or count. Among them I want to thank Rebecca Fuhrer, Amy Alt, Nicholas Dew, Martine Dias, Pernille Due, Eva and Myron Echenberg, Elizabeth Elbourne, Randi Epstein, Elham Freiha, Hannah Gilbert, Janet Golden, Hugh Gusterson, Sam Harper, Michelle Hartman, Lesley Husbands, Daniel Kleinman, Wendy Kline, Nicholas Kluge, Judy Leavitt, Abby Lippman, Chris Lockhart, Alison Macfarlane, Eric Michot, Sue Morton, Shree Mulay, Greg Nobles, Marion Olynyk, Joy Parr, Laila Parsons, Carol Patterson, Carrie Rentschler, Naomi Rogers, Barbara Seaman, Jonathan Sterne, Alison Waldenberg, Erica Wood, Mike Zaitsoff, and Eric Zinner. Jo McMillan, Simon Sykes, Thomas Hughes, Claudia Serpa Hughes, Coleen Grace Asmin, Michal Waldfogel, Hannah Gilbert, and especially Lesley Husbands arranged countless play dates to give me extra writing time; my mother, Elke Kluge, and stepfather, John Aitchison, gave me coveted weekends that left my daughter cheerfully exhausted and me a bit more caught up.

At Basic Books, Jo Ann Miller gave this project's launch the benefit of her seasoned input. I count myself extraordinarily lucky to have had Amanda Moon take over when Jo Ann retired. Amanda has been a fantastic editor, giving me untold time, access, steady but unstinting support and, at a critical juncture, a fruit and chocolate basket that kept my daughter smiling for weeks. She is the kind of editor who I suspect has become a rarity in the publishing world, and I feel privileged to have had the pleasure of working with her. I am also appreciative of the help and endless patience of her assistant, Whitney Casser, and of the press's editorial production group, particularly Sandra Beris. As always, my agent Emma Parry gave me a pitch-perfect combination of sage advice and abundant enthusiasm.

Samuel Barondes, James Delbourgo, William Hefland, Lesley Husbands, Kristen Keerma, John Lynch, Christopher Lyons, Greg Nobles, Oakley Ray, John Tone, Gil Troy, and Liz Watkins gave constructive feedback on portions of this book. I am especially grateful to the few intrepid souls who tackled the manuscript from beginning to end, including Tom Ban (who reviewed whole chapters and responded to questions on everything from mouse testing in the 1950s to the chemical properties of alpha-phenylglycerol ether, in record time and with trademark thoroughness), David Healy, Brian Lewis, Amanda Moon, Emma Parry, Lana Povitz, Jason Szabo, Thomas Schlich, and George Weisz.

I consider myself particularly fortunate to count George as a colleague and friend. His unflinching candor, practical advice, wise words—an assemblage of which, hastily scrawled on a napkin during an engaging cocktail get-together, helped me reframe the entire book—and creative incentive schemes for meeting deadlines (which usually involved eating cake) kept me on track.

Jason Szabo materialized in my life as this book was inching toward completion and its author was sliding toward exhaustion. Even as he rushed to meet his own deadline on a book on the history of suffering and incurability, care for his patients, and look after his children, he found time to read it through repeatedly, refining my arguments and ironing out my prose with a skill and finesse born of years of practicing medicine and with a sensitivity to historical accuracy and linguistic precision. For his unfailing generosity and patience, and for restoring my faith in many things in life that had gotten lost along the way, I am beyond grateful.

My daughter Sophia, age eight, has been with this book from its beginning without knowing or caring to ask what, precisely, tranquilizers are. When her mommy began to disappear into her study too often, she began to write books of her own (fifty-nine and counting), and had the good sense to post a "laughter chart" on the fridge to counter what she rightly declared to be a surplus of household seriousness. For her capacious curiosity, bountiful laughter, daily morning song, and for her uncanny ability to keep me grounded in all the right ways, I dedicate this to her with thanks and love.

NOTES

PREFACE

1. Andrea Tone, "Listening to the Past: History, Psychiatry, and Anxiety," *Canadian Journal of Psychiatry* 50 (June 2005): 378; "Valium Celebrates 40th, but Not with a Bang," *Victoria Times Colonist,* July 21, 2003, D4; Nick Paumgarten, "Little Helper," *New Yorker,* June 16, 2003, 70.

2. To date, there has been one book tracing the rise and commercial popularity of minor tranquilizers: *A Social History of the Minor Tranquilizers* by Mickey Smith, a pharmacist. An excellent academic overview of the subject, the book is now out of print. Drawing largely from published sources, it concludes in the 1980s at a time when the full cultural and political effects of the tranquilizer backlash could not be assessed. See Mickey C. Smith, *A Social History of the Minor Tranquilizers: The Quest for Small Comfort in the Age of Anxiety* (New York: Pharmaceutical Products Press, 1985). For an excellent analysis of cultural concerns regarding America's overmedication, including its use of tranquilizers, see Susan Lynn Speaker, "Too Many Pills: Patients, Physicians, and the Myth of Overmedication in America, 1955–1980" (Ph.D. diss., University of Pennsylvania, 1992). As my book was going to press, Patricia Pearson's *A Brief History of Anxiety: Yours and Mine* (New York: Random House, 2008) was published, not a history of psychopharmacology but a moving and poignant account of one woman's struggle to understand the meaning and place of anxiety in her own life and the broader world.

3. Kierkegaard, quoted in Richard Restak, *Poe's Heart and the Mountain Climber: Exploring the Effects of Anxiety on Our Brains and on Our Culture* (New York: Harmony, 2004), 31. James, quoted in William James, *The Varieties of Religious Experience: A Study in Human Nature* (New York: Wilder, 2007), 109. Morley, quoted in George Rosen, "Emotion and Sensibility in Ages of Anxiety: A Comparative Historical Review," *American Journal of Psychiatry,* Dec. 6, 1967, 772; Schlesinger, quoted in Sam Tanenhaus, "History, Written in the Present Tense," *New York Times,* Mar. 4, 2007, Week in Review section. W. H. Auden, *The Age of Anxiety: A Baroque Eclogue* (New York: Random House, 1947).

4. Allan Young, *The Harmony of Illusions: Inventing Post-Traumatic Stress Disorder* (Princeton: Princeton University Press, 1995), 5. Also see Joseph E. Davis, *Accounts of Innocence: Sexual Abuse, Trauma, and the Self* (Chicago: University of Chicago Press, 2005); Restak, *Poe's Heart and the Mountain Climber.* Kierkegaard penned memorable quips about anxiety in his published writings and journal. On Kierkegaard, see Joakim Garff, *Søren Kierkegaard: A Biography,* trans. Bruce H. Kirmmse (Princeton: Princeton University Press, 2005).

5. I am often asked who was more anxious: men in the Crusades or breadwinners in the Depression? There's an epistemological hollowness to such questions, which assume, incorrectly, that the anxiety under investigation has been the same thing all along. See Joan Jacobs Brumberg, *Fasting Girls: The History of Anorexia* (New York: Plume, 1989), 1–8; and Ian Hacking, *The Social Construction of What?* (Cambridge: Harvard University Press, 1999), 100–124. Diseases and disorders are an amalgam of biological states and social definitions. Inextricably bound, the two have evolved in tandem. See Charles Rosenberg, "Framing Disease: Illness, Society, and History," in *Framing Disease: Studies in Cultural History,* ed. Charles Rosenberg and Janet Golden (New Brunswick, NJ: Rutgers University Press, 1992), xiii–xxvi. On the inseparability of culture and biology in disease construction and symptom reportage, see Margaret Lock and Patricia Kaufert, "Menopause, Local Biologies, and Cultures of Aging," *American Journal of Human Biology* 13 (May 2001): 494–504.

6. On the political importance of engaging the reality of illness and suffering, while acknowledging the epistemological obstacles of the effort, see Allan Brandt, "Global Governance: The Framework Convention for Tobacco Control" (lecture given to the Department of Social Studies of Medicine, McGill University, Mar. 5, 2008). Virginia Woolf, "On Being Ill," *Criterion* 4 (Jan. 1926): 34.

7. As Ian Hacking suggests, people act "under description": their interactions with psychiatric classifications change the classifications themselves. Hacking, *The Social Construction of What?* 100–124.

8. M. Lader, "Benzodiazepines—The Opium of the Masses?" *Neuroscience* 3 (Feb. 1978): 159–165. On global psychopharmacology, see, for instance, Andrew Lakoff, "The Anxieties of Globalization: Antidepressant Sales and Economic Crisis in Argentina," *Social Studies of Science* 34 (April 2004): 247–269; Lakoff, *Pharmaceutical Reason: Knowledge and Value in Global Psychiatry* (Cambridge: Cambridge University Press, 2005); Adriana Petryna, Andrew Lakoff, and Arthur Kleinman, eds., *Global Pharmaceuticals: Ethics, Markets, Practices* (Chapel Hill, NC: Duke University Press, 2006); Nikolas Rose, "Becoming Neurochemical Selves," in *Biotechnology Between Commerce and Civil Society,* ed. N. Stehr (Piscataway, NJ: Transaction, 2003), 89–126; Laurence J. Kirmayer, "Psychopharmacology in a Globalizing World: The Use of Antidepressants in Japan," *Transcultural Psychiatry* 39 (Sept. 2002): 295–322.

9. As the late historian Roy Porter has suggested, we must "'defamiliarize' ourselves with the assumptions of modern-physician-focused history and sociology of medicine and hack our way into the empirical forests of the past in all their strangeness and diversity." Roy Porter, "The Patient's View: Doing Medical History From Below," *Theory and Society* 14 (1985): 176.

10. On the importance of patient experience in the creation of medical economies, see Porter, "The Patient's View," 189; see also Nancy Tomes, "The Great American Medicine Show Revisited," *Bulletin of the History of Medicine* 79 (Winter 2005): 627–663; and Tomes, "Merchants of Health: Medicine and Consumer Culture in the United States, 1900–1940," *Journal of American History* 88 (Sept. 2001): 519–547. In one sense, anxiety remained a by-product of attempts to treat it. On the complexities of disease diagnosis and therapeutics, see Charles E. Rosenberg, "The Tyranny of Diagnosis: Specific Entities and Individual Experience," *Milbank Quarterly* 80 (2002): 237–260; and Rosenberg, "Contested Boundaries: Psychiatry, Disease, and Diagnosis," *Perspectives in Biology and Medicine* 49 (Summer 2006): 407–424.

11. On the importance of a therapeutic ethos of self-improvement that has served to individualize problems, particular those of women, see Elaine Tyler May, *Homeward Bound: American Families in the Cold War Era* (New York: Basic, 1999*);* Beth Haiken, *Venus Envy: A*

History of Cosmetic Surgery (Baltimore: Johns Hopkins University Press, 1997); Mari Jo Buhle, *Feminism and Its Discontents: A Century of Struggle with Psychoanalysis* (Cambridge: Harvard University Press, 1998); Susan J. Douglas, *Where the Girls Are: Growing Up Female with the Mass Media* (New York: Random House, 1995); Ruth Cooperstock, "Sex Differences in Psychotropic Drug Use," *Social Science Medicine* 12 (July 1978): 179–186; Ruth Cooperstock and Henry L. Lennard, "Some Social Meanings of Tranquilizer Use," *Sociology of Health and Illness* 14 (Dec. 1979): 331–347.

12. On this, see Susan Reynolds Whyte, Sjaak van der Geest, and Anita Hardon, *Social Lives of Medicines* (Cambridge: Cambridge University Press, 2002).

13. Tone, "Listening to the Past," 373–379; Erika Dyck, "Flashback: Psychiatric Experimentation with LSD in Historical Perspective," *Canadian Journal of Psychiatry* 50 (June 2005): 381–387; Sjaak van der Geest, Susan Reynolds Whyte, and Anita Hardon, "The Anthropology of Pharmaceuticals: A Biographical Approach," *Annual Review of Anthropology* 25 (Oct. 1996): 153–178; Susan Speaker, "From 'Happiness Pills' to 'National Nightmare': Changing Cultural Assessments of Minor Tranquilizers in America, 1955–1980," *Journal of the History of Medicine and Allied Sciences* 52 (July 1997): 338–376; David Herzberg, "The Pill You Love Can Turn on You: Feminism, Tranquilizers, and the Valium Panic of the 1970s," *American Quarterly* 58 (2006): 79–103; Brumberg, *Fasting Girls*, 3.

CHAPTER 1

1. J. M. Da Costa, "On Irritable Heart: A Clinical Study of a Form of Functional Cardiac Disorder and Its Consequences," *American Journal of Medical Sciences*, January 1871, 2–52. Lee quoted in Winston Groom, *Shrouds of Glory: From Atlanta to Nashville: The Last Great Campaign of the Civil War* (New York: Grove, 1996), 31.

2. Da Costa, "On Irritable Heart." Also see De Witt C. Peters, "Remarks on the Evils of Youthful Enlistments and Nostalgia," *American Medical Times*, Feb. 14, 1863, 75–76; Saul Jarcho, "Functional Heart Disease in the Civil War," *American Journal of Cardiology* 4 (Dec. 1959): 809–817; Robert Dawson Fudolf, "The Irritable Heart of Soldiers," *Canadian Medical Association Journal* 6 (1916): 796–810; Kenneth C. Hymans, Stephen Wignall, and Robert Roswell, "War Syndromes and Their Evaluation: From the U.S. Civil War to the Persian Gulf War," *Annals of Internal Medicine*, Sept. 1, 1996, 398–405; Charles F. Wooley, *The Irritable Heart of Soldiers and the Origins of Anglo-American Cardiology: The US Civil War to World War I* (Aldershot, U.K.: Ashgate, 2002), 8–20. On nineteenth-century therapeutic orientations, see John Harley Warner, *The Therapeutic Perspective: Medical Practice, Knowledge, and Identity in America, 1820–1855* (Cambridge: Harvard University Press, 1986).

3. J. A. Den Boer, "Defining Panic: A Diagnostic Dilemma," *Human Psychopharmacology* 12 (1997): S3–S6; Allen Frances et al., "The Classification of Panic Disorders," *Journal of Psychiatric Research* 27 (1993): suppl. 1, pp. 3–10; Solomon Snyder, *Drugs and the Brain* (New York: Scientific American Books, 1986), 153–154; David Healy, "Mandel Cohen and the Origins of the Diagnostic and Statistical Manual of Mental Disorders, 3rd ed., DSM-III: Interview with David Healy," *History of Psychiatry* 13 (2002): 209–230.

4. Psychiatrists are medical doctors with extended training and licensing in psychiatry. Clinical psychologists possess a doctoral degree in psychology from an accredited university or a professional school and are licensed to work in a clinical setting with patients. Therapists without a Ph.D. or M.D. are generally referred to as counselors. Contemporary psychoanalysts are usually therapists trained at a recognized psychoanalytic institute who rely on recognized

psychoanalytic techniques to treat mental health problems. For a thoughtful examination of the effect of brain imagery and the fashioning of self-identity, see Joseph Dumit, "Is It Me or My Brain? Depression and Neuroscientific Facts," *Journal of Medical Humanities,* Summer 2003, 35–47; and Joseph Dumit, "When Explanations Rest: 'Good-Enough' Brain Science and the New Sociomedical Disorders," in *Living and Working with the New Medical Technologies: Intersections of Inquiry,* ed. Margaret Lock, Allan Young, and Alberto Cambrosio (Cambridge: Cambridge University Press, 2000), 209–232. Details on the APA's mission and membership can be found at www.psych.org (accessed Dec. 5, 2007).The third DSM, published in 1980 and commonly called DSM-III, is recognized as a turning point in the classification of anxiety disorders. It embraced a symptom-based scheme that discounted the earlier emphasis on the psychodynamic origins of mental illness. Since 1980, DSM has been revised and expanded, and descriptions of anxiety disorders have been refined accordingly. The most recent DSM is DSM-IV-TR, published in 2000 as a revision of DSM-IV, published in 1994. DSM-IV-TR's fifty-six-page chapter on anxiety disorders details the symptoms of several disorders: panic attacks, agoraphobia, panic disorder without agoraphobia, panic disorder with agoraphobia, agoraphobia without history of panic disorder, specific phobia, social phobia (also called social anxiety disorder), obsessive-compulsive disorder, posttraumatic stress disorder, acute stress disorder, generalized anxiety disorder, anxiety disorder due to a general medical condition, substance-induced anxiety disorder, and anxiety. Despite this proliferation, the primary anxiety disorders are considered panic disorders, generalized anxiety disorder, posttraumatic stress disorder, obsessive compulsive disorder, and phobia. See, for instance, the National Institute of Mental Health's anxiety guide at www.nimh.nih.gov/health/topics/anxiety-disorders/index.shtml (accessed Dec. 5, 2007).

5. Quoted in Jeanne Jordan and Julie Pedersen, *The Panic Diaries: The Frightful, Sometimes Hilarious Truth About Panic Attacks* (Berkeley: Ulysses, 2004), 145. National Institutes of Mental Health, "Anxiety Disorders," www.nimh.nih.gov/health/publications/anxiety-disorders/introduction.shtml (accessed Dec. 5, 2007).

6. Pichot, "Panic: Attack and Disorder. History of the Word and Concepts," *Encephale,* Dec. 22, 1996, 3–8. Although its first use in the English language dates to the sixteenth century, the concept of anxiety goes back earlier. In Greek mythology, sudden attacks of fear—panic—were attributed to Pan, the god of the woods and fields. Fay Bound, "Keywords in the History of Medicine: Anxiety," *Lancet,* Apr. 24, 2004, 1407; *Oxford English Dictionary,* 2d ed. (1989).

7. Edward Shorter, *A History of Psychiatry: From the Era of the Asylum to the Age of Prozac* (New York: Wiley, 1997), 2–5; Roy Porter, "Madness and Its Institutions," in *Medicine in Society: Historical Essays,* ed. Andrew Wear (Cambridge: Cambridge University Press, 1992), 277–301; Roy Porter and David Wright, eds., *The Confinement of the Insane: International Perspectives, 1800–1965* (Cambridge: Cambridge University Press, 2003); Andrew Scull, *The Most Solitary of Afflictions: Madness and Society in Britain, 1700–1900* (New Haven: Yale University Press, 1993); and Scull, *Madhouses, Mad Doctors, and Madmen* (Philadelphia: University of Pennsylvania Press, 1981); Shomer S. Zwelling, *Quest for a Cure: The Public Hospital in Williamsburg, Virginia, 1773–1885* (Williamsburg, VA: Colonial Williams Foundation, 1990), 5; Gerald N. Grob, *The Mad Among Us: A History of the Care of America's Mentally Ill* (New York: Free Press, 1994), 5–17. As Grob has argued, madness, while not yet a medical or political problem, still had to be handled on an informal, ad hoc basis.

8. Zwelling, *Quest for a Cure,* 1, 10–11. Nancy Tomes, *The Art of Asylum-Keeping: Thomas Story Kirkbride and the Origins of American Psychiatry* (Philadelphia: University of Pennsylvania Press, 1994); and David J. Rothman, *The Discovery of the Asylum: Social Order and Disor-*

der in the New Republic (Boston: Little, Brown, 1971); Scull, *Most Solitary of Afflictions;* Anne Digby, *Madness, Morality, and Medicine: A Study of the York Retreat, 1796–1914* (Cambridge: Cambridge University Press, 1985). For an important reconsideration of psychiatry's presence at the bedside and evolution outside the asylum, see Akihito Suzuki, *Madness at Home: The Psychiatrist, the Patient, and the Family in England, 1820–1860* (Berkeley: University of California Press, 2006).

9. Quoted in Roy Porter, *The Greatest Benefit to Mankind: A Medical History of Humanity from Antiquity to the Present* (New York: HarperCollins, 1997), 494. For a critical analysis of Rush's treatment of psychiatric patients, see Shorter, *History of Psychiatry*, 16. Nancy C. Andreasen, *The Broken Brain: The Biological Revolution in Psychiatry* (New York: Harper & Row, 1984), 189–190. On Rush, see Alvyn Brodsky, *Benjamin Rush: Patriot and Physician* (New York: Truman Talley, 2004).

10. Elizabeth Lunbeck, *The Psychiatric Persuasion: Knowledge, Gender, and Power in Modern America* (Princeton: Princeton University Press, 1994), 6, 20–23; 26–28; Jack D. Pressman, *Last Resort: Psychosurgery and the Limits of Medicine* (Cambridge: Cambridge University Press, 1998), 18–21; George Weisz, *Divide and Conquer: A Comparative History of Medical Specialization* (New York: Oxford University Press, 2006); George Weisz, "Medical Directories and Medical Specialization in France, Britain, and the United States," *Bulletin of the History of Medicine* 71 (1997): 23–68; George Weisz, "Mapping Medical Specialization in Paris in the Nineteenth and Twentieth Centuries," *Social History of Medicine* 7 (1994): 177–211; Suzuki, *Madness at Home.* The *Oxford English Dictionary* (OED) offers 1828 as date when psychiatry is first defined. The word "alienist," meaning "one who treats mental diseases; a mental pathologist; a mad-doctor," is first identified in 1864, whereas psychiatrist, defined as "an expert or specialist in psychiatry; *spec.* a medical practitioner qualified in psychiatry," appears later in 1874. See the *Oxford English Dictionary*, http://dictionary.oed.com (accessed Dec. 7, 2007).

11. Weisz, *Divide and Conquer*, 67; Lunbeck, *Psychiatric Persuasion*, 3.

12. Noga Arikha, *Passions and Tempers: A History of the Humours* (New York: Harper-Collins, 2007); Roy Porter, *Blood and Guts: A Short History of Medicine* (New York: Norton, 2003), 25–30; Peter Bart, "Makers Worried on Tranquilizers," *New York Times*, Aug. 28, 1960, F1. For an illuminating study of humoral medicine and the boundaries of therapeutics in the practice of a Maine midwife, see Laurel Thatcher Ulrich, *The Life of Martha Ballard: Based on Her Diary, 1785–1812* (New York: Vintage, 1991). Roy Porter, *Blood and Guts*, 25–30.

13. Letter to the editor, *Columbian Magazine*, Nov. 1786, 110.

14. Bound, "Keywords in the History of Medicine"; Edward Shorter, *A Historical Dictionary of Psychiatry* (New York: Oxford University Press, 2005), 27.

15. Weisz, *Divide and Conquer;* Janet Oppenheim, *Shattered Nerves: Doctors, Patients, and Depression in Victorian England* (New York: Oxford University Press, 1991); Weisz, "Mapping Medical Specialization"; Diana Martin, "The Rest Cure Revisited," *American Journal of Psychiatry*, May 2007, 737–738.

16. George M. Beard, "Neurasthenia, or Nervous Exhaustion," *Boston Medical and Surgical Journal* 3 (1869): 217–221; Charles E. Rosenberg, "The Place of George M. Beard in Nineteenth-Century Psychiatry," *Bulletin of the History of Medicine* 36 (1962): 245–259; F. G. Gosling, *Before Freud: Neurasthenia and the American Medical Community, 1870–1910* (Chicago: University of Illinois Press, 1987); Tom Lutz, *American Nervousness, 1903: An Anecdotal History* (Ithaca, NY: Cornell University Press, 1991); David G. Schuster, "Personalizing Illness and Modernity: S. Weir Mitchell, Literary Women, and Neurasthenia,

1870–1914," *Bulletin of the History of Medicine* 79 (2005): 696; Edward Shorter, *From Paralysis to Fatigue: A History of Psychosomatic Illness in the Modern Era* (New York: Free Press, 1992), 220–232, 277–280. Schuster, "Personalizing Illness and Modernity," 696; Oppenheim, *Shattered Nerves*, 3–6.

17. Barbara Sicherman, "The Uses of a Diagnosis: Doctors, Patients, and Neurasthenia," *Journal of the History of Medicine and Allied Sciences,* Jan. 1977, 34. Schuster, "Personalizing Illness and Modernity," 696. Beard, "Neurasthenia, or Nervous Exhaustion," 217–221; Rosenberg, "Place of George M. Beard in Nineteenth-Century Psychiatry," 245–259; Brad Campbell, "The Making of 'American': Race and Nation in Neurasthenic Discourse," *History of Psychiatry* 18 (2007): 157–178; Philip P. Wiener, "G.M. Beard and Freud on 'American Nervousness,'" *Journal of the History of Ideas*, Apr. 1956, 269–274. On neurasthenia in Germany, see Joachim Radkau, "The Neurasthenic Experience in Imperial Germany: Expeditions into Patient Records and Side-looks upon General History," in *Cultures of Neurasthenia from Beard to the First World War*, ed. Marijke Gijswijt-Hofstra and Roy Porter (Amsterdam: Rodopi, Clio Medica Series), 199–217. On neurasthenia in Victorian England, see Oppenheim, *Shattered Nerves*; on neurasthenia in Russia, see Laura Goering, "Russian Nervousness: Neurasthenia and National Identity in Nineteenth-Century Russia," *Medical History,* Jan. 2003, 23–46; on the meanings of different cultural interpretations of the illness, see Arthur Kleinman, *Social Origins of Distress and Disease: Depression, Neurasthenia, and Pain in Modern China* (New Haven: Yale University Press, 1986); and Anson Rabinbach, *The Human Motor: Energy, Fatigue, and the Origins of Modernity* (Berkeley: University of California Press, 1990); Tom Lutz, *American Nervousness, 1903*. On neurasthenia and the working classes, see Sicherman, "Uses of a Diagnosis," 32–34. Schuster, "Personalizing Illness and Modernity," 701.

18. Henry G. Cole, quoted in Stephen R. Kandall, *Substance and Shadow: Women and Addiction in the United States* (Harvard: Harvard University Press, 1996), 28. See advertisements in *Medical News*, June 28, 1980, 3; *National Police Gazette*, Mar. 6, 1880, 15; *The Cosmopolitan: A Monthly Illustrated Magazine*, Apr. 1904, 36, 6, 762; postcard for Dr. Miles's Nervine, 1918, in author's possession; Barbara Hodgson, *In the Arms of Morpheus: The Tragic History of Laudanum, Morphine, and Patent Medicines* (Buffalo, NY: Firefly, 2001); Annabel Hecht, "Tranquilizers: Use, Abuse, and Dependency," *FDA Consumer*, Oct. 1978; Matt Clark, "Drugs and Psychiatry: A New Era?" *Newsweek*, Nov. 12, 1979, 100–104; Charles Medawar, *Power and Dependence: Social Audit on the Safety of Medicines* (London: Bath, 1992*)*, 38–39. The Pure Food and Drug Act of 1906, also known as the Wiley Act, did not prohibit the inclusion of alcohol or opiates in over-the-counter medications but focused on the adulteration or misbranding of drugs. As such, it did little to restrict consumers' access to medications and upheld the principle of caveat emptor: let the buyer beware. In 1914, passage of the Anti-Narcotics Law pushed the regulation of opiates and cocaine to the national level. See John Swann, "FDA and the Practice of Pharmacy: Prescription Drug Regulation Before the Durham-Humphrey Amendment of 1951," *Pharmacy in History* 36 (1994): 59; and Willis Emmons and Jeremiah O'Regan, Monica Brand, and James Bradford, "Note on Pharmaceutical Industry Regulation," *Harvard Business School*, 9–792–002, rev. Aug. 11, 1994, 1–4.

19. *Merck's 1899 Manual of the Materia Medica* (1899; New York: Merck, 1999), 139, 149–150; Da Costa, "On Irritable Heart," 2–52; Charlotte Perkins Gilman, *The Yellow Wallpaper and Other Stories* (New York: Dover, 1997), originally published in *New England Magazine*, Jan. 1892. Also see Medawar, *Power and Dependence*, 43–55. Pharmacological

nostrums for frazzled nerves could also include stimulating substances. See Nicolas Rasmussen, *On Speed: The Many Lives of Amphetamine* (New York: New York University Press, 2008).

20. Advertisement for Bryan's electric belts, *Saturday Evening Post*, May 7, 1881, 14; Lutz, *American Nervousness*, 47. On the medical uses of electric vibrators to treat hysteria, see Rachel Maines, *The Technology of Orgasm: "Hysteria," the Vibrator, and Women's Sexual Satisfaction* (Baltimore: Johns Hopkins University Press, 1999).

21. Jackson Sanatorium ad, *Lippincott's Monthly Magazine*, June 1897, 33. Schuster, "Personalizing Illness and Modernity," 700–701; Martin, "The Rest Cure Revisited," 737–738; Carla B. Frye, "Using Literature in Health Care: Reflections on the 'Yellow Wallpaper,'" *Annals of Pharmacotherapy* 32 (July-Aug. 1998): 830–831; S. Weir Mitchell, *Fat and Blood: And How to Make Them*, 2nd ed. (Philadelphia: Lippincott, 1878); E. Earnest, *S. Weir Mitchell: Novelist and Physician* (Philadelphia: University of Pennsylvania Press, 1950).

22. Advertisement in *Outlook*, Apr. 4, 1896, 646. Lutz, *American Nervousness*, 63.

23. Schuster, "Personalizing Illness and Modernity." As Schuster argues, Mitchell was no advocate of female emancipation and equality, but he was also no misogynist monster as he has sometimes been portrayed. The rest cure was a therapy he reserved for patients, including Gilman, he considered to be extreme cases; his treatment of other affluent women embraced a more variegated and less ostracizing approach. Gilman, *Yellow Wallpaper;* Gilman, "Why I Wrote 'The Yellow Wallpaper,'" *Forerunner*, 1913. On the gendered nature of care, also see Lutz, *American Nervousness, 1903;* Edmund Morris, *The Rise of Theodore Roosevelt* (1979; New York: Modern Library, 2001).

24. On the evolution of psychiatric disease diagnosis, see Mark S. Micale, "On the 'Disappearance' of Hysteria: A Study in the Clinical Deconstruction of a Diagnosis," *ISIS*, Sept. 1993, 496–526. Weisz, *Divide and Conquer*, 67–68, 75; Oppenheim, *Shattered Nerves;* Rosenberg, "The Place of George M. Beard in Nineteenth-Century Psychiatry"; Lunbeck, *Psychiatric Persuasion*, 6, 20–23; 26–28; Pressman, *Last Resort*, 18–21; Sicherman, "Uses of a Diagnosis," 40. Ironically, before his death in 1868, German neurologist and psychiatrist Wilhelm Griesinger, a firm believer in neurobiology, had written that "psychiatry and neuropathology are not merely two closely related fields; they are but one field in which only one language is spoken and the same laws rule." Quoted in W. A. Lishman, "Psychiatry and Neuropathology: The Maturing of a Relationship," *Journal of Neurology, Neurosurgery, and Psychiatry* 58 (1995): 284–292.

25. In Europe, the pioneering work of German Emil Kraeplin, often regarded as the architect of modern psychiatric science, created an important intellectual foundation from which a subsequent generation of biologically oriented psychiatrists would draw. As historian Edward Shorter notes, Kraeplin's careful long-term observations of the course of psychiatric disorders in patients, and his insistence that there are indeed different types of psychiatric illness that can be classified according to common patterns of symptoms, established modern psychiatric nosology. See Shorter, *History of Psychiatry*, 1–109; Shorter, *A Historical Dictionary of Psychiatry*, 156–157; Andreasen, *Broken Brain*, 27–30. Shorter, *History of Psychiatry*, 103. For an interesting examination of how English psychiatrists negotiated the boundaries between madhouse and home, see Suzuki, *Madness at Home*. Franklin G. Ebaugh, "The Importance of Introducing Psychiatry into the General Internship," *Journal of the American Medical Association*, Mar. 31, 1934, 982–986; Silas Weir Mitchell, "Address Before the Fiftieth Annual Meeting of the American Medico-Psychological Association, Held in Philadelphia, May 16, 1894," *Journal of Nervous and Mental Disease* 21 (1894): 413–437; quoted in

Shorter, *History of Psychiatry*, 67–68. Shorter, *History of Psychiatry*, 46. On the history of psychiatric care in late nineteenth- and early twentieth-century asylums, see Jeffrey L. Geller, "A History of Private Psychiatric Hospitals in the USA: From Start to Almost Finished," *Psychiatric Quarterly*, Spring 2006, 1–41; Joel Braslow, *Mental Ills and Bodily Cures: Psychiatric Treatment in the First Half of the Twentieth Century* (Berkeley: University of California Press, 1997) is an important and illuminating analysis of somatic treatments at two state hospitals in California; Ellen Dwyer, *Homes for the Mad: Life Inside Two Nineteenth-Century Asylums* (New Brunswick: Rutgers University Press, 1987); Gerald Grob, *From Asylum to Community: Mental Health Policy in Modern America* (Princeton: Princeton University Press, 1991); Grob, *The Mad Among Us*; Grob, *Mental Institutions in America: Social Policy to 1875* (New York: Free Press, 1973); Tomes, *The Art of Asylum-Keeping*; Jeffrey L. Geller, *Women of the Aslyum: Voices from Behind the Walls, 1840–1945* (New York: Anchor, 1995); Pressman, *Last Resort.* Lunbeck's insightful *Psychiatric Persuasion* deftly analyzes the case records of Boston's Psychopathic Hospital to trace the rising cultural credibility of psychiatry in twentieth-century America. For an important overview of the meanings attached to psychiatric therapies, see Andrew Scull, "Somatic Treatments and the Historiography of Psychiatry," *History of Psychiatry* 5 (1994): 1–12.

26. Quoted in Shorter, *History of Psychiatry*, 119.

27. Lunbeck, *Psychiatric Persuasion*, 3–4. Anne Harrington, *The Cure Within: A History of Mind-Body Medicine* (New York: Norton, 2008), 69–70.

28. Quoted in Claudia Kalb, "The Therapist as Scientist," *Newsweek*, Mar. 27, 2006, 50. Harrington, *Cure Within*, 68–69; Peter Gay, *Freud: A Life for Our Time* (New York: Norton, 2006), 49–53.

29. Shorter, *History of Psychiatry*, 149. Freud quoted in Gay, *Freud*, 62. Jeffrey Moussaief Masson, ed., *The Complete Letters of Sigmund Freud to Wilhelm Fliess, 1887–1904* (Cambridge: Harvard University Press, 1985), 378; Gay, *Freud*, 53.

30. The comment, made in his fifth lecture at Clark University, correctly credits Carl Jung with this observation. Freud's full comment reads: "Let me give at this point the main result at which we have arrived by the psychoanalytic investigation of neurotics, namely, that neuroses have no peculiar psychic content of their own, which is not also to be found in healthy states; or, as C. G. Jung has expressed it, neurotics fall ill of the same complexes with which we sound people struggle. It depends on quantitative relationships, on the relations of the forces wrestling with each other, whether the struggle leads to health, to a neurosis, or to compensatory over-functioning." Jung and Freud maintained a close friendship until the two parted over doctrinal differences. The text of Freud's fifth lecture was first published in Sigmund Freud, "The Origin and Development of Psychoanalysis," *American Journal of Psychology* 21, no. 2 (Apr. 1910): 213–218.

31. Sigmund Freud, "On the Grounds for Detaching Particular Syndrome from Neurasthenia Under the Description Anxiety Neurosis," *The Standard Edition of the Complete Psychological Works of Sigmund Freud*, vol. 3 (1893–1899), *Early Psycho-Analytic Publication*, 85–115. Allen Frances et al., "The Classification of Panic Disorders: From Freud to DSM-IV," *Journal of Psychiatric Res.* 27 (1993): suppl. 1, pp. 3–10.

32. Porter, *Greatest Benefit to Mankind*, 515. Freud, *Selected Papers on Hysteria*, 113–114. Andreasen, *Broken Brain*, 21.

33. Freud, *Selected Papers on Hysteria*, 88, 113; Shorter, *History of Psychiatry*, 151.

34. Shorter, *A Historical Dictionary of Psychiatry*, 113.

35. Shorter, *History of Psychiatry*, 145.

36. T. A. Ross, *The Common Neuroses* (London: Edward Arnold, 1923), quoted in *The Nervous Breakdown* (Garden City, NY: Doubleday, Doran, 1935), 10. *Nervous Breakdown*, 10; William Campbell, "The Mind: Science's Search for a Guide to Sanity," *Newsweek*, Oct. 24, 1955, 11.

37. American Psychiatry Association, *Diagnostic and Statistical Manual* (1952), 31.

38. Joel Paris, *The Fall of an Icon: Psychoanalysis and Academic Psychiatry* (Toronto: University of Toronto Press, 2005); Nathan G. Hale Jr., *The Rise and Crisis of Psychoanalysis in the United States: Freud and the Americans, 1917–1985* (New York: Oxford University Press, 1995); John C. Burnham, *Psychoanalysis and American Medicine, 1894–1917: Medicine, Science, and Culture* (New York: International Universities Press, 1967). Nathan G. Hale Jr., "From Berggasse XIX to Central Park West: The Americanization of Psychoanalysis, 1919–1940," *Journal of the History of the Behavioral Sciences* 14 (1979): 299–315; F. H. Matthews, "The Americanization of Sigmund Freud: Adaptations of Psychoanalysis before 1917," *Journal of American Studies* 1, no. 1 (Apr. 1967): 39–62; Shorter, *History of Psychiatry*, 160–189; Mari Jo Buhle, *Feminism and Its Discontents: A Century of Struggle with Psychoanalysis* (Cambridge: Harvard University Press, 1998); Campbell, "The Mind," 60, 65. *The Nervous Breakdown*, 10.

39. *Nervous Breakdown*, iii, 75; Campbell, "The Mind," 65.

40. Virginia Berridge and Griffith Edwards, *Opium and the People: Opiate Use in Nineteenth-Century England* (New York: St. Martin's, 1981), 58–59, 65; Medawar, *Power and Dependence*, 28–29. On the nomenclature of a soldier's heart, see Healy, "Mandel Cohen," 209–230. Aldous Huxley, "The History of Tension," *Annals of New York Academy of Sciences*, May 9, 1957, 675–684. William Sargant, "Discussion on Sedation and Stimulation in Man," *Proceedings of the Royal Society of Medicine* 51 (1958): 13–18; quoted in Medawar, *Social Audit*, 49.

41. Osler, quoted in Michael Bliss, *William Osler: A Life in Medicine* (New York: Oxford University Press, 2007), 189.

42. Gelett Burgess, *Are You a Bromide? Or, the Sulphitic Theory* (New York: Huebsch, 1906). The book went through multiple printings and has since been reissued.

43. Committee on Public Health, Subcommittee on Barbiturates, "Report on Barbiturates," *New York Academy of Medicine*, June 1956, 474–475; Charles Grutzner, "Grave Peril Seen in Sleeping Pills," *New York Times*, Dec. 16, 1951, 1; "Veronal and Its Uses," *New York Times*, Jan. 23, 1906, 8; Medawar, *Power and Dependence*, 56–58. As one 1939 article observed, a "decade or so ago" the "average insomniac . . . might have requested bromides, but today the barbiturates . . . are the most popular sleep-inducers, forming an important part of the nation's annual $360,000,000 patent medicine bill." See "The 'Lullaby Pill' Peril: Barbiturates, Taken for Binges As Well As Sleep, Attacked," *Newsweek*, Mar. 13, 1939, 36. In the 1920s, deep sleep therapy, induced by intravenous injections of barbiturates, was a somatic treatment used in psychiatric institutions to treat depression, schizophrenia, and catatonia. See Braslow, *Mental Ills and Bodily Cures*, 37–38; Shorter, *A Historical Dictionary of Psychiatry*, 38–39. On the expanding field of neuropsychiatry, see Nicolas Rasmussen, "Making the First Anti-Depressant Amphetamine in American Medicine, 1929–1950," *Journal of the History of Medicine and Allied Science* 61, no. 3 (2006): 292–293; Lunbeck, *Psychiatric Persuasion;* W. A. Lishman, "What Is Neuropsychiatry?" *Neurology, Neurosurgery, and Neuropsychiatry*, Nov. 1992, 983–985; W. A. Lishman, "Psychiatry and Neuropathology: The Maturing of a Relationship," *Journal of Neurology, Neurosurgery, and Psychiatry* 58 (1995): 284–292. Irving J. Sands, "Barbital (Veronal) Intoxication," *Journal of the American Medical Association*, Nov. 3,

1923, 1519–1520; William H. Leake and E. Richmond Ware, "Barbital (Veronal) Poisoning," *Journal of the American Medical Association*, Feb. 7, 1925, 434–436; "Sleeping Pill Racket Drive by City, State Snares Eight," *New York Times*, Sept. 23, 1949, 1; "Four Druggists Guilty: They Offer Pleas to Unlawful Sales of Barbiturates," *New York Times*, Oct. 18, 1949, 21.

44. "Weinstein Warns of New Controls to Check Sales of Sleeping Pills," *New York Times*, Oct. 15, 1946, 35. "Edward Germann's Death: Veronal Prescribed by a Physician Who Had Never Heard of It," *New York Times*, June 22, 1906, 6. "Topics of the Times," *New York Times*, Jan. 23, 1906.

45. *Merck's Index: An Encyclopedia for the Chemist, Pharmacist, and Physician*, 4th ed. (Rahway, NJ: Merck, 1930), 102. *Merck's Index*, 4th ed., 102; Shorter, *History of Psychiatry*, 203.

46. Committee on Public Health, New York Academy of Medicine, "Report on Barbiturates," 456; John P. Swann, "FDA and the Practice of Pharmacy: Prescription Drug Regulation Before the Durham-Humphrey Amendment of 1951," *Pharmacy in History* 36, no. 2 (1994): 55–70; Richard D. Lyons, "Science's Knowledge on the Misuse of Drugs and How They Act Is Found to Lag," *New York Times*, Jan. 9, 1968; Grutzner, "Grave Peril," 1; "'Lullaby Pill' Peril," 36. Charles Medawar has suggested that barbiturates be considered among the earliest me-too drugs because of the ease with which they could be chemically modified. Medawar, *Social Audit*, 55–57.

47. Charles O. Jackson, "Before the Drug Culture: Barbiturate/Amphetamine Abuse in American Society," *Clio Medica*, 11, no. 1 (1976): 50; Grutzner, "Grave Peril," 1. William L. Laurence, "War, Social Strife Test Psychiatrist," *New York Times*, May 12, 1937, 12; William L. Laurence, "General Metcalfe Says Giving Barbiturates to Wounded Men Will Mean Many Lives: Tells Men Method to Cut War Shock," *New York Times*, Oct. 24, 1940, 30. As Nick Rasmussen has shown, amphetamines were also employed to keep soldiers on their toes and combat fatigue. See Rasmussen, *On Speed*, 56–57.

48. "Army Drops Label of Psychoneurotic," *Los Angeles Examiner*, May 16, 1944; "Tension Tops U.S. Disorders," *Los Angeles Examiner*, Mar. 5, 1952; and Chris Clausen, "1 Out of 3 Held Victims of Anxiety," *Los Angeles Examiner*, all in *Los Angeles Examiner* Clippings File, Special Collections Division, University of South California, Los Angeles; Ben Shepard, *A War of Nerves: Soldiers and Psychiatrists in the Twentieth Century* (Cambridge: Harvard University Press, 2000), 325–335; Hans Binneveld, *From Shell Shock to Combat Stress: A Comparative History of Military Psychiatry* (Amsterdam: Amsterdam University Press, 1997); Hans Pols, "War Neurosis, Adjustment Problems in Veterans, and an Ill Nation: The Disciplinary Project of American Psychiatry During and After World War II," *Osiris* 22 (2007): 76; Allan Young, *The Harmony of Illusions: Inventing Post-Traumatic Stress Disorder* (Princeton: Princeton University Press, 1995); Hale, *The Rise and Crisis of Psychoanalysis in the United States*, 188–210; Ellen Herman, *The Romance of American Psychology: Political Culture in the Age of Experts* (Berkeley: University of California Press), chap. 4. The fifty-eight-minute film *Let There Be Light* aided the cause. Filmed by John Huston at Edgewood State Hospital in Long Island, it showed veterans' remarkable psychological recovery via talk therapy and facilitating drugs such as sodium pentothal. Although the film showcased the successful treatment of war-induced neurosis, soldiers' return to a fully functional state, and their reintegration into mainstream America, the U.S. War Department banned it for thirty-five years, presumably because it showed the psychological scars war could inflict. U.S. Army Pictorial Services, *Let There Be Light*, 1946 (issued for the public

in 1981). Committee on Public Health, Subcommittee on Barbiturates, "Report on Barbiturates," 457–458.

49. Victor H. Vogel quoted in Grutzner, "Grave Peril," 1; Richard D. Lyons, "Science's Knowledge on the Misuse of Drugs and How They Act Is Found to Lag," *New York Times*, Jan. 9, 1968; Committee on Public Health, Subcommittee on Barbiturates, "Report on Barbiturates," 458; "Barbiturates and Barbiturate-Like Drugs: Considerations in Their Medical Use," *Journal of the American Medical Association*, Dec. 9, 1974; Medawar, *Social Audit*, 58–69; "U.N. Voices Concerns on Barbiturate Use," *New York Times*, Feb. 13, 1966.

50. "Academy Endorses Sleeping Pill Curb," *New York Times*, 8.

51. "Academy Endorses Sleeping Pill Curb," 8; Grutzner, "Grave Peril," 1. David Courtwright, *Dark Paradise: A History of Opiate Addiction in America* (Cambridge: Harvard University Press, 2001), 146–147.

52. "The 'Lullaby Pill' Peril," 36; Jackson, "Before the Drug Culture," 48; Rasmussen, *On Speed*, pp. 100–101; Jim Hogshire, *Pills-a-Go-Go: A Fiendish Investigation into Pill Marketing, Art, History, and Consumption* (Los Angeles: Feral House, 1999), 94. James Toolan quoted in Grutzner, "Grave Peril," 1.

53. "Barbiturate Curb Backed by Doctors," *New York Times*, Apr. 3, 1947, 26. Grutzner, "Grave Peril," 1.

54. "Sleeping Pill Racket Drive by City, State Snares Eight"; "Four Druggists Guilty: They Offer Pleas to Unlawful Sale of Barbiturates," *New York Times*, Oct. 18, 1949, 21.

55. Jackson, "Before the Drug Culture," 50, 52; Shorter, *History of Psychiatry*, 203. Grutzner, "Grave Peril," 1.

CHAPTER 2

1. Carl Elliott, *Better Than Well: American Medicine Meets the American Dream* (New York: Norton, 2003), 131.

2. Elliott, *Better Than Well*, xvi. Karl Rickels, interview by David Healy, Dec. 14, 1988, 7. Transcript in author's possession, with special thanks to David Healy for transcribing and sending it to me. Emphasis is mine. Tom Ban, "They Used to Call It Psychiatry," in David Healy, ed., *The Psychopharmacologists: Interviews by David Healy* (London: Arnold, 2001), 597–598.

3. "Spare-Time Research Triumph for Czech Refugee: Penicillin Made at Cost of a Few Shillings," *Reynolds News*, Mar. 4, 1945, 3. Frank Berger, interview by Andrea Tone, New York City, July 10, 2003.

4. Frank Berger, interview by Brian Pierce, July 14, 2004, New York City. Berger autobiography, 3, Frank Berger Manuscript Collection, International Archives of Neuro-Psychopharmcology, Vanderbilt University. Berger autobiography, 6.

5. Berger autobiography, 8–9.

6. Berger autobiography, 11–12. The relevant articles were "Besonders hohe Wirksamkeit des Follikelhormons bei vaginaler Installation" ["The particularly high efficacy of the female sexual hormone on vaginal administration"], *Klinische Wochenschrift*, Nov. 9, 1935, 1601–1602. This study, Berger's first article, was supplemented by "Forgesezte Studien über vaginal Anwendung des Follikelhormones" ["Continued investigations concerning the vaginal administration of estrogenic hormone"], *Klinische Wochenschrift*, Oct. 9, 1937, 1428–1431. Frank Berger Collection, Publications 1935–1951, Vol. 1, Box 1, International Archives of Neuro-Psychopharmacology. Berger autobiography, 23–24.

7. Berger autobiography, 13. *A Dictionary of Modern History,* ed. A. W. Palmer (New York: Penguin, 1962), 227. Berger autobiography, 24–26.

8. Berger, interview by Pierce. Berger autobiography, 28.

9. Peter Neushul, "Fighting Research: Army Participation in the Clinical Testing and Mass Production of Penicillin During the Second World War," in *War, Medicine, and Modernity,* ed. Roger Cooter, Mark Harrison, and Steve Sturdy (Gloucestershire, U.K.: Sutton, 1999), 205; Robert Bud, *Penicillin: Triumph and Tragedy* (London: Oxford University Press, 2007), 24–27. Edward Shorter, *The Health Century* (New York: Doubleday, 1987), 37. On penicillin and Fleming, see Ronald Hare, "New Light on the History of Penicillin, *Medical History* 26 (1982); 1–24; and Gwyn Macfarlane, *Alexander Fleming: The Man and the Myth* (Cambridge: Harvard University Press: 1984). On the social construction of penicillin, see Wai Chen, "The Laboratory as Business: Sir Almroth Wright's Vaccine Programme and the Construction of Penicillin," in *The Laboratory Revolution in Medicine,* ed. Andrew Cunningham and Perry Williams (Cambridge: Cambridge University Press, 1992), 245–292.

10. Bud, *Penicillin,* 28–30; E. P. Abraham et al., "Further Observations on Penicillin," *Lancet,* Aug. 16, 1941, 177–189; "Penicillin in Action," *Lancet,* Aug. 16, 1941, 192. This elaborated on Chain and Florey's claims regarding the chemotherapeutic properties of penicillin on infected animals in E. Chain et al., "Penicillin as a Chemotherapeutic Agent," *Lancet,* Aug. 24, 1940, 226–228.

11. Rogert Cooter, "War and Modern Medicine," in *Companion Encyclopedia of the History of Medicine,* ed. W. F. Bynum and Roy Porter (New York: Routledge, 2007), 1541–1544; Roger Cooter, "Medicine in War," in *Medicine Transformed: Health, Disease, and Society in Europe, 1800–1930,* ed. Deborah Brunton (Manchester University Press, 2004), 334–339; Neushul, "Fighting Research," 204.

12. Shorter, *Health Century,* 37, 40. Neushul, "Fighting Research," 209. Bud, *Penicillin,* 31–35; H. Sutcliffe, "County Council Now Making Penicillin: New Method of Extraction and Purification," *Wharefedale and Airedale Observer,* Oct. 22, 1944; Berger Scrapbook, Vol. 1, Frank Berger Family Archives, New York City. John L. Smith of Pfizer quoted on the American Chemical Society website, http://acswebcontent.acs.org/landmarks/landmarks/penicillin/scaleup.htlml (accessed Dec. 31, 2007). The P-patrol was the name of the Oxford bike team that would retrieve patients' urine from the hospital and transport it to the laboratory. See Bud, *Penicillin,* 32; Dee Unglab Silverthorn, *Human Physiology: An Integrated Approach,* 3rd ed. (New Jersey: Benjamin Cummings, 2004).

13. John P. Swann, "The Search for Synthetic Penicillin During World War 2," *British Journal for the History of Science* 16 (1983): 154–188; Bud, *Penicillin,* 37–41. As Bud argues, the infusion of money and personnel, as well as the involvement of government and big business, made penicillin a bellwether for a new pattern of scientific work grounded in large-scale, collaborative industrial research. H. Sutcliffe, "County Health Work Helped by New Drug: Instance of Penicillin Saving Lives," *Wharfedale & Airedale Observer,* Oct. 27, 1944; Berger Scrapbook, Vol. 1, Frank Berger Family Archives; "Spare-Time Research Triumph for Czech Refugee: Penicillin Made at Cost of a Few Shillings," *Reynolds News,* Mar. 4, 1945, 3; Frank Berger, "Extraction and Purification of Penicillin," *Nature* (London), Oct. 7, 1944, 459; F. M. Berger, "Preparation of Purified Penicillin," *British Medical Journal,* Jan. 27, 1945, 116–117.

14. H. Sutcliffe, "County Council Now Making Penicillin"; Berger Scrapbook, Vol. 1, Frank Berger Family Archives, New York City. On a comparable controversy regarding in-

tellectual property, public health, and the discovery of insulin, see Michael Bliss, *The Discovery of Insulin* (Chicago: University of Chicago Press, 1982). Berger, "Extraction and Purification of Penicillin," 459; and Berger, "Preparation of Purified Penicillin," 116–117.

15. David Healy, *The Antidepressent Era* (Cambridge: Harvard University Press, 1997), 23; Bud, *Penicillin,* 44–45; Shorter, *Health Century;* Neusheul, "Fighting Research"; Peter Temin, *Taking Your Medicine: Drug Regulation in the United States* (Cambridge: Harvard University Press), 65–66.

16. Dilip Ramchandani, Francisco Lopez-Munoz, and Cecilio Alamo, "Meprobamate—Tranquilizer or Anxiolytic? A Historical Perspective," *Psychiatric Quarterly* 77, no. 1 (Spring 2006): 45–46; Frank M. Berger, "As I Remember," in *The Rise of Psychopharmacology,* ed. T. A. Ban, D. Healy, and E. Shorter (Budapest: Animula, 1998), 59; Alfred Berger, "History," in *Psychotherapeutic Drugs,* ed. Carl Usdin and Irene Forrest (New York: Marcel Dekker, 1976), 38–39. Mephenesin (3-o-toloxy 1,2-propanediol) was the result of the condensation of o-cresol with glycerine in 1908. Tom Ban, *Psychopharmacology* (Baltimore: Williams & Wilkins, 1969), 313. Frank M. Berger, "Anxiety and the Discovery of the Tranquilizers," in *Discoveries in Biological Psychiatry,* ed. Frank Ayd and Barry Blackwell (Philadelphia: Lippincott, 1970), 121; F. M. Berger and W. Bradley, "The Pharmacological Properties of alpha, beta-dihydroxy-gamma-)(2-methylphenoxy)-propane (myanesin)," *British Journal of Pharmacology and Chemotherapy* 1 (Dec. 1946): 265–272; Thomas Whiteside, "Onward and Upward with the Arts: Getting There First with Tranquility," *New Yorker,* May 3, 1958, 112.

17. Frank Berger and W. Bradley, "The Pharmacological Properties of alpha:beta dihydrozy-gamma-(2 methylphenoxy) propane (Myanesin)," 265. In 1800, English novelist and diarist Frances Burney wrote, "I find, however, *useful* employment the best tranquilliser & I have less of the violent emotions which have hitherto torn me." Thomas De Quincey also referenced a "tranquilliser of nervous and anomalous sensation" in his famous tome, *Confessions of an English Opium-Eater.* See *Oxford English Dictionary Online,* 2nd ed., 1989, http://dictionary.oed.com (accessed Jan. 2, 2008).

18. Berger, "Anxiety and the Discovery of the Tranquilizers," 121. Anonymous, "For and Against Myanesin," *Lancet,* Mar. 27, 1948, 487. F. M. Berger and R. P. Schwartz, "Oral 'Myanesin' in Treatment of Spastic and Hyperkinetic Disorders," *Journal of the American Medical Association,* June 26, 1948, 772–774; G. D. Gammon and J. A. Churchill, "Effects of Myanesin upon the Central Nervous System," *American Journal of the Medical Sciences,* Feb. 1949, 143–148. Berger, "As I Remember," 60; Birger R. Kaada, "Site of Action of Myanesin (Mephenesin, Tolserol) in the Central Nervous System," *Journal of Neurophysiology* 13 (Jan. 1950): 89–104 .

19. Berger, autobiography, 38–39.

20. Berger, autobiography, 45–46.

21. Marcia Angell, *The Truth About Drug Companies: How They Deceive Us and What to Do About It* (New York: Random House, 2004), 3; Greg Critser, *Generation RX: How Prescription Drugs Are Altering American Lives, Minds, and Bodies* (New York: Houghton Mifflin, 2005), 2. "Competition Keen in 'Wonder Drugs,'" *New York Times,* Jan. 11, 1953, F6. "Rx for Prosperity: More Druggists Play Up Prescriptions, Cash In on Swift Sales Climb," *New York Times,* July 30, 1958, 1. Also see Nancy Tomes, "The Great American Medicine Show Revisited," *Bulletin of the History of Medicine* 79 (Winter 2005): 627–663.

22. Temin, *Taking Your Medicine,* 66; Robert E. Bedingfield, "Drug Makers View '52 As a Tough Year," *New York Times,* Apr. 5, 1953, F5. Sydney B. Self, "World Drugstore: Showboats

and Sound Trucks Help U.S. Firms Gain a Global Market," *Wall Street Journal*, Aug. 3, 1948, 1.

23. Arthur C. Emelin, president of Schenley Laboratories, quoted in "Drug Makers View '52 as a Tough Year."

24. Healy, *Let Them Eat Prozac: The Unhealthy Relationship between the Pharmaceutical Industry and Depression* (New York: New York Univeristy Press, 2004), 33; David Healy, *The Creation of Psychopharmacology* (Cambridge: Harvard University Press, 2002), 77–79. Researchers at Rhône-Poulenc screened phenothiazines to determine if they had antihistamine effects. Antihistamines were regarded as breakthrough drugs in the 1940s and 1950s, and were used to treat a number of conditions, including allergies but also hypothermia, wounds, insomnia, and eventually psychosis.

25. Angel, "Truth About Drug Companies," 3; Douglas N. Cray, "Drug Industry Seeks Ways to Make Up for a New-Product Lag," *New York Times*, June 4, 1967, F1.

26. Testimony of Henry Hoyt, *Administered Prices: Hearings Before the Subcommittee on Antitrust and Monopoly of the Committee on the Judiciary*, United States Senate, pt. 16 (Washington, DC: Government Printing Office, 1960), 9108; Carter Products Memorandum, Oct. 21, 1957, Berger Scrapbooks, Vol. 3; Henry Hoyt, address to the New York Society of Security Analysts, June 9, 1958, Berger Scrapbooks, Vol. 3, Frank Berger Family Archives; John N. Wilford, "Old-Time Remedies: From Eagle-Eye Salve to Stomach Bitters, They Still Sell Well," *Wall Street Journal*, Oct. 9, 1959, 1. Whiteside, "Onwards and Upwards with the Arts," 114; "Henry Hoyt, 96, Dies," *New York Times*, Nov. 8, 1990, D25.

27. FDA memorandum, June 18, 1965, Manufacturers Files, AF 19–503, Wallace Laboratories, FDA History Office; Testimony of Henry Hoyt, *Administered Prices*, 9108; Berger, interview by Tone; Frank M. Berger, "The 'Social-Chemistry' of Pharmacological Discovery: The Miltown Story," *Social Pharmacology* 2, no. 3 (1988): 1389. Paul Starr, *The Social Transformation of American Medicine* (New York: Basic, 1982); Andrea Tone, *Devices and Desires* (New York: Hill & Wang, 2001).

28. "What's in a Name? FTC-Carter Squabble Drags into 15th Year," *Wall Street Journal*, May 28, 1957, 1; "Carter's Liver Pills Don't Help Liver, Federal Court Rules," *Wall Street Journal*, June 18, 1959, 3. "Court Upsets FTC Ban on Carter Firm's Use of the Word 'Liver,'" *Wall Street Journal*, Jan. 21, 1953, 8.

29. "Henry Hoyt, 96, Dies." Testimony of Henry Hoyt, *Administered Prices: Hearings Before the Committee on Antitrust and Monopoly of the Committee on the Judiciary*, United States Senate, pt. 16 (Washington, DC: Government Printing Office, 1960), 9108; Whiteside, "Onward and Upward with the Arts," 114; FDA Establishment Inspection Report, Mar. 11, 1955, FDA Establishment Inspection Report, May 6, 1960, and FDA Establishment Inspection Report, June 18, 1965, all in Manufacturers Files, AF 19–503, FDA History Office; Berger, "As I Remember," 60.

30. Berger autobiography, 23, 46.

31. Berger autobiography, 33.

32. Berger, interview by Tone; Frank Berger, interview by Leo Hollister, 1999, IANP Archives, Vanderbilt University.

33. Whiteside, "Onward and Upward with the Arts," 114; Berger autobiography, 50–53, 56–57; "Tolserol, the Drug that Relaxes You," *Pageant Magazine*, Oct. 1952, 31, Berger Scrapbooks, Vol. 1, Berger Family Archives, New York City. The original patent, serial number 176,764, was filed July 29, 1950. It was abandoned and superseded by patent application 2,724,720, "Dicarbamates of Substituted Propanediols," U.S. Patent Office, patented Nov. 22, 1955.

34. Louis S. Schlan, "Some Effects of Myanesin in Psychiatric Patients," *Journal of the American Medical Association,*" June 25, 1949, 672–673. Dixon et al., "Clinical Observations on Tolserol in Handling Anxiety Tension States," *American Journal of the Medical Sciences,* July 1950, 24. Dixon et al., "Clinical Observations on Tolserol," 27, 29.

35. Arthur O. Hecker, Margaret M. Mercer, and Mark A. Griffin, "Further Clinical Investigation of Tolserol (Myanesin)," *Diseases of the Nervous System* 12 (Apr. 1951): 101, 102.

36. Hecker, Mercer, and Griffin, "Further Clinical Investigation of Tolserol (Myanesin)," 104.

37. John P. Swann, "FDA and the Practice of Pharmacy: Prescription Drug Regulation Before the Durham-Humphrey Amendment of 1951," *Pharmacy in History* 36 (1994): 60; Temin, *Taking Your Medicine,* 51–53.

38. Swann, "FDA and the Practice of Pharmacy," 55–70; Temin, *Taking Your Medicine,* 51–53; Dennis B. Worthen, "Carl Thomas Durham (1892–1974): Pharmacy's Representative," *Journal of the American Pharmacists Association* 45 (Mar.-Apr. 2005): 295–298. "Prescription Curbs Hailed as Helpful," *New York Times,* Apr. 29, 1952, 20; "Drug Bill Scored at Meeting Here," *New York Times,* Sept. 6, 1951; "Truman Signs Rules Limiting Drug Sales," *New York Times,* Oct. 27, 1951. On the evolving relationship between doctors, patients, and prescription drugs, see Nancy Tomes, "The Great American Medicine Show Revisited," *Bulletin of the History of Medicine* 79 (Winter 2005): 627–663.

39. "Proprietary Group Assails Drug Bill," *New York Times,* May 15, 1951, 56.

40. See, for instance, J. Maurice Rogers, "Drug Abuse: Just What the Doctor Ordered," *Psychology Today,* Sept. 1971, 16.

41. Temin, *Taking Your Medicine.* Berger, autobiography, 57–58.

42. Crosby, quoted in Nathan G. Hale, "From Berggasse XIX to Central Park West: The Americanization of Psychoanlysis, 1919–1940," *Journal of the History of Behavioral Sciences* 14 (1978): 307.

43. Berger, interview by Tone. Berger, "Anxiety and the Discovery of the Tranquilizers," 115.

44. Joseph C. Borrus, "Study of Effect of Miltown (2-Methyl-2-n-Propyl-1,3-Propoanediol Dicarbamate) on Psychiatric States," *Journal of the American Medical Association,* Apr. 30, 1955, 1596–1598.

45. Cited in Whiteside, "Onward and Upward with the Arts," 115. Lowell S. Selling, "Clinical Use of a New Tranquilizing Drug," *Journal of the American Medical Association,* Apr. 30, 1955, 1594–1596.

46. Selling, "Clinical Use of a New Tranquilizing Drug," Whiteside, "Onward and Upward with the Arts," 115; U.S. Food and Drug Evaluation and Research, Center for Drug Evaluation and Research, *From Test Tube to Patient: Improving Health Through Human Drugs,* DHHS Publication (FDA) 99–3168 (Washington, DC: Department of Health and Human Services, 1999), 19–21. Although the designs of these trials were later found to be deficient and problematic, they were consistent with how clinical trials in this era were conducted. Leo Hollister remembers that in the mid-1950s, running trials—getting the drugs, enrolling patients, setting up an experiment—made it "so much simpler to do clinical research than it is today." See David Healy, *The Psychopharmacologists II* (London: Altman, 1998), 216–217. As historians have shown, what is recognized as "scientific fact" has varied dramatically over time. In 1953 and 1954, nothing about the design of the meprobamate trials—neither the number of participants nor the absence of blinding or a control group—worried regulators or researchers. Informed consent was not required; indeed, it was not discussed in the same

terms as it is today. Theirs was a research world bracketed by different ethical codes. On the evolution of clinical trials, pharmaceutical regulation, and the assertion of scientific fact, see Harry Marks, *The Progress of Experiment* (Cambridge: Cambridge University Press); Steven Epstein, *Impure Science: AIDS, Activism, and the Politics of Knowledge* (Berkeley: University of California Press, 1998); Arthur A. Daemmrich, *Pharmacopolitics: Drug Regulation in the United States and Germany* (Chapel Hill: University of North Carolina Press, 2004); Lara Marks, "A Cage of Ovulating Females: The History of the Early Oral Contraceptive Pill Clinical Trials, 1950–1959," in *Molecularizing Biology and Medicine: New Practices and Alliances, 1930s–1970s,* ed. S. de Chaderevian and H. Kamminga (Amsterdam: Harwood Academic, 199), 221–247; Suzanne White Junod and Lara Marks, "Women's Trials: The Approval of the First Oral Contraceptive Pill in the United States and Great Britain," *Journal of the History of Medicine* 57 (Apr. 2002): 117–160.

47. Whiteside, "Onward and Upward with the Arts," 115.

48. Eric J. Hobsbawm and Terence Ranger, *The Invention of Tradition* (Cambridge: Cambridge University Press, 1992); Whiteside, "Onward and Upward with the Arts," 99. "Leo Sternbach, the Father of Mother's Little Helpers," USNEWS.com, accessed Mar. 12, 2003. On the ways in which images were harnessed to promote one vision of pharmaceutical history, see Jonathan Metzl and Joel Howell, "Making History: Lessons from the Great Moments Series of Pharmaceutical Advertisements," *Academic Medicine* 79 (Nov. 2004): 1027–1032; and Jacalyn Duffin and Alison Li, "Great Moments: Parke, Davis and Company and the Creation of Medical Art," *Isis* 86 (1995): 1–29.

49. Whiteside, "Onward and Upward with the Arts," 116.

50. Whiteside, "Onward and Upward with the Arts," 116; H. Rodney Luery, A. S. Barnes & Company for the Borough of Miltown, *The Story of Milltown* (South Brunswick and New York, 1971), 231–223; *Milltown Tales* 1, no. 1 (1964): 1; William Michelfelder, "Tranquilizing Drugs Have the U.S. Agog: How Good Are They?" *New York World-Telegram,* Apr. 7, 1956, 6.

51. Frank M. Berger, Charles D. Hendley, and Thomas E. Lynes, *Effect of Meprobamate (Miltown) on Animal Behavior* (New Brunswick, NJ: Wallace Labs). The film is described in the Berger Scrapbooks, Vol. 1, Berger Family Archives; Berger Manuscript Collection, Vol. 2, Box 1, p. 347, International Archives of Neuro-Psychopharmacology.

52. Dixon testimony, *Administered Prices,* 9146–9151.

53. Dixon testimony, *Administered Prices,* 9146–9151. Although Wyeth began selling meprobamate as Equanil in the fall of 1955, the formal licensing agreement between the two firms was not signed until Dec. 5, 1955.

54. Paul Janssen, interview, in "From Haloperidol to Risperidone," in David Healy, ed., *The Psychopharmacolgists II* (London: Chapman & Hall, 1998), 59. Healy, *The Creation of Psychopharmacology,* 104–105.

CHAPTER 3

1. "Texts of Surgeon General's Statements on the Polio Inoculation Program," *New York Times,* May 9, 1955, 14.

2. Thomas Whiteside, "Onward and Upward with the Arts: Getting There First with Tranquility," *New Yorker,* May 3, 1958, 117.

3. Whiteside, "Onward and Upward," 117. John Carson, "Meprobamate Revisited," *New York State Journal of Pharmacy* 9 (1989): 45.

4. *Gone with the Wind* and *Lawrence of Arabia* are discussed in Jim Hogshire, *Pills a Go-Go* (Venice, CA: Publisher's Group West, 1999), 105. On Garland's history of drug use, see

"Judy Garland, 47, Found Dead," *New York Times,* June 23, 1969, 1; Doris Grumbach, "Neurosis and Rainbows: The Garland Legend Grows," *New York Times,* Aug. 17, 1975, 93; and David Shipman's more controversial *Judy Garland: The Secret Life of an American Legend* (New York: Little, Brown, 1993).

5. Horace Sutton, "A Traveller's Diary," *Los Angeles Times,* June 3, 1956, D11. Dorothy Kilgallen, "The Voice of Broadway," *New York Journal American,* Mar. 26, 1956, Berger Scrapbooks, Vol. 2, Berger Family Archives, New York City. "Don't-Give-a-Damn Pills," *Time,* Feb. 27, 1956, 98; Ken Schessler, *This Is Hollywood: An Unusual Movieland Guide* (Redlands, CA: Ken Schessler, 1978), 41. Jack Geyer, "New Fad in Pill Town," *Los Angeles Times,* April 5, 1956, A5; Jim Cook, "The Happy Pills: Are They?" *New York Post,* Jan. 22, 1957, 36.

6. Kendis Rochlen, "Movie Ulcer Crowd Goes for New 'Tranquil Pill,'" *Los Angeles Mirror-News,* Feb. 8, 1956, sec. 2, p. 6; "Pill vs. Worry: How Goes the Frantic Quest for Calm in Frantic Lives?" *Newsweek,* May 21, 1956, 68. Thrifty Drug Store ad, *Los Angeles Times,* Dec. 18, 1955, 26. "Don't-Give-a-Damn-Pills," 98; FDA Memo, Henry B. Packscher, Feb. 28, 1956, Manufacturers Files, AF19–503, Wallace Laboratories, FDA History Office.

7. Quoted in Victor Schmidt, "What You Should Know About Those New Happiness Pills," *Uncensored,* Oct. 25, 1957, 62. Kendis Rochlen, "Movie Ulcer Crowd Goes for New 'Tranquil Pill,'" 2–6.

8. Quoted in Cook, "Happy Pills," 36.

9. Coyne Steven Sanders and Tom Gilbert, *Desilu: The Story of Lucille Ball and Desi Arnaz* (New York: HarperCollins, 2001), 141. Lauren Bacall, *By Myself and Then Some* (New York: HarperCollins, 2005), 302. Lewis Funke and John E. Booth, "Williams on Williams," *Theatre Arts,* Jan. 1962, 17–19, 72–73; Edmund White, "Playwright's Diary," *New York Times,* Mar. 4, 2007, 20.

10. Quoted in Schmidt, "What You Should Know," 37, 60. Rudolf Flesch, "A Troubled Writer," *Los Angeles Times,* Nov. 15, 1959, B5. Mansfield, quoted in Cook, "Happy Pills," 36; on the importance of media coverage of celebrity experience to changing perceptions of illness, see Barron H. Lerner, *When Illness Goes Public: Celebrity Patients and How We Look at Medicine* (Baltimore: Johns Hopkins University Press, 2006).

11. A. E. Hotchner, "Can Mood Pills Really Help You?" *This Week Magazine, Los Angeles Times,* Aug. 19, 1956, N8. Schmidt, "What You Should Know," 62.

12. Cook, "Happy Pills," 4. Quoted in David Sears Houston, "Hollywood's Latest Pill Kick: 'Don't-Give-a-Damn Drugs,'" *Hollywood Magazine,* 60.

13. Hotchner, "Can Mood Pills Really Help?" 8. Jim Cook, "The Happy (?) Pills: Sex and Tranquility," *New York Post,* Jan. 24, 1957, 4. Tranquilease is discussed in *False and Misleading Advertisements (Prescription Tranquilizing Drugs): Hearings before a Subcommittee of the Committee of the Committee on Government Operations,* Eighty-fifth Congress, 2nd sess. (Washington, DC: Government Printing Office, 1958), 143. Dorothy Kilgallen, "The Voice of Broadway," 26; "Cityside with Gene Sherman," June 12, 1957, 2; Cook, "Happy Pills," 4.

14. See, for instance, the Baskin-Robbins advertisements in the *Los Angeles Times* on May 18, 1957, B5; Mar. 2, 1957, 2; and Dec. 1, 1956, 15.

15. Domeliner ad in *Los Angeles Times,* Sept. 14, 1956, 23. Advertisement for Holiday Motor in the *Los Angeles Times,* Apr. 21, 1957, 39.

16. "Teary Film on View," *Los Angeles Times,* June 4, 1957, B7. *Feliz Año, Amor Mio* was a Spanish-speaking movie filmed in Mexico. Portofino discussed in Ken Mandelbaum, *Not Since Carrie: Forty Years of Broadway Musical Flops* (New York: St. Martin's Griffin, 1991), 28.

17. "'Behavior' Drugs Now Envisioned: Aldous Huxley Predicts They Will Bring Re-Examining of Ethics and Religion," *New York Times,* Oct. 19, 1956, 29; Orville Prescott, "Two Aldous Huxleys," *New York Times,* Nov. 24, 1963, 22; "Aldous Huxley Dies of Cancer on Coast," *New York Times,* Nov. 24, 1963, 1. By 1956 the skeptical materialism of Huxley's earlier years had yielded to a fascination with mysticism and the experiences of chemical mind-bending. Aldous Huxley, "Brave New World Revisited," *Esquire,* July 1956. Aldous Huxley, "The History of Tension," *Annals of the New York Academy of Sciences,* May 9, 1957, 675–684; Frank M. Berger, "As I Remember," in *The Rise of Psychopharmacology and the Story of CINP,* ed. T. A. Ban, D. Healy, E. Shorter (Budapest: Animula, 1998), 61. Huxley later wrote a friend that the symposium had been intellectually stimulating but physically strenuous, for "I found no less than seven radio and TV appearances lined up for me, at hours ranging from six thirty in the morning to eleven fifteen at night." Aldous Huxley to Dr. Humphry Osmond, Oct. 20, 1956, in *Letters of Aldous Huxley,* ed. G. Smith (London: Chatto & Windus, 1969), 809–810.

18. Aldous Huxley, "Pleasures," *Esquire,* Feb. 1957; reprinted in Robert S. Baker and James Sexton, eds., *Aldous Huxley: Complete Essays,* vol. 6, *1956–1965* (Chicago: Ivan R. Dee, 2002), 209–215.

19. William Boddy, *Fifties Television: The Industry and Its Critics* (Urbana: University of Illinois Press, 1990), 187. Graham, quoted in Cook, "Happy Pills."

20. James L. Baughman, *The Republic of Mass Culture: Journalism, Filmmaking, and Broadcasting in America Since 1941* (Baltimore: Johns Hopkins University Press, 1992), 30; David Halberstam, *The Fifties* (New York: Ballantine, 1993), 199; "Population: 1900 to 2002," U.S. Census Bureau, *Statistical Abstract of the United States,* 2003.

21. Milton Berle and Haskel Frankel, *Milton Berle: An Autobiography* (New York: Applause Theatre and Cinema, 1974), 294. "Don't-Give-a-Damn Pills," 100. On Berle, see Tim Brooks and Earle Marsh, *The Complete Directory to Prime Time Network and Cable TV SHOWS 1946–Present,* 7th ed. (New York: Ballantine, 1999), 665–666. Berle script, n.d., Jay Burton Collection, Box 5, Vol. 3, Manuscripts Division, Cinema-Television Library, University of Southern California.

22. "Uncle Miltie's Mrs. Loves That New 4-a-Year Schedule," *New York Post,* Mar. 20, 1956, Berger Scrapbooks, Vol. 1, Frank Berger Family Archives. Quoted in Cook, "Happy Pills," 42. See the Jay Burton Collection, Manuscripts Division, Cinema and Television Library, University of Southern California. Burton was one of Milton Berle's scriptwriters, and the collection comprises eleven volumes of monologues that Burton wrote for Berle's variety shows.

23. Cook, "Happy Pills," 42. Hope, quoted in "Nick Kenny's T.V. Viewing and Radio," *Los Angeles Daily Mirror,* June 7, 1956. Whiteside, "Onward and Upward," 119.

24. Hope script from Whiteside, "Onward and Upward," 119, 122.

25. "Gridiron Fete Pokes Fun at Notables," *Los Angeles Times,* Mar. 3, 1957, 21. Whiteside, "Onward and Upward," 128.

26. "Walter Winchell of New York," *Daily Mirror,* Sept. 5, 1956, 10. FDA Memorandum, Los Angeles District, Mar. 26, 1956; FDA Memorandum, Aug. 14, 1957; "Counterfeit Miltown & Equanil Tablets," and "Miami Drug Exchange: Report of R.T. Piper," Aug. 22, 1958, and "Memorandum of Meeting," Aug. 27, 1958, all in Manufacturers Files, AF19–503, Wallace Laboratories, FDA History Office. Letters to FDA, May 14, May 25, and June 20, 1960, and FDA reply of June 27, 1960, Manufacturers Files, AF19–503, Wallace Laboratories, FDA History Office. Schmidt, "What You Should Know About Those New 'Happiness Pills,'" 37.

27. Memo of A. E. Rayfield, Mar. 26, 1956, Manufacturers Files, AF 19–503, Wallace Laboratories, FDA History Office. Memo of Feb. 28, 1956, from Henry B. Packscher, and Memo of A. E. Rayfield, Mar. 26, 1956, both in Manufacturers Files, AF 19–503, Wallace Laboratories, FDA History Office.

28. Philip K. Scheuer, "Oscar Audience Sheds Real Tears—It's Smog," *Los Angeles Times,* Mar. 28, 1957, 2.

29. Whiteside, "Onward and Upward," 111, 119, 120. "It got to the point where all a . . . press agent had to do to get mention of a client in a column was to link the name up somehow with Miltown. . . . Our press clippings on Miltown so far fill eight huge, heavy scrapbooks, and they don't even include most of the wire service stories that appeared in a whole raft of papers," a Bates publicist recalled.

30. Berger, quoted in "The 'Social-Chemistry' of Pharmacological Discovery: The Miltown Story," *Social Pharmacology* 2 (1988): 189–204; Berger, interview by Andrea Tone.

CHAPTER 4

1. James Harvey Young, *The Toadstool Millionaires: A Social History of Patent Medicines in America Before Federal Regulation* (Princeton: Princeton University Press, 1961); Nancy Tomes, "The Great American Medicine Show Revisited," *Bulletin of the History of Medicine* 79 (2005): 633; Jeremy A. Greene, *Prescribing by Numbers: Drugs and the Definition of Disease* (Baltimore: Johns Hopkins University Press, 2007), 36–37; Jeremy A. Greene, "Attention to 'Details': Etiquette and the Pharmaceutical Salesman in Postwar America," *Social Studies of Science* 34 (Apr. 2004): 272.

2. Tomes, "Great American Medicine Show," 634.

3. John N. Wilford, "Medicine Men: Drug Makers Defend High Promotion Costs Against Senate Probers," *Wall Street Journal,* Jan. 27, 1960, 1; Greene, "Attention to 'Details,'" 271–272; Leo Bartemeier testimony, *False and Misleading Advertisements (Prescription Tranquilizing Drugs): Hearings Before a Subcommittee of the Committee of the Committee on Government Operations,* Eighty-fifth Congress, 2nd sess. (Washington, DC: Government Printing Office, 1958), 67–68; Mike Gorman testimony, *Study of Administered Prices in the Drug Industry,* Eighty-seventh Congress (Washington, DC: Government Printing Office, 1961), 8989–8993; Tomes, "Great American Medicine Show," 635. Alvin G. Brush testimony, *Administered Prices in the Drug Industry,* 9243–9244.

4. See, for instance, Daniel Carlat, "Dr. Drug Rep," *New York Times,* Nov. 25, 2007, 64–99; David Healy, *Let Them Eat Prozac* (New York: New York University Press, 2004). Mike Gorman, "Pharmaceutical Industry Must Join America," 12–13, U.S. Senate Antitrust and Monopoly Subcommittee, Washington, DC, Jan. 22, 1960. Mike Gorman Papers, 1946–1989. Speeches and Public Appearances, Box 11, Folder 7, Modern Manuscripts Collection, History of Medicine Division, National Library of Medicine, Bethesda, MD; MS C 462.

5. Frank Berger, autobiography, 60–61, 63–64, Frank Berger Manuscript Collection, International Archives of Neuro-Psychopharmacology, Vanderbilt University; Frank Berger, interview by Andrea Tone, July 2003.

6. Berger, autobiography, 61.

7. In 1965 Carter Products and Wallace Laboratories, a subsidiary of Carter since 1938, merged. H. P. Cragin, "Factory Visit," Apr. 13, 1955, Carter Products, Manufacturers Files, AF19–503, Wallace Laboratories, FDA History Office; Berger, interview by Andrea Tone.

8. Quoted in Thomas Whiteside, "Onward and Upward with the Arts: Getting There First with Tranquility," *New Yorker,* May 3, 1958, 120. As was customary for the time, the company had not engaged in the kind of premarketing blitz that today typically precedes a drug launch, whereby patients and doctors often learn about new drugs months or even years before they are approved for sale.

9. Whiteside, "Onward and Upward," 121. Barbara Moulton and Frank Berger, memorandum of telephone conversation, Feb. 7, 1956, Manufacturers Files, AF19–503, Wallace Laboratories, FDA History Office. Joseph A. Loftus, "Costs Held Small in Making Drugs: But the Miltown Producers Cite the Expense of Samples, Ads, and Promotions," *New York Times,* Jan. 27, 1960, 22.

10. Whiteside, "Onward and Upward," 111.

11. William Shakespeare, *Macbeth* 5.3; Whiteside, "Onward and Upward," 108.

12. Hoyt testimony, 9206; John N. Wilford, "Medicine Men: Drug Makers Defend High Promotion Costs Against Senate Probers," *Wall Street Journal,* Jan. 27, 1960, 1. Berger testimony, 9197; Carter Products, *Annual Report for the Year Ending Mar. 31, 1961,* AF19–503, Wallace Laboratories FDA History Office, Manufacturers Files, p. 12.

13. Whiteside, "Onward and Upward," 121.

14. Miltown ad in *American Journal of Psychiatry,* 116 (July 1959). On the recognized compatibility of pharmaceutical psychiatry and talk therapy, see also Nicolas Rasmussen, *On Speed,* chap. 5; and Jonathan Metzl, *Prozac on the Couch* (Durham, NC: Duke University Press, 2003).

15. Thomas Maier, *Dr. Spock: An American Life* (New York: Harcourt, Brace, 1998). Berger, interview by Andrea Tone.

16. "Tranquil Pills Stir Up Doctors," *Business Week,* June 28, 1958, 28–30; Eli Meyer and James Levin, "Tranquility Emphasis Growing in Dali's Work," *Sunday Star-Ledger,* May 31, 1959; John N. Wilford, "Medicine Men: Drug Makers Defend High Promotion Costs Against Senate Probers," *Wall Street Journal,* Jan. 27, 1960; Salvador Dali, *Crisalida,* Apr. 1958, Berger Scrapbooks, Vol. 3, Frank Berger Family Archives, New York City.

17. James Smart, "Dali and the Journey to Tranquility," n.d., Berger Scrapbooks, Vol. 3, Frank Berger Family Archives. Meyer and Levin, "Tranquility Emphasis."

18. "Tranquilizers—Successors to Aspirin?" *Chemical Week,* Aug. 25, 1956, 18. *Study of Administered Prices in the Drug Industry,* 8945, 8949, 9293; John Troan, "Best U.S. Money Makers: Drug Firms Lead Field," *Memphis Press,* Jan. 22, 1960.

19. On earlier somatic therapies for psychiatric illness, see Joel Braslow, *Mental Ills and Bodily Cures: Psychiatric Treatment in the First Half of the Twentieth Century* (Berkeley: University of California Press, 1997); and Edward Shorter, *A History of Psychiatry: From the Era of the Asylum to the Age of Prozac* (New York: Wiley, 1997), chaps. 3, 6–7; on the scientific credibility of lobotomy, see Jack Pressman, *Last Resort: Psychosurgery and the Limits of Medicine* (Cambridge: Cambridge University Press, 1988).

20. Andrea Tone, "Heinz Lehmann: There at the Revolution," *Collegium Internatinale Neuro-Psychopharmacologicum,* Mar. 2004, 16–17; Charles Cahn, "Heinz Edgar Lehmann, 1911–1999," *Proceedings of the Royal Society of Canada,* 6th series, vol. 12, 2001.

21. Heinz E. Lehman Manuscripts, Box 1, File 27, Box 4, File 3, and Box 39, File 5, International Archives of Neuro-Psychopharmacology; Tone, "Heinz Lehmann"; Heinz Lehmann, "Psychopharmcotherapy," in *The Psychopharmacologists,* ed. David Healy (London: Arnold, 1996), 159–186; Heinz Lehmann, "Reflections on a Career in Psychiatry," *Canadian Psychiatric Association Bulletin* 12, no. 4 (1980): 14–16.

22. Tone, "Heinz Lehmann"; Smith Kline & French Laboratories, *Ten Years' Experience with Thorazine* (Philadelphia: Smith Kline & French, 1964).

23. John W. Robinson, "A Chance for the Mentally Ill," *Science News Letter,* Apr. 27, 1957, 266; Matt Clark with Marina Gosnell, Dan Shapiro, Janet Huck, and William D. Marbath, "Drugs and Psychiatry," *Newsweek,* Nov. 12, 1979, 98. As Earl Ubell, science editor of the *New York Herald Tribune,* explained in a story that he wrote on the 1955 American Psychiatric Association meeting: "There is a revolution in psychiatry: a change of emphasis from psychology to biology. And the biological approach seems to be working." Ubell, quoted in Gorman, *Every Other Bed* (Cleveland: The World Publishing Company, 1956), 121.

24. European practitioners referred to drugs such as chlorpromazine and resperine as neuroleptics; in the United States they were called major tranquilizers and were less likely to be called antipsychotics. Semantic convergence—recognizing that both major tranquilizers and neuroleptics could be considered antipsychotics—occurred only in the 1990s. See David Healy, *The Creation of Psychopharmacology* (Cambridge: Harvard University Press, 2002), 99.

25. Gorman, *Every Other Bed,* 24. Sydney B. Self, "Tranquilizers: Mental Drug Use Grows Fast; Scientists Seek New, Better Products," *Wall Street Journal,* May 7, 1956, 1; Harold D. Watkins, "Probing the Mind: Scientists Speed New Drugs That May Help the Mentally Ill," *Wall Street Journal,* Mar. 5, 1959, 1. Cook, "The Happy Pills: Are They?"

26. Andrea Tone and Elizabeth Siegel Watkins, introduction, *Medicating Modern America: Prescription Drugs in History* (New York: New York University Press, 2007), 2–3.

27. Tone and Watkins, *Medicating Modern America,* 2–3.

28. Exhibit 10B, *False and Misleading Advertisements (Prescription Tranquilizing Drugs): Hearings Before a Subcommittee of the Committee of the Committee on Government Operations,* 215; Edward Shorter, *A Historical Dictionary of Psychiatry* (New York: Oxford University Press, 2005), 186–187. Mike Gorman, testimony, "Nationwide Evaluation of New Psychiatric Drugs is Urgent Need," Senate Appropriations Subcommittee on Labor-H.E.W.: Hearings on Fiscal 1957 Budget, May 9, 1956, Mike Gorman Papers, 1946–1989, Speeches and Public Appearances, Box 10, Folder 12, Modern Manuscripts Collection, History of Medicine Division, National Library of Medicine, Bethesda, MD; MS C 462. Watkins, "Probing the Mind," 1–2.

29. Testimony of Nathan S. Kline, *False and Misleading Advertisements (Prescription Tranquilizing Drugs): Hearings Before a Subcommittee of the Committee of the Committee on Government Operations,* 4.

30. See John Marks, *The Search for the Manchurian Candidate: The CIA and Mind Control, The Secret History of the Behavioral Sciences* (New York: Norton, 1979); Harvey Weinstein, *A Father, a Son, and the CIA* (Toronto: Lorimer, 1988); Anne Collins, *In the Sleep Room: The Story of the CIA Brainwashing Experiments in Canada* (Toronto: Lester & Orpen Dennys, 1988); Don Gilmore, *I Swear by Apollo: Dr. Ewen Cameron and the CIA-Brainwashing Experiments* (Montreal: Eden, 1987). Harold D. Watkins, "Drugs Sharpen Thinking, Lessen Anxieties: A New Weapon for Battlefield?" *Wall Street Journal,* Mar. 5, 1959, 1–2. Psychiatric engineering remains important to the U.S. military, especially since 9/11 and the war against terror. See Chapter 9 of this book. Jonathan D. Moreno, *Mind Wars: Brain Research and National Defense* (New York: Dana, 2006); Martin A. Lee and Bruce Shlain, *Acid Dreams: The Complete Social History of LSD, The CIA, The Sixties, and Beyond* (New York: Grove, 1985), 23–24.

31. Frank Ayd, "Discovery of Antidepressants," in *The Psychopharmacologists*, ed. David Healy (London: Chapman & Hall, 1996) 88; David Healy, *The Antidepressant Era* (Cambridge: Harvard University Press, 1997), 65. Ayd, quoted in Shorter, *History of Psychiatry*, 316.

32. Wallace Laboratories, *Miltown, The Tranquilizer with Muscle Relaxant Action: Physicians' Reference Manual*, 4th ed. (Wallace Laboratories, 1958), 49; Charles Brutzner, "Grave Peril Seen in Sleeping Pills," *New York Times*, Dec. 16, 1951, 1. Frank Ayd testimony, in *False and Misleading Advertising*, 48.

33. Francis Bello, "The Tranquilizer Question," *Fortune*, May 1957, 164. "Sobering Up," *Newsweek*, Jan. 9, 1956, 64–65.

34. Frank Ayd testimony, in *False and Misleading Advertising*, 49. Kline, quoted in "Soothing, But Not for Businessmen," *Business Week*, Mar. 10, 1956, 32.

35. Raymond B. Cattell and Ivan H. Scheier, "The Nature of Anxiety: A Review of Thirteen Multivariate Analyses Comprising 814 Variables," *Psychological Reports* 4 (1958): 351.

36. New York Academy of Medicine, Committee on Public Health Minutes, 1956, 174–175, 179, 181–184, 200–202, 210–213. "Report on Tranquilizing Drugs by the Committee on Public Health of the New York Academy of Medicine," *Bulletin of Academy of Medicine*, Apr. 1957, 282–289. "Tranquilizers and Ethics," *America*, Oct. 11, 1958, 32.

37. "Tranquilizers Threat Cited," *Los Angeles Examiner*, Nov. 4, 1957. Kennedy, quoted in A. E. Hotchner, "Can Mood Pills Really Help You?" *Los Angeles Times*, Aug. 19, 1956, 28.

38. Biochemist Paul Saltman, quoted in "Dash of Anxiety Plays Part in Genius, Scientist Declares," *Los Angeles Examiner*, Mar. 23, 1958.

39. Lehmann, quoted in *Administered Prices*, 9029, 9053.

40. "The American Forum" (NBC): "Tranquilizer Drugs: Blessing or Danger?" July 8, 1956, Mike Gorman Papers, 1946–1989. Speeches and Public Appearances, Box 10, Folder 15, Modern Manuscripts Collection, History of Medicine Division, National Library of Medicine, Bethesda, MD; MS C 462. Thomas Doherty, *Cold War, Cool Medium: Television, McCarythism, and American Culture* (New York: Columbia University Press, 2003), 17.

41. Healy, *Creation of Psychopharmacology*, 98–99.

42. "The Mind: Science's Search for a Guide to Sanity," *Newsweek*, Oct. 24, 1955, 61; Nathan G. Hale Jr., "From Berggassee XIX to Central Park West: The Americanization of Psychoanalysis, 1919–1940," *Journal of the History of the Behavioral Sciences* 14 (1978): 299–315; Lehmann, "Psychopharmacotherapy," 159–186.

43. Stephen Stahl, interview by Andrea Tone, Dec. 13, 2004, transcript of oral history in International Archives of Neuro-Psychopharmacology.

44. "The Mind: Science's Search for a Guide to Sanity," *Newsweek*, Oct. 24, 1955, 61. Solomon H. Snyder, *Drugs and the Brain* (New York: Scientific American Library, 1986), 155.

45. Donald G. Cooley, "The New Nerve Pills and Your Health," *Cosmopolitan*, Jan. 1956, 70–74.

46. Bernard D. Nossiter, "Two Tranquilizer Firms Face Antitrust Charges," *Washington Post*, A18. The pattern of having nonpsychiatrists prescribe tranquilizers intensified with the advent of benzodiazepines. See Deborah Larned, "Do You Take Valium," *Ms.* 4 (1975): 27; "Tightening the Lid on Legal Drugs," *Science News*, June 14, 1975, 382.

CHAPTER 5

1. Anthony Leviero, "U.S. Reaction Firm: President Does Not Say Soviet Union Has an Atomic Bomb, Picks Words Carefully, But He Implies Our Absolute Dominance in New

Weapons Has Virtually Ended," *New York Times,* Sept. 24, 1949, 1–2; David Halberstam, *The Fifties* (New York: Villard, 1993), 24–30.

2. Leviero, "U.S. Reaction Firm," 1–2.

3. Leviero, "U.S. Reaction Firm," 1–2. Paul Boyer, *By the Bomb's Early Light: American Thought and Culture at the Dawn of the Atomic Age* (New York: Pantheon, 1985), 336.

4. Paul S. Boyer, Clifford E. Clark Jr., Joseph F. Kett, Neal Salisbury, Harvard Sitkoff, and Nancy Woloch, *The Enduring Vision: A History of the American People* (Boston: Houghton Mifflin, 2000), 2:798.

5. George Gallup, "7,000,000 in U.S. Use 'Happy Pills,'" *Los Angeles Times,* Mar. 18, 1957; George H. Gallup, *The Gallup Poll: Public Opinion 1935–1971,* vol. 2, *1949–1958* (New York: Random House, 1972), 1475–1476. Francis Bello, "The Tranquilizer Question," *Fortune,* May 1957, 162–188. *New York Post,* Jan. 22, 1957, 36.

6. "Ideal in Tranquility," *Newsweek,* Oct. 29, 1956. *New York Post,* Jan. 24, 1957, 4.

7. Andrea Tone and Elizabeth Siegel Watkins, introduction to *Medicating Modern America* (New York: New York University Press, 2007), 6–7. Roy Porter, "The Patient's View: Doing Medical History From Below," *Theory and Society* 14 (1985): 189. Also see Nancy Tomes, "The Great American Medicine Show Revisited," *Bulletin of the History of Medicine* 79 (2005); and Nancy Tomes, "Merchants of Health: Medicine and Consumer Culture in the United States, 1900–1940," *Journal of American History* 88 (Sept. 2001): 519–547. Hoyt, quoted in Thomas Whiteside, "Onward and Upward with the Arts: Getting There First with Tranquility," *New Yorker,* May 3, 1958, 122.

8. Chapman Pincher, "Here—the Drug that Swept America," *London Daily Press,* July 5, 1956, Berger Scrapbooks, Vol. 1, Frank Berger Family Archives, New York City. Whiteside, "Onward and Upward," 109. "Happiness by Prescription," *Time,* Mar. 11, 1957, 59. Letter from Harvey J. Sachs to Ms. Magazine Corporation, Dec. 10, 1975, Carton 3. Folder 66. Letters to *Ms.* Magazine. Schlesinger Library, Radcliffe Institute, Harvard University.

9. "'Miltown' Drug Output Raised," *Journal of Commerce,* May 8, 1956, 12; "Pill vs Worry—How Goes the Frantic Quest for Calm in Frantic Lives," *Newsweek,* May 21, 1956, 68–70; "Don't-Give-a-Damn Pills," *Time,* Feb. 27, 1956, 68–70; "The Tranquilizer Question," 162–188. Weldon Wallace, "Doctors See Peace-of-Mind Pills As No Final Solution," *Baltimore Sun,* May 22, 1956; Whiteside, "Onward and Upward," 118. Quoted in La Fay, "All Wound Up? Here's a New Drug to Calm You Down," *Town Journal,* May 1956, 72.

10. David Sears Houston, "Hollywood's Latest Pill Kick: 'Don't-Give-a-Damn' Drugs," *Top Secret,* July 1956, 12.

11. Elaine Tyler May, *Homeward Bound* (New York: Basic, 1999), 23.

12. "Radio Listeners in Panic, Taking War Drama as Fact: Many Flee Homes to Escape 'Gas Raid from Mars,'" *New York Times,* Oct. 31, 1938, 1; Orrin E. Dunlap Jr., "Message from Mars: Radio Learns That Melodrama Dressed Up as a Current Event Is Dangerous," *New York Times,* Nov. 6, 1938, 184. For a an insightful and illuminating analysis and rendition of the cold war political theater of panic management, see Jackie Orr, *Panic Diaries: A Genealogy of Panic Disorder* (Durham, NC: Duke University Press, 2006), 33–78.

13. Andrew D. Grossman, *Neither Dead Nor Red: Civilian Defense and American Political Development During the Early Cold War* (New York: Routledge, 2001), 59–62. Also see Guy Oakes, *The Imaginary War: Civil Defense and American Cold War Culture* (New York: Oxford University Press, 1994).

14. Kenneth D. Rose, *One Nation Underground: The Fallout Shelter in American Culture* (New York: New York University Press, 2001), 126–140.

15. Federal Civil Defense Administration, *Bert the Turtle Says Duck and Cover,* Archer Productions, 1951; Rose, *One Nation Underground,* 128–129. The film can be viewed at the Internet Archive, www.archive.org/details/DuckandC1951.

16. Grossman, *Neither Dead Nor Red,* pp. 62–65.

17. Whiteside, "Onward and Upward," 104. "Baby Pup Tent," *Newsweek,* Jan. 9, 1956, 64.

18. Rose, *One Nation Underground,* 79; civil defense film referenced in Devin Rafferty, Jayne Loader, and Pierce Raferty, *The Atomic Café* (The Archives Project: 1982), produced and directed by Kevin Rafferty, Jayne Lodern, Pierce Rafferty. I am grateful to Liz Watkins for this reference. *Dr. Strangelove or: How I Learned to Stop Worrying and Love the Bomb* (1964).

19. Paul S. Boyer et al., *The Enduring Vision: A History of the American People* (Boston: Houghton Mifflin, 2000), vol. 2:822–823.

20. Lizabeth Cohen, *A Consumers' Republic: The Politics of Mass Consumption in Postwar America* (New York: Vintage, 2003); James T. Patterson, *Grand Expectations: The United States, 1945–1974* (New York: Oxford University Press, 1996), 315–316.

21. Antonia Zerbisias, "Why Do Women Turn to Pills so Often?" *Toronto Star,* July 9, 2007.

22. "The Mind: Science's Search for a Guide to Sanity," *Newsweek,* Oct. 24, 1955, 61. Of the country's approximately 200,000 practicing doctors in 1955, fewer than 9,500 were psychiatrists. Of these, more than half were devoted full-time to institutional care. That left about 4,000 private-practice psychiatrists to care for the mental health needs of more than 100 million adults. Safeway prices from the *New York Post,* Jan. 3, 1967, 3F; *Weekly Pharmacy Reports,* Feb. 8, 1960, Berger Scrapbooks, Vol. 4, Frank Berger Family Archives. Testifying in 1960 before the Senate Subcommittee on Administered Prices in the Drug Industry (Tranquilizers), Henry Hoyt calculated that the cost of a single tablet of Miltown was about 10.6 cents, "about the price of a cup of coffee or a candy bar. The average dose of three tablets a day, or a total cost of 31.8 cents a day, is comparable to the price of a pack of cigarettes or a gallon of gasoline." Hoyt, *Hearings before the Subcommittee on Antitrust and Monopoly of the Committee on the Judiciary,* pt. 16, *Administered Prices in the Drug Industry: Tranquilizers* (Washington, DC: Government Printing Office, 1960), 9110.

23. Elizabeth Haiken, *Venus Envy: A History of Cosmetic Surgery* (Baltimore, MD: Johns Hopkins University Press, 1997), 134–155; May, *Homeward Bound,* 14, 24, 27.

24. Walter C. Alvarez, "Do You Worry Too Much?" *Ladies Home Journal,* July 1956, 51.

25. Roland Berg, "The Unhappy Facts About 'Happy Pills,'" *Look,* July 24, 1956. In one study conducted by Frank Ayd, frigid women "who abhorred marital relations reported they responded more readily to their husbands' advances." Quoted in Cooley, "The New Nerve Pills and Your Health," *Cosmopolitan,* Jan. 1956, 70. Also see Jonathan Metzl, "Mother's Little Helper: The Crisis of Psychoanalysis and the Miltown Resolution," *Gender and History* 15, no. 2 (Aug. 2003): 240–267.

26. George Gallup, "7,000,000 in U.S. Use 'Happy Pills,'" *Los Angeles Times,* Mar. 18, 1957. "Sedative Keeps Junior Quiet in Dental Chair," *Oakland Tribune,* Apr. 25, 1956.

27. Peter D. Kramer, *Listening to Prozac: A Psychiatrist Explores Anitdepressant Drugs and the Remaking of the Self* (New York: Viking, 1993), 39. "Tranquilizers were developed in the 1950s in response to a need that physicians explicitly saw as female," historian Stephanie Coontz writes in her otherwise careful analysis of 1950s family ideals and gender roles. Stephanie Coontz, *The Way We Never Were: American Families and the Nostalgia Trap* (New York: Basic Books, 2000), 36. Also see Metzl, "Mother's Little Helper," 240–267, which focuses on the feminization of tranquilizer use in the 1950s. Andrea Tone, "Listening to the

Past: History, Psychiatry, and Anxiety," *Canadian Journal of Psychiatry* 50, no 7 (June 2005): 376–377.

28. Because comprehensive surveys of tranquilizer use were not done until the 1960s, we cannot be certain of the exact demographic breakdown of tranquilizer consumption.

29. W. H. Auden, *The Age of Anxiety: A Baroque Eclogue* (New York: Random House, 1947), 4. In Auden's poem, four strangers—Malin, Rosetta, Emble, and Quant—meet by chance in a Manhattan bar during World War II on the Night of All Souls. After passing the night exploring possible routes to psychological fulfillment and spiritual meaning, they go their separate ways at daybreak. K. A. Cuordileone, *Manhood and American Political Culture in the Cold War* (New York: Routledge, 2005), 138. David Riesman, Nathan Glazer, and Reuel Denney, *The Lonely Crowd: A Study of the Changing American Character* (New York: Doubleday Anchor, 1950), 32–45, 133–141, 348–349; quote is on p. 139. On anxiety as a cultural idiom of the 1950s, see Cuordileone, *Manhood*, ix, 97–110, 134–145; K. A. Cuordileone, "Politics in the Age of Anxiety: Cold War Political Culture and the Crisis in American Masculinity, 1949–1960," *Journal of American History*, Sept. 2000; and James Gilbert, *Men in the Middle: Searching for Masculinity in the 1950s* (Chicago: University of Chicago Press, 2005).

30. Bello, "Tranquilizer Question," 164.

31. Henry Hoyt testimony, *Hearings Before the Subcommittee on Antitrust and Monopoly of the Committee on the Judiciary United States Senate*, pt. 16, *Administered Prices in the Drug Industry* (Washington, DC: Government Printing Office, 1960), 9110. Roche Laboratories, *Aspects of Anxiety*, 2nd and enl. ed. (Philadelphia: Lippincott, 1965), 88. J. B. Roerig, *The Relaxed Wife*, 1957.

32. Bello, "Tranquilizer Question." "Pill vs. Worry: How Goes the Frantic Quest for Calm in Frantic Lives?" *Newsweek*, May 21, 1956, 162–188. Victor Schmidt, "What You Should Know About Those New 'Happiness' Pills," *Uncensored*, Oct. 25, 1957, 60–62.

33. Howard La Fay, "All Wound Up? Here's a New Drug to Calm You Down," *Town Journal*, May 1956, 72.

34. "Report: JFK Suffered More Pain, Ailments Than Revealed; President Took as Many as 8 Medications a Day," *Washington Post*, Nov. 18, 2002, A3; "The J.F.K. File," *New York Times*, Nov. 19, 2002, A30; Tracy Connor, "JFK Popped Lots of Pills," *New York Daily News*, Nov. 17, 2002, 3; Tim Reid, "JFK Had to Fight Pain Every Day," *London Times*, Nov. 18, 2002, 15.

35. "Happiness by Prescription," *Time*, Mar. 11, 1957. "Tranquil Tales: Senate Hears of Valium Woes," *Time*, Sept. 24 1979, 78.

36. "'Ideal' in Tranquility," *Newsweek*, Oct. 29, 1956, 63–64. Jess Raley, "That Wonderful Frustrated Feeling," *American Mercury* 85, no. 402 (July 1957: 22; "Army Grounds Aviators for Using Tranquilizers," *Los Angeles Times*, Apr. 21, 1957, 15. A few years later, after a tranquilized pilot flying a Piedmont Airlines DC-33 crashed into a Virginia mountainside killing twenty-three passengers and three crewmen, the Federal Aviation Agency ruled that commercial pilots taking tranquilizers must be automatically grounded. "What You Should Know About Tranquilizers," *Reader's Digest*, July 1962.

37. Military Medical Supply Agency report, Subcommittee on Antitrust and Monopoly of the Committee on the Judiciary, U.S. Senate, *Administered Price in the Drug Industry (Tranquilizers)* (Washington: Government Printing Office, 1960), 16:9188. VA data from Subcommittee on Antitrust and Monopoly of the Committee on the Judiciary, U.S. Senate, *Administered Price in the Drug Industry (Tranquilizers)* (Washington, DC: Government Printing Office, 1960), 16:9189.

38. Athletes have long used prescription and nonprescription agents to enhance performance. Keith Wailoo, "Old Story, Updated: Better Living Through Pills," *New York Times,* Nov. 13, 2007, F5.

39. Jack Pickering, "Happy Pills: Use with Care, Say Physicians," May 19, 1957, in Berger Scrapbooks, Vol. 3, Frank Berger Family Archives.

40. Pickering, "Happy Pills."

41. Oscar Fraley, "Tension-Easing Miltowns Relax Major Leagues," *New York Daily News,* May 18, 1957. Pickering, "Happy Pills." "Sugar Ray's Aide Confirms Injury," *Los Angeles Times,* Apr. 28, 1957, D4.

42. Pickering, "Happy Pills"; "Sports Medicine Group to Probe Pep Pill Use," *Los Angeles Times,* June 9, 1957, D2. Fraley, "Tension-Easing Miltowns."

43. Kefauver testimony, *Hearings Before the Subcommittee on Antitrust and Monopoly of the Committee on the Judiciary United States Senate,* pt. 16, *Administered Prices in the Drug Industry: Tranquilizers,* 9188, 9421.

CHAPTER 6

1. Edward Shorter, *A History of Psychiatry: From the Era of the Asylum to the Age of Prozac* (New York: Wiley, 1997): 202–203, 315. Irvin Cohen, "The Benzodiazepines," in *Discoveries in Biological Psychiatry,* ed. Frank J. Ayd and Barry Blackwell (Philadelphia: Lippincott, 1970), 130. Andrea Tone, "Listening to the Past: History, Psychiatry, and Anxiety," *Canadian Journal of Psychiatry* 50, no. 7 (June 2005): 377.

2. Hans Conrad Peyer, *Roche: A Company History, 1896–1996* (Basel: Roche, 1996), 15–30; Philip Revzin and Margaret Studer, "Hoffman-La Roche Bid Aims at Growth," *Wall Street Journal,* Jan. 7, 1988, 8, www.roche/com/home/company/com_hist.htm (accessed Apr. 23, 2008); "Hoffmann-La Roche World-Wide Results Given for First Time," *Wall Street Journal,* June 10, 1974, 6.

3. Peyer, *Roche,* 29, 45, 48–49, 61–63, 88, 382; Revzin and Studer, "Hoffmann-La Roche Bid," 8, www.roche/com/home/company/history (accessed Jan. 31, 2007).

4. Peyer, *Roche,* 61–63, 382, 385; Rezin and Studer, "Hoffmann-La Roche Bid," 8, www.roche/com/home/company/history (accessed Jan. 31, 2007).

5. Rima A. Apple, *Vitamania: Vitamins in American Culture* (Piscataway, NJ: Rutgers University Press, 1996), 2–11. Peyer, *Roche,* 121–127; 382–383; 385–388, www.roche/com/home/company/history (accessed Jan. 31, 2007); Leo H. Sternbach, interview by Tonja Koeppel, Mar. 12, 1986, Hoffmann-La Roche, Nutley, NJ; Oral History Collection of the Beckman Center for the History of Chemistry, 19.

6. Peyer, *Roche,* 146–150.

7. Peyer, *Roche,* 146–153; Lois Redisch, "Nutley," *New Jersey Sunday Herald,* Oct. 22, 1989, 18; Paul J. Cardinal, "Hoffmann-La Roche Inc.," in *Nutley: Yesterday and Today,* 330–333 (with thanks to the Nutley New Jersey Chamber of Commerce for their help in identifying this source); Alex Baenninger et al., *Good Chemistry: The Life and Legacy of Valium Inventor Leo Sternbach* (New York: McGraw-Hill, 2004), 34–35, www.roche/com/home/company/history (accessed Jan. 31, 2007).

8. Baenninger et al., *Good Chemistry,* 9. Leo Sternbach, interview by Andrea Tone, May 18, 2005, Chapel Hill, NC; Baenninger et al., *Good Chemistry,* 16. Leo Sternbach, interview by Koeppel, 5–6.

9. The quote is from Dr. Joseph Hellerbach.

10. Alex Baenninger et al., *Good Chemistry*, 12. Maureen Rouhi, "At 90, Inventor of Librium, Valium Is Still in Love with Chemistry," *Chemical and Engineering News*, June 29, 1988, 83. Sternbach, interview by Koeppel, 12.

11. Baenninger et al., *Good Chemistry*, 26; Lloyd Shearer, "Dr. and Mrs. Leo Sternbach—He's the Man Who Invented Valium," *Parade*, June 27, 1976, 8–10. Julia Flynn, "In Two Generations, Drug Research Sees a Big Shift," *Wall Street Journal*, Feb. 11, 2004, 1.

12. Baenninger et al., *Good Chemistry*, 28–29.

13. Rouhi, "Inventor of Librium," 83. Sternbach, interview by Koeppel, 22.

14. Sternbach, interview by Tone, 11, 44–45. Peyer, *Roche*, 130. Quote is from B. D. Colen, "Adventurous Chemist and His Pill," *Washington Post*, Jan. 20, 1980, A18. Also see Leo Sternbach, "The Benzodiazepine Story," *Journal of Medicinal Chemistry*, Jan. 1979, 1. Dilip Ramchandani, "The Librium Story," *Psychiatric News* 5 (Oct. 2, 1998): 21; Cohen, "Benzodiazepines," 132; "Leo Sternbach, 1908–2005," *Montreal Gazette*, Sept. 29, 2005, 7; Rouhi, "Inventor of Librium"; Sternbach, interview by Koeppel, 24–25.

15. Marcia Angell, *The Truth About the Drug Companies: How They Deceive Us and What to Do About It* (New York: Random House, 2004), xvi, 16–17, 73–76, 79–80. Quote is from page 73. Also see Ray Moynihan and Alan Cassels, *Selling Sickness: How the World's Biggest Pharmaceutical Companies Are Turning Us All into Patients* (Vancouver: Greystone, 2005). Stephen S. Hall, "Prescription for Profit," *New York Times Magazine*, Mar. 11, 2001, 40–45, 59, 91–92, 100. The recent case of Nexium illuminates the corporate choreography involved. AstraZeneca introduced Nexium when its top-selling heartburn medication, Prisolec, which had earned the company $26 billion in a single five-year stretch, was scheduled to go off patent in Apr. 2001. Prisolec was made up of two "isomers," two parts of the same omeprazole molecule. Company scientists cut the molecule into two. The single-isomer offspring was christened Nexium and began to be sold in Mar. 2001, at the whopping price of $125 for a month's supply. The price signaled state-of-the-art innovation, and the company spent half a billion dollars to promote its new purple pill as a powerful weapon in the war against erosive esophagitis and acid reflux disease. In fact, Nexium offered patients no clear health advantage over its predecessor but was widely purchased at more than twice the price. Malcolm Gladwell, "High Prices: How to Think About Prescription Drugs," *New Yorker*, Oct. 25, 2004, 86–90; Angell, *Truth*, 76–79.

16. Sternbach, quoted in Colen, "Adventurous Chemist," A18; Angell, *Truth*, 80. Sternbach, "The Benzodiazepine Story," *Journal of Medicinal Chemistry*, Jan. 1979. Sternbach, interview by Koeppel, 39.

17. Milton Moskowitz, "Librium: A Marketing Case History," *Drug and Cosmetic Industry* 87 (Oct. 1960): 4, 460; Thomas Whiteside, "Onward and Upward with the Arts: Getting There First with Tranquility," *New Yorker*, May 3, 1958, 104.

18. Flynn, "Big Shift Two Generations Drug Research," 1. Sternbach, interview by Koeppel, 39.

19. Sternbach, interview by Tone, 11, 13; "Benzodiazepine Story," 1; Colen, "Adventurous Chemist"; Rouhi, "Inventor of Librium," 83; Sternbach, interview by Koeppel, 25, 26. Shearer, "Dr. and Mrs. Leo Sternbach," June 27, 1976.

20. Sternbach, quoted in Colen, "Adventurous Chemist." Cohen, "Benzodiazepines," 132; Sternbach, interview by Koeppel, 25–26. "Amine," *Encyclopedia Brittanica 2007*, www.britannica.com/eb/article-9007181.

21. Sternbach, interview by Koeppel, 26; Colen, "Adventurous Chemist." Cohen, "Benzodiazepines," 132; Stephen Miller, "Valium Inventor, Earl Reeder, 79," *New York Sun*, Oct. 20, 2003, 9.

22. Sternbach, "Benzodiazepine Story," 2. Miller, "Valium Inventor," 9; Cohen, "Benzodiazepines," 132; Colen, "Adventurous Chemist," A18.

23. "Mental Drug Shows Promise," *New York Times*, Apr. 7, 1957, 195; David Healy, *Let Them Eat Prozac* (Toronto: Lorimer, 2003), 37–38; "Hoffman-La Roche Discovers New Drug for Mental Patients," *Wall Street Journal*, Apr. 8, 1957, 10. In 1957, Swedish neuroscientist Arvid Carlsson submitted work on the role of dopamine as a neurotransmitter. In the same year, Bernard Brodie and Parkhurst Shore suggested that serotonin might have a similar role to play in the regulation of mental illness. Edward Shorter, *A Historical Dictionary of Psychiatry* (New York: Oxford University Press, 2005), 195. Letter from V.W. Smart, assistant director of Division of Regulatory Management, Bureau of Enforcement, Dec. 13, 1961, Manufacturers Files, AF14–324, Hoffman-La Roche, FDA History Office; "Hoffman-La Roche Discovers New Drug," 10; "Hoffman-La Roche, Inc., Drops Anti-Depression Drug from its Line," *Wall Street Journal*, Feb. 7, 1961, 21; Peyer, *Roche*, 172.

24. Randall, quoted in Lowell O. Randall, "Pharmacology of Methaminodiazepoxide," *Diseases of the Nervous System*, Mar. 1960, 7, 8; Sternbach, "Benzodiazepine Story," 2; Note from Max Fink to Andrea Tone, June 6, 2005, in author's possession; Cohen, "Benzodiazepines," 132; Colen, "Adventurous Chemist," A18. Nick Paumgarten, "Little Helper," *New Yorker*, June 16, 2003, 70. Solomon H. Snyder, *Drugs and the Brain* (New York: Scientific American Books, 1986), 160.

25. Edmond H. Drummond, *Benzo Blues: Overcoming Anxiety Without Tranquilizers* (New York: Plume, 1998), 85–86.

26. See, for instance, Peter Keating and Alberto Cambrosio, *Biomedical Platforms: Realigning the Normal and the Pathological in Late-Nineteenth-Century Medicine* (Cambridge: MIT Press, 2003); and Thomas Schlich, "The Art and Science of Surgery: Innovation and Concepts of Medical Practice in Operative Fracture Care, 1960s–1970s," *Science, Technology & Human Values* 32, no. 1 (Jan. 2007): 1–23. Alfred Pletscher, interview by Andrea Tone, June 2004; transcript in International Archives of Neuro-Psychopharmacology, Vanderbilt University. For further perspectives on novelty and the importance of historicizing innovation, see Keating and Cambrosio, *Biomedical Platforms*; Jennifer R. Fishman, "Making Viagra: From Impotence to Erectile Dysfunction," in Andrea Tone and Elizabeth Siegel Watkins, eds., *Medicating Modern America: Prescription Drugs in History* (New York: New York University Press, 2007), 229–252; and Nicholas B. King, "Infectious Disease in a World of Goods" (Ph.D. diss., Harvard University, 2001). Although psychopharmacologists have acknowledged Randall's importance, they have ignored Earl Reeder's contributions. The New Jersey–born Reeder attended school in Norway and spent time in a Nazi labor camp before returning to the United States and enrolling in college on the GI Bill. Hired in 1952 without a Ph.D., he worked at Sternbach's side for decades and considered himself Librium (and later Valium's) coinventor. His name appears on thirty patents, including the patent for Valium. Still, Roche did not value Reeder's laboratory or public relations contributions enough to retain him. Projecting diminished revenues from the loss of Valium's patent protection, Hoffman-La Roche announced in Jan. 1985 that it would dismiss about 1,000 employees to trim operations costs by $50 million. Reeder was one of those laid off. He was incensed. "I made Librium. I made Valium," he fumed. "Do you call this a reward?" The sixty-one-year-old filed a lawsuit against Roche for age discrimination. The company settled, agreeing to pay Reeder his normal salary until his regular retirement date. Reeder died in relative obscurity on Oct. 13, 2003. His story shows that how we tell

the history of pharmaceutical innovation can have profound consequences for those who find themselves marginalized in narratives of medical and technological discovery. Miller, "Valium Inventor, Earl Reeder," 9; Reeder's commentary on his relationship with Sternbach is documented in Baenninger et al., *Good Chemistry*, 59–60; "Hoffmann-La Roche to Cut Work Force by 9% in Bid to Lower Operating Costs," *Wall Street Journal*, Jan. 29, 1985, 10; "Dr. Lowell O. Randall Honoured on the Occasion of his 80th Birthday," *Roche International Information*, July 1991, 1, 7. I am grateful to John Randall to sharing this article with me.

27. See, for instance, Erika Dyck, "Flashback: Psychiatric Experimentation with LSD in Historical Perspective," *Canadian Journal of Psychiatry* 50 (June 2005): 381–387. Flynn, "In Two Generations," 1. Sternbach's self-experiment is detailed in Colen, "Adventurous Chemist," A18. U.S. Patent and Trademark Office, patent 2,893,992, patented July 7, 1959.

28. Moskowitz, "Librium," 461.

29. David Armstrong, "The Rise of Surveillance Medicine," in *The Sociology and Politics of Health: A Reader*, ed. M. Purdy and D. Banks (New York: Routledge, 2001); Noeimi R. Tousignant, "Pain and the Pursuit of Objectivity: Pain-Measuring Technologies in the United States, c. 1890–1975" (Ph.D. diss., McGill University, 2006); Geoffrey Bowker, *Sorting Things Out: Classification and Its Consequences* (Cambridge: MIT Press, 1999); Lorraine Daston, "Objectivity and the Escape From Perspective," *Social Studies of Science* 22 (Nov. 1992): 597–618; Harry M. Marks, "Trust and Mistrust in the Marketplace: Statistics and Clinical Research, 1945–1960," *History of Science* 38 (Sept. 2000): 343–355; George Weisz and Annick Opinel, eds., *Body Counts: Medical Quantification in Historical and Sociological Perspective* (Montreal: Foundation Merieux/McGill-Queen's University Press, 2005). Earlier well-known anxiety scales included Janet Taylor's *Scale of Manifest Anxiety* published in 1953 and Cattell's *Institute for Personality and Ability Testing* (IPAT) anxiety scale, published in 1957. See Janet A. Taylor, "A Personality Scale of Manifest Anxiety," *Journal of Abnormal and Social Psychology* 48 (1953): 285–290; and R. B. Cattell, *Handbook for the IPAT Anxiety Scale* (Champaign, IL: Institute for Personality and Ability Testing, 1957); Max Hamilton, "The Assessment of Anxiety States by Rating," *British Journal of Medical Psychology* 32 (1959): 50–55; M. Roth, "Max Hamilton: A Life Devoted to Psychiatric Science," in *The Hamilton Scales*, ed. Per Bech and Alec Coppen (Berlin: Springer-Verlag, 1990), 4–5; Tom Ban, personal communication with Andrea Tone, Jan. 25, 2008; David Healy, personal communication with Andrea Tone, Mar. 30, 2006. Hoffman-La Roche, *Aspects of Anxiety* (Philadelphia: Lippincott, 1965), 62–69.

30. Cohen, "Benzodiazepines," 133.

31. Joseph M. Tobin, Ivan F. Bird, and Daniel E. Boyle, "Preliminary Evaluation of Librium (Ro 5–0690) in the Treatment of Anxiety Reactions," *Diseases of the Nervous System* 21 (Mar. 1960): 11–19; H. Angus Bowes, "The Role of Librium in an Out-Patient Psychiatric Setting," *Diseases of the Nervous System* 21 (Mar. 1960): 20–22; John Kinross-Wright, Irvin M. Cohen, and James A. Knight, "The Management of Neurotic and Psychotic States with Ro 5–0690 (Librium)," *Diseases of the Nervous System* 21 (Mar. 1960): 23–26; Harry H. Farb, "Experience with Librium in Clinical Psychiatry," *Diseases of the Nervous System* 21 (Mar. 1960): 27–35; Titus H. Harris, "Methaminodiazepoxide," *Journal of the American Medical Association*, Mar. 12, 1960, 1162–1164; Titus H. Harris and Irvin M. Cohen, "Effects of Chlordiazepoxide on Psychoneurotic Symptoms," *American Practitioner and Digest of Treatment* 11 (Dec. 1960): 999–1002; David C. English, "Librium, A New Non-Sedative Neuroleptic Drug: A Clinical Evaluation," *Current Therapeutic Research* 2 (Mar. 1960): 38–91. On the capacity

of pharmaceutical firms to create drug markets in advance of FDA approval, see Jennifer Fishman, "Manufacturing Desire: The Commodification of Female Sexual Dysfunction," *Social Studies of Science* 34 (Apr. 2004): 187–218.

32. Kinross-Wright, Cohen, and Knight, "Management of Neurotic and Psychotic States," 23–26. David J. Rothman, *Strangers at the Bedside* (New York: Basic, 1991), 53; Allen M. Hornblum, "They Were Cheap and Available: Prisoners as Research Subjects in Twentieth Century America," *British Medical Journal*, Nov. 29, 1997, 1437–1441. Pharmaceutical company quote is from page 1439. Cohen, "Benzodiazepines," 135.

33. New Drug Application 12–249 for Librium Hydrochloride Tablets, FDA Records, discussed in Suzanne White Junod and Lara Marks, "Approval of the First Oral Contraceptive," *Journal of the History of Medicine* 57 (Apr. 2002): 149–150; William D'Aguanno of the FDA Division of Pharmacology to J. D. Archer, FDA New Drug Branch, Apr. 7, 1961, Manufacturers Files, AF14–324, Hoffman-La Roche, FDA History Office. William L. Laurence, "Help for Mental Ills: Reports on Tests of Synthetic Drug Say the Results Are Promising," *New York Times*, Feb. 28, 1960, E9; Moskowitz, "Librium," 461.

34. Bowes, "Role of Librium," 21. Farb, "Experience with Librium in Clinical Psychiatry," 28–30.

35. Kinross-Wright et al., "Management of Neurotic and Psychotic States," 25. Laurence, "Help for Mental Ills," E9. Hoffman-La Roche, *Aspects of Anxiety* (Philadelphia: Lippincott, 1965).

36. Junod and Marks, "Approval of the First Oral Contraceptive," 149. Titus M. Harris, "Methaminodiazepoxide," *Journal of the American Medical Association*, Mar. 12, 1960, 1162.

37. For a discussion of studies that enabled scientists to understand the mechanisms of benzodiazepines, see Chapter 8.

38. Moskowitz, "Librium," 461, 566; Stuart Elliott, "McAdams Forms Division on Latest Drugs," *New York Times*, Dec. 16, 1991, D9.

39. Herbert G. Lawson, "New-Drug Slowdown," *Wall Street Journal*, Mar. 26, 1963, 1; Andrea Tone, "Tranquilizers on Trial: Psychopharmacology in the Age of Anxiety," in *Medicating Modern America: Prescription Drugs in History*, ed. Andrea Tone and Elizabeth Siegel Watkins (New York: New York University Press, 2007), 167; Moskowitz, "Librium," 460–461, 566. Librium package insert, Manufacturers Files, AF14–324, Hoffman-La Roche, FDA History Office; William D'Aguanno of the FDA Division of Pharmacology to J. D. Archer, FDA New Drug Branch, Apr. 7, 1961, Manufacturers Files, AF14–324, Hoffman-La Roche, FDA History Office.

40. FDA History Office, Librium package insert, Manufacturers Files, AF14–324, Hoffman-La Roche, FDA History Office. Tone, "Tranquilizers on Trial," 167; Moskowitz, "Librium," 461.

41. Moskowitz, "Librium," 460–461, 566–567.

42. Sternbach, interview by Tone, 17–18, 34.

43. Shearer, "Dr. and Mrs. Leo Sternbach." Gerhard Satzinger, "Drug Discovery and Commercial Exploitation," *Drug News Perspective* 14, no. 4 (May 2001): 197.

44. Shearer, "Dr. and Mrs. Leo Sternbach." Sternbach, interview by Tone, 18, 34. Sternbach, interview by Koeppel.

45. Miller, "Valium Inventor Earl Reeder," 9. Early reported adverse side effects included slurred speech and ataxia. See Ramchandani, "The Librium Story," and Lemere, "Toxic Reactions to CDZ," *Journal of the American Medical Association* 174 (Oct. 1960):

493; I. M. Ingram and Gerald C. Timbury, "Side-effects of Librium," letter to the editor, *Lancet*, Oct. 1, 1960; A. A. Bartholomew, "A Dramatic Side Effect of a New Drug, Librium," *Medical Journal of Australia* 48 (Sept. 1961): 436–438. Colen, "Adventurous Chemist," A18.

46. My thanks to Faith Wallis for her help with the Latin translation.

CHAPTER 7

1. Andrea Tone, "Hollister in History," *Collegium Internationale Neuro-Psychopharmcologicum Newsletter*, July 2003, 5–6; Leo Hollister, interview by David Healy, "From Hypertension to Psychopharmacology—A Serendipitous Career," in *The Psychopharmacologists II* (London: Chapman & Hall, 1998), 225–226; Leo Hollister, "How to Succeed as a Clinical Psychopharmacologist Without Trying," typed manuscript, Jan. 5, 2000, Box 9a, Folder 4, Leo Hollister Collection, International Archives of Neuro-Psychopharmacology, Vanderbilt University; Charles Medawar, *Power and Dependence: Social Audit on the Safety of Medicines* (London: Social Audit Limited, 1992), 60–69.

2. Leo Hollister, Francis P. Motzenbecker, and Roger O. Degan, "Withdrawal Reactions from Chlordiazepoxide (Librium)," *Psychopharmacologia* 2 (1961): 63–68.

3. Hollister, "From Hypertension to Psychopharmacology," 226. Hollister, Motzenbecker, and Degan, "Withdrawal Reactions," 63–68. L. E. Hollister, J. L. Bennet, I. Kimbell et al., "Diazepam in Newly Admitted Schizophrenics," *Diseases of the Nervous System*, Dec. 1963, 746–750. Also see Medawar, *Power and Dependence*, 86–88.

4. David Herzberg, "The Pill You Love Can Turn on You: Feminism, Tranquilizers, and the Valium Panic of the 1970s," *American Quarterly* 58 (2006): 82–83.

5. Letter of July 7, 1956, Manufacturers Files, AF19–503, Carter-Wallace, FDA History Office.

6. Patients also wrote the FDA and other organizations in the 1960s for information on medications such as birth control and hormone replacement therapy. See Andrea Tone, *Devices and Desires* (New York: Hill & Wang, 2001); Elizabeth Siegel Watkins, *On the Pill: A Social History of Contraceptives, 1950–1970* (Baltimore: Johns Hopkins University Press, 1998); Watkins, *The Estrogen Elixir: A History of Hormone Replacement Therapy in America* (Baltimore: Johns Hopkins University Press, 2007); and Judith A. Houck, "'What Do These Women Want?' Feminist Responses to *Feminine Forever*, 1963–1980," *Bulletin of the History of Medicine* 77 (Spring 2003): 103–132.

7. Letter of Mar. 11, 1958, Manufacturers Files, AF19–503, Carter-Wallace, FDA History Office.

8. Letter of Nov. 7, 1961, Ralph G. Smith, director, Division of New Drugs, Bureau of Medicine, Food and Drug Administration, Manufacturers Files, AF14–324, Hoffman-La Roche Manufacturers Files, FDA History Office. FDA letter of Nov. 9, 1961, Manufacturers Files, AF14–324, Hoffman-La Roche, FDA History Office.

9. Letter of Mar. 31, 1958, N. E. Cook, assistant to the director, Bureau of Enforcement, Manufacturers Files, AF19–503, Carter-Wallace, FDA History Office.

10. "Suspected Dependence on Chlordiazepoxide Hydrochloride (Librium)," and reply from Ronald M. Fyfe, *Canadian Med Ass. J.*, Aug. 27, 1966, 416. Indeed, Roche's 1964 mailings to doctors about Valium suggested that there had been *no* reports of withdrawal symptoms when recommended dosages had been used. The *Physicians' Desk Reference*, the standard guide to drug prescribing in the United States, relayed the same information; no surprise,

268

Notes

given that this information was supplied by manufacturers directly to the publisher, which was not obligated to perform tests to verify its accuracy before the manual went to press. Librium product information, Jan. 1961, Manufacturers Files, AF14–324, Hoffman-La Roche, FDA History Office; Product information for Valium, Apr. 1964, Manufacturers Files, AF 14–324, Hoffman-La Roche, FDA History Office; *Physicians' Desk Reference* (1975), 1261–1263; *Physicians' Desk Reference* (1979), 1466–1469; Miltown product information, Nov. 1955 and Oct. 1963, Manufacturers Files, AF19–503, Carter-Wallace, FDA History Office. Also see *Barbara Muney Libertelli vs. Hoffman-La Roche, Inc. and Medical Economics Co.*, 1981 U.S. Dist. LEXIS 11049, a case in which a woman unsuccessfully tried to sue the publisher of the *PDR* for gross negligence in refusing to run independent tests on Valium before publishing company-supplied information.

11. The World Health Organization's recommendation that the term "addiction" be replaced by "drug dependence"—acknowledging a more nuanced physical or psychological state—reflected both the fluidity of medical language and the rising interest among medical organizations to investigate and codify such distinctions. "Senate Unit Accused of Misleading Public about Miltown Drug," *Wall Street Journal*, Jan. 27, 1960, 7. Lydia McLean, "A Psychiatrist Discusses What's Good About Tranquilizers," *Vogue*, Apr. 1976, 221. It should be noted that the author misidentified Berger as a psychiatrist. Berger's scalpel comment from Harold M. Schmeck, "Sedative and Stimulant Drugs Pose a Problem for Physicians," *New York Times*, June 23, 1965, 63.

12. FDA Manufacturers Files, AF19–503, Carter-Wallace, FDA History Office. Studies published in widely read and respected journals such as *Journal of the American Medical Association* and *American Journal of Psychiatry* reported that some meprobamate users were experiencing all the markers of addiction, including psychological dependence, withdrawal symptoms upon abstinence (anxiety, insomnia, hyperirritability, and convulsions), and a physiological tolerance requiring steadily higher doses to maintain a therapeutic benefit. Researchers were careful to point out that meprobamate's addictiveness did not mean that all patients who took it would be susceptible or that the drug lacked medicinal value. As researcher Carl F. Essing of the Lexingon-based Addiction Research Center observed in 1957, "as is true of barbiturates, addiction to meprobamate will probably occur in only a very small proportion of persons who receive the drug therapeutically." It was at the physician's discretion to decide how much and to whom the drug should be prescribed. H. Isbell, "Addiction to Barbiturates and the Barbiturates Abstinence Syndrome," *Annals of Internal Medicine* 33 (July 1950): 108–121; Carl F. Essig and John D. Ainslie, "Addiction to Meprobamate," *JAMA*, July 20 1957, 1382; Council on Drugs, "Potential Hazards of Meprobamate (Equanil, Miltown)," *JAMA*, July 20 1957, 1332; John A. Ewing and Thomas H. Maizlip, "A Controlled Study of the Habit Forming Propensities of Meprobamate," *American Journal of Psychiatry* 114 (Mar. 1958): 835; Havelock F. Fraser, "Problems Resulting from the Use of Habituating Drugs in Industry," *American Journal of Public Health* 48 (May 1958): 561–570; Carl F. Essig, "Withdrawal Convulsion in Dogs Following Chronic Meprobamate Intoxication," *American Medical Association Archives of Neurology and Psychiatry* 80 (Oct. 1958): 414–417; H. M. Cann and H. L. Verhulst, "Accidental Ingestion and Overdosage Involving Psychopharmacologic Drugs," *New England Journal of Medicine*, Oct. 13 1960, 719–724; Frank J. Ayd Jr., "Meprobamate: A Decade of Experience," *Psychosomatics* 5 (Mar.-Apr. 1964): 892–897; Carl F. Essig, "Addiction to Nonbarbiturate Sedative and Tranquilizing Drugs," *Clinical Pharmacology and Therapeutics* 5 (May-June 1964): 334–343.

13. Arthur Daemmrich, "A Tale of Two Experts: Thalidomide and Political Engagement in the United States and West Germany," *Society for the Social History of Medicine* 15 (Apr. 2002): 138.

14. This interpretation borrows heavily from Daemmrich, "Tale of Two Experts," 137–143. Linda Bren, "Frances Oldham Kelsey: FDA Medical Reviewer Leaves Her Mark on History," *FDA Consumer Magazine,* Mar.-Apr. 2001, 24–29; Morton Mintz, "'Heroine' of FDA Keeps Bad Drug Off of Market," *Washington Post,* July 15, 1962, A1; Trent Stephens and Rocky Brynner, *Dark Remedy: The Impact of Thalidomide and Its Revival as a Vital Medicine* (Cambridge: Perseus, 2001).

15. Bren, "Frances Oldham Kelsey"; Morton Mintz, "'Heroine' of FDA Keeps Bad Drug Off of Market," *Washington Post,* July 15, 1962, A1; www.nlm.nih.gov/changingtheface-ofmedicine/physicians/biologray (accessed July 16, 2007).

16. Letter from Frances Oldham Kelsey, May 18, 1962, Manufacturers Files, AF14–324, Hoffman-La Roche, FDA History Office; Bren, "Frances Oldham Kelsey"; Mintz, "'Heroine' of FDA," A1; www.nlm.nih.gov/changingthefaceofmedicine/physicians/biologray (accessed July 16, 2007).

17. Kelsey quoted in Bren, "Frances Oldham Kelsey," 24.

18. Mintz, "'Heroine' of FDA," A1. Daemmrich, "Tale of Two Experts," 155–156; "Access Before Approval—A Right to Take Experimental Drugs?" *New England Journal of Medicine,* Aug. 3, 2006; FDA, Center for Drug Evaluation and Research, *From Test Tube to Patient: Improving Health Through Human Drugs,* 37; Mintz, "'Heroine' of FDA," 1. William H. Helfand, *Medicine Avenue: The Story of Medical Advertising in America* (Huntington, NY: Medical Advertising Hall of Fame, 1999), 45.

19. Daemmrich, "Tale of Two Experts," 137–158; Steven Epstein, "Activism, Drug Regulation, and the Politics of Therapeutic Evaluation in the AIDS Era: A Case Study of ddC and the 'Surrogate Markers' Debate," *Social Studies of Science* 27 (Oct. 1997): 691–726.

20. Letter of Sept. 27, 1964, to Frances Kelsey, Manufacturers Files, AF14–324, Hoffman-La Roche, FDA History Office.

21. Letter of Aug. 25, 1962, to Frances Kelsey, Manufacturers Files, AF14–324, Hoffman-La Roche, FDA History Office.

22. Letter of Aug. 11, 1962, to Frances Kelsey, Manufacturers Files, AF14–324, Hoffman-La Roche, FDA History Office.

23. FDA letters of Sept. 28 and Oct. 17, 1962, and Apr. 3, 1963, Manufacturers Files, AF14–324, Hoffman-La Roche, FDA History Office. Letter of Apr. 3, 1963, Jules S. Orloff, assistant to the director, Division of Advisory Opinions, Bureau of Enforcement, Manufacturers Files, AF14–324, Hoffman-La Roche, FDA History Office.

24. Letters of June 24, 29, Aug. 5, 28, Oct. 6, Nov. 3, 1964, Manufacturers Files, AF14–324, Hoffman-La Roche, FDA History Office.

25. Helfand, *Medicine Avenue,* 47. Andrea Tone, "Listening to the Past: History, Psychiatry, and Anxiety," *Canadian Journal of Psychiatry* 50 (June 2005): 378; "Valium Celebrates 40th, But Not with a Bang," *Victoria Times Colonist,* July 21, 2003, D4; Nick Paumgarten, "Little Helper," *New Yorker,* June 16, 2003, 70. Linda Murray, "Why Users of Valium, Librium Aren't So Tranquil," *Chicago Daily News,* Feb. 4, 1976.

26. "Hoffman-La Roche Moves to Protect Librium Sales Rights," *Wall Street Journal,* Jan. 21, 1975, 6; "Government to Control 2 Major Tranquilizers," *Cleveland Plain Dealer,* Monday June 2, 1975, 6B. B. D. Colen, "America's Psychic Aspirin," *Washington Post,* Jan. 21, 1980, A20; Edward Shorter, *A Historical Dictionary of Psychiatry* (New York: Oxford

University Press, 2005), 41; Gilbert Cant, "Valiumania," *New York Times Magazine,* Feb. 1, 1976, 34–41; Hoffman-La Roche Bid Aims at Growth," *Wall Street Journal,* Jan. 1988, 8; "Facts About Valium," Manufacturers Files, AF14–324, Hoffman-La Roche, FDA History Office.

27. Manufacturers Files, AF14–324, Hoffman-La Roche, FDA History Office; Hans Conrad Peyer, *Roche: A Company History, 1896–1996* (Basel: Roche, 1996), 178–179.

28. Peyer, *Roche,* 174–175, 178–179.

29. John Pekkanen, "The Tranquilizer War: Controlling Librium and Valium," *New Republic,* July 19, 1975, 17–19; Stuart Elliott, "McAdams Forms Division on Latest Drugs," *New York Times,* Dec. 16, 1991, D9; Carter Products, *Annual Report,* 1961, 2, Berger Scrapbooks, Vol. 3, Frank Berger Family Archives, New York City.

30. Helfand, *Medicine Avenue,* 45–47, 53–55; Nancy Tomes, "The Great American Medicine Show Revisited," *Bulletin of the History of Medicine* 79 (2005): 645–649; Jeremy A. Greene, "Attention to 'Details': Etiquette and the Pharmaceutical Salesman in Postwar America," *Social Studies of Science* 34 (Apr. 2004): 271–292.

31. FDA Division of Pharmacology Memo to Frances Kelsey, Division of New Drugs, Jan. 23, 1962, Manufacturers Files, AF14–324, Hoffman-La Roche, FDA History Office. Hoffman-LaRoche, Western Region Plan, Valium, 1977, quoted in *The Use and Misuse of Benzodiazepines: Hearing Before the Subcommittee on Health and Scientific Research of the Committee on Labor and Human Resources,* United States Senate, Ninety-sixth Congress (Washington, DC: Government Printing Office, Sept. 10, 1979), 173–175.

32. *Use and Misuse,* 205. The company's largesse sprang from its determination to undercut its competition, which included about a dozen rival firms, permitted under Canadian law to manufacture diazepam. Following a year-long trial instigated in 1979, Hoffman-La Roche became the first corporation to be convicted for predatory pricing under Canada's Combines Investigation Act, an antimonopoly measure some legal experts had previously denounced as "toothless." Anthony Whittingham, "Downer for the Downers," *Maclean's,* Feb. 18, 1980.

33. John R. Lion et al., "Psychiatrists' Opinions of Psychotropic Drug Advertisements," *Social Science & Medicine* 13A (Jan. 1979): 123. "Valiumania," *New York Times Magazine,* Feb. 1, 1976; Dr. Hendler testimony, *Use and Misuse,* 29. Although scholars often use ads as stand-alone evidence to index broader changes in the history of psychiatry, they must be used with methodological caution and care. Ads are but one part of a complicated process by which medical markets are created, negotiated, and transformed, and an ad itself doesn't "reveal" how doctors or consumers respond to it. That information must be corroborated with other sorts of evidence. On this point, see Andrea Tone, review of Jonathan Michel Metzl, *Prozac on the Couch: Prescribing Gender in the Era of Wonder Drug, Transcultural Psychiatry* 44 (2007): 302–304. Manufacturers Files, AF14–324, Hoffman-La Roche, FDA History Office.

34. *Archives of Internal Medicine* 126, no. 3 (Sept. 1970). "Thirty-five, Single, and Psychoneurotic," *Archives of General Psychiatry* 22 (1970): 481–482.

35. For an excellent analysis of gender and pharmaceutical advertising, see Jonathan Metzl, *Prozac on the Couch: Prescribing Gender in the Era of Wonder Drugs* (Durham, NC: Duke University Press, 2003); and Metzl, "Mother's Little Helper: The Crisis of Psychoanalysis and the Miltown Revolution," *Gender and History* 15 (Aug. 2003): 240–267. Also see Joellen W. Hawkins and Cynthia S. Aber, "The Content of Advertisements in Medical Journals: Distorting the Image of Woman," *Women and Health* 14 (1988): 45–51; P. Haberman

and D. E. Sexton, "Women in Magazine Advertisements," *Journal of Advertising Research* 14 (1976); R. Seidenberg, "Drug Advertising and Perception of Mental Illness," *Mental Hygiene* 55 (1971): 21–31; Michey C. Smith and Lisa Griffin, "Rationality of Appeals Used in the Promotion of Psychotropic Drugs: A Comparison of Male and Female Models," *Social Science & Medicine* 11 (Apr. 1977): 409–414; Gerry V. Stimson, "The Message of Psychotropic Drug Ads," *Journal of Communication Studies* 25 (Summer 1975): 153–160. Ad, *Archives of Internal Medicine* 126, no. 5 (Nov. 1970).

36. Jane Prather and Linda S. Fidell, "Sex Differences in the Content and Style of Medical Advertisements," *Social Science and Medicine* 9 (Jan. 1975): 23–26.

37. Roche Laboratories, *Aspects of Anxiety*, 2nd ed. (Philadelphia: Lippincott, 1968), 88.

38. Roche Laboratories, *Aspects of Anxiety*, 88.

39. Roche Laboratories, *Aspects of Anxiety*, 88–90. "Excessive Anxiety in the Hypertensive Patient," Librium ad, *Archives of Internal Medicine* 129 (Apr. 1972).

40. Letter of Aug. 29, 1979, assistant vice president, Hoffman-La Roche; "Program to Help Public to Understand Stress Is Announced at Cornell," public relations release, Dudley-Anderson-Yutzy, n.d.; Clinical Roundtables, The Consequences of Stress: The Medical and Social Implications of Prescribing Tranquilizers; Theodore Cooper, "The Consequences of Stress: The Medical and Social Implications of Prescribing Tranquilizers," in *Use and Misuse of Benzodiazepines*, 210–211, 213, 215–255; 272–288. Also, memorandum of Nov. 27, 1979 of Thomas W. Cavanaugh, consumer safety officer to director of drug advertising, Manufacturers Files, AF 14–324, Hoffman-La Roche, FDA History Office. "Stress Drive Held Promotion for Valium," *Washington Post*, Jan. 12, 1979, A4.

41. Clinical Roundtables, "The Consequences of Stress: The Medical and Social Implications of Prescribing Tranquilizers," in *Use and Misuse of Benzodiazepines*, 281. For a discussion of the relationship between psychosocial factors and disease, see "The Great Debate: Psychosocial Interventions Can Improve Clinical Outcomes in Organic Disease," *Psychosomatic Medicine* 64 (July-Aug. 2002): 549–570.

42. Letters of Apr. 4 and May 3, 1977 to Peter Bourne; UPI press statement, "Carter May Pull Sedatives Off Market," n.d., all in Peter Bourne Collection, Box 13, Folders 1977–1978, Jimmy Carter Library, National Archives. Victor Cohn, "Barbiturate Ban Eyed by White House," *Washington Post*, Mar. 30, 1977, A1.

43. Letter of Mar. 31, 1977, to Peter Bourne, Peter Bourne Collection, Box 12, Folder 1977–1978, Jimmy Carter Library, National Archives.

44. Don Colburn, "Valium in an Age of Anxiety," *Washington Post*, Feb. 17, 1987, 29–31; James Dietch, "The Nature and Extent of Benzodiazepine Abuse: An Overview of Recent Literature," *Hospital and Community Psychiatry* 34 (Dec. 1983): 1139–1145; Bryan S. Finkle, Devin L. McCloskey, Louis S. Goodman, "Diazepam and Drug-Associated Deaths," *JAMA*, Aug. 3, 1979, 429–434; David Greenblatt, Marcia D. Allen, Barbara J. Noel, and Richard I. Shader, "Acute Overdosage with Benzodiazepine Derivatives," *Clinical Pharmacology and Therapeutics* 21 (1977): 497–514; J. Hojer, S. Baehrendtz and L. Gustaffson, "Benzodiazepine Poisoning: Experience of 702 Admissions to an Intensive Care Unit During a 14-Year Period," *Journal of Internal Medicine* 226 (Aug. 1989): 117–122. Harold M. Schmeck Jr., "Valium: Often a Suicide Step, Seldom Works," *New York Times*, Feb. 11, 1987, A17; Philip Shabecoff, "Washington Talk: The Capital Limelight; Stress and the Lure of Harmful Remedies," *New York Times*, Oct. 14, 1987, B6; Tone, "Listening to the Past," 378.

45. Gerald L. Klerman, "The Psychiatric Patient's Right to Effective Treatment: Implications of *Osheroff v. Chestnut Lodge*," *American Journal of Psychiatry* 147 (Apr. 1990): 409–418;

Miriam Shuchman and Michael S. Wilkes, "Dramatic Progress Against Depression," *New York Times Magazine*, Oct. 7, 1990, 12.

46. Osheroff, quoted in Schuchman and Wilkes, "Dramatic Progress Against Depression," 12; Gerald L. Klerman, "The Psychiatrist Patient's Right to Effective Treatment, 409–418.

47. Karl Menninger, *The Vital Balance* (New York: Viking, 1963), 325; Gerald Grob, "The Forging of Mental Health Policy in America: World War II to New Frontier," *Journal of the History of Medicine and Allied Sciences* 42 (Oct. 1987): 410–446; Grob, "Origins of DSM–1: A Study in Appearance and Reality," *American Journal of Psychiatry* 148 (Apr. 1991): 421–431; Mitchell Wilson, "DSM-III and the Transformation of American Psychiatry: A History," *American Journal of Psychiatry* 150 (Mar. 1993): 399–410; Shorter, *A Historical Dictionary*, 178. *Diagnostic and Statistical Manual: Mental Disorder. Prepared by the Committee on Nomenclature and Statistics of the American Psychiatric Association* (Washington, DC: American Psychiatric Association, 1952), 31–34.

48. Wilson, "DSM-III and the Transformation of American Psychiatry," 400, 407; Gerald L. Klerman, "The Advantage of DSM-III," *American Journal of Psychiatry* 141, no. 4 (Apr. 1984): 539–541.

49. Tone, "Listening to the Past"; Klerman, "Advantage of DSM-III," 540; Wilson, "DSM-III," 407; Shorter, *Historical Dictionary*, 91.

50. Shorter, *A Historical Dictionary of Psychiatry*, 91; Klerman, "Advantage of DSM-III," 540.

51. Tone, "Hollister in History," 6.

52. Klerman, "Advantage of DSM-III," 540; Erik R. Kandel, "A New Intellectual Framework for Psychiatry," *American Journal of Psychiatry* 1554 (Apr. 1998): 457–459.

53. As Leo Hollister observed, "The new classification of anxiety disorders has vastly broadened the scope of drugs used to treat them." See Hollister, *Journal for Drug Therapy and Research* 9, no. 8 (1984): 418. Gerry V. Stimson, "The Message of Psychotropic Drug Ads," *Journal of Communication* 25 no. 3 (Summer 1975): 153.

54. Solomon H. Snyder, *Drugs and the Brain* (New York: Scientific American Books, 1986), 4.

55. Snyder, *Drugs and the Brain*, 166–167.

56. Harold M. Schmeck Jr., "The Biology of Fear and Anxiety: Evidence Points to Chemical Triggers," *New York Times*, Sept. 7, 1982, C1. Peter Tyrer, "Classification of Anxiety Disorder: A Critique of DSM III," *Journal of Affective Disorders* 11 (1986), 99–104. As Klein said, "One could hardly believe that the panic attack was simply the quantitative extreme of chronic anxiety since imipramine could dispel the apparently worse anxiety but had little effect on the chronic minor form." Donald F. Klein, "Anxiety Reconceptualized," in *Anxiety: New Research and Changing Concepts*, ed. D. F. Klein and J. G. Rabkin (New York: Raven, 1981), 235–263. Also see Donald F. Klein, "Delineating of Two Drug-Responsive Anxiety Syndromes," *Psychopharmacology* 5 (Nov. 1964): 397–408. On how depression could be diagnosed as an observed response to antidepressants, see Laura Hirshbein, "Science, Gender, and the Emergence of Depression in American Psychiatry, 1952–1980," *Journal of the History of Medicine and Allied Sciences* 61 (Apr. 2006): 200–201. Allen Frances et al., "The Classification of Panic Disorders: From Freud to DSM-IV," *Journal of Psychiatric Research* 27 (1993): suppl. 1, pp. 3–10; Kandel, "New Intellectual Framework," 457–459; Ross, quoted in Linda A. Johnson, "Mother's Little Helper Not So Little: Valium Is 40 Years Old This Year," *Southeast Missourian*, July 16, 2003. Michael L. Radelet, "Health Beliefs, Social Networks, and Tranquilizer Use," *Journal of Health and Social Behavior* 22 (June 1981): 165–173.

57. Nikolas Rose, "Becoming Neurochemical Selves," in *Biotechnology: Between Commerce and Civil Society*, ed. Nico Stehr (Piscataway, NJ: Transaction, 2004), 100.

58. Celebrity drug taking is more likely to be relegated to the realm of tabloids. See, for instance, A. J. Hammer and Brooke Anderson, "Special Edition: 'Prescription for Rehab': Celebrities Coping with Addictions, Those Who Make It Through Recovery," *CNN Headline News*, Aug. 17, 2007; Nina Burleigh and Frank Swertlow, "Tammy Faye Messner, 1942–2007," *People*, Aug. 6, 2007. Brendan I. Koerner, "Leo Sternbach: The Father of Mother's Little Helpers," Dec. 27, 1999, www.usnews.com/usnews/culture/articles/991227/archive_004705.htm (accessed 04/28/2008). John G. Hubbell, "Danger! Prescription-Drug Abuse," *Reader's Digest*, Apr. 1980. Lawrence K. Altman and Todd S. Purdum, "In J.F.K. File, Hidden Illness, Pain and Pills," *New York Times*, Nov. 17, 2002, sec. 1, p. 1; "The J.F.K. File," *New York Times*, Nov. 19, 2002, A30; Tim Reid, "JFK Had to Fight Pain Every Day," *London Times*, Nov. 18, 2002, 15; "Report: JFK Suffered More Pain, Ailments Than Revealed; President Took as Many as 8 Medication a Day," *Washington Post*, A3.

59. Barbara Gordon, interview by Andrea Tone, July 18, 2006, New York City.

60. Richard Tessler, Randall Stokes, and Marianne Pietras, "Consumer Responses to Valium," *Drug Therapy* 8 (Feb. 1978): 178–183. "V is for Valium," *Sunday Independent* (London), Nov. 23, 2003, 1–2.

61. Letter of Oct. 26, 1975, to Deborah Larned, *Ms.* Magazine letters. Carton 3. Folder 66. Schlesinger Library, Radcliffe Institute, Harvard University.

62. Letter of July 18, 1980, Manufacturers Files, AF14–324, Hoffman-La Roche, FDA History Office. Memorandum of telephone conversation, Aug. 28, 1963, Frederick A. Knoblich, supervisory inspector, Manufacturers Files, AF14–324, Hoffman-La Roche, FDA History Office.

63. Letter of Sept. 12, 1979, to Senator Howard H. Baker Jr., Manufacturers Files, AF14–324, Hoffman-La Roche, FDA History Office. Letter of July 18, 1980, Manufacturers Files, AF14–324, Hoffman-La Roche, FDA History Office. Murray, "Why Users of Valium, Librium Aren't So Tranquil."

64. Letter to the editors, Oct. 28, 1975, *Ms.* Magazine letters. Carton 3. Folder 66. Schlesinger Library, Radcliffe Institute, Harvard University.

65. Letters to the editors, Nov. 17, 1975, *Ms.* Magazine letters. Carton 3. Folder 66. Schlesinger Library, Radcliffe Institute, Harvard University.

66. Susan Lynn Speaker, "Too Many Pills: Patients, Physicians, and the Myth of Overmedication in America, 1955–1980" (Ph.D. diss., University of Pennsylvania, 1992), 25. Department of Health, Education, and Welfare, Food and Drug Administration, "Report Including Recommended Findings and Conclusions Re: Potential for Abuse of the Drugs Librium and Valium," Apr. 7, 1967, Manufacturers Files, AF14–324, Hoffman-La Roche, FDA History Office; letter of Robert C. Wetherell, July 14, 1975, Manufacturers Files, AF14–324, Hoffman-La Roche, FDA History Office.

67. Department of Health, Education, and Welfare, Food and Drug Administration, "Report Including Recommended Findings and Conclusions Re: Potential for Abuse of the Drugs Librium and Valium," Apr. 7, 1967, Manufacturers Files, AF14–324, Hoffman-La Roche, FDA History Office; testimony of Robert Clark, in *Use and Misuse of Benzodiazepines*. FDA letter of Apr. 4, 1975, Manufacturers Files, AF14–324, Hoffman-La Roche, FDA History Office; letter of Robert C. Wetherell Jr., director, Office of Legislative Services, Department of Health, Education, and Welfare, to Honorable Sam Nunn, Sept. 22, 1977, Manufacturers Files, AF14–324, Hoffman-La Roche, FDA History Office; William Celis 3d, "As Computer Track Drugs, Fears of Abuse Arise," *New York Times*, Jan. 17, 1972, 12.

68. FDA letter, Nov. 6, 1979, Manufacturers Files, AF14–324, Hoffman-La Roche, FDA History Office. The FDA's careful review of the promotional materials related to the Roche-sponsored CME program, The Consequences of Stress, reflected each organization's jockeying for semantic clarity. See, for instance, FDA memo of consumer safety officer Thomas W. Cavanaugh to the FDA director's Division of Drug Advertising, Nov. 27, 1979, Manufacturers Files, AF14–324, Hoffman-La Roche, FDA History Office.

69. Telegram to the FDA, Sept. 11, 1979, and FDA reply, Nov. 6, 1979, Manufacturers Files, AF14–324, Hoffman-La Roche, FDA History Office.

70. Testimony of Leo Hollister, *Use and Misuse of Benzodiazepines*, 209.

CHAPTER 8

1. *NBC Evening News* broadcast, May 22, 1978, Television News Archives, Vanderbilt University, Nashville, Tennessee. For a more extended discussion of Maginnis's experience, as well as her efforts to help women with similar difficulties through grassroots organizing, see her testimony before the Select Committee on Narcotics Abuse and Control, *Women's Dependency on Prescription Drugs*, Ninety-sixth Congress, 1st sess., Sept. 13, 1979 (Washington, DC: Government Printing Office, 1979), 4–18.

2. Maginniss testimony, *Women's Dependency on Prescription Drugs*, 4–18.

3. *The Use and Misuse of Benzodiazepines: Hearing Before the Subcommittee on Health and Scientific Research of the Committee on Labor and Human Resources*, United States Senate, Ninety-sixth Congress, 1st sess. on the Examination of the Use and Misuse of Valium, Librium, and other Minor Tranquilizers (Washington, DC: Government Printing Office, 1979), 1; David Herzberg, "The Pill You Love Can Turn on You: Feminism, Tranquilizers, and the Valium Panic of the 1970s," *American Quarterly* 58 (2006): 79–103.

4. Edward Shorter, *A Historical Dictionary of Psychiatry* (New York: Oxford University Press, 2005), 42.

5. Edwin Diamond, "Young Wives," *Newsweek*, Mar. 7, 1960, 58. Stephanie Coontz, *The Way We Never Were: American Families and the Nostalgia Trap* (New York: Basic, 1992), 32. For a fascinating analysis of the importance of sex and cultural expectations of women in psychiatrists' decisions to lobotomize patients, see Joel Braslow, *Mental Ills and Bodily Cures: Psychiatric Treatment in the First Half of the Twentieth Century* (Berkeley: University of California Press, 1997), 152–170. Joanne Meyerowitz, "Beyond the Feminine Mystique: A Reassessment of Postwar Mass Culture, 1946–1958," in *Not June Cleaver: Women and Gender in Postwar America, 1945–1960*, ed. Joanne Meyerowitz (Philadelphia: Temple University Press, 1994), 229–262.

6. Betty Friedan, preface to *The Feminine Mystique* (1963; New York, Norton, 1981); Nancy Woloch, *Women and the American Experience*, 2nd ed. (New York: McGraw-Hill: 1994), 482–485.

7. Friedan, *Feminine Mystique*, 20–21.

8. Friedan, *Feminine Mystique*, 30–31.

9. Hugh J. Parry, "Use of Psychotropic Drugs by U.S. Adults," *Public Health Reports* 83 (Oct. 1968): 799. Parry was interested in elucidating patterns of everyday prescription drug use among noninstitutionalized Americans. Since their introduction in the 1950s, mild tranquilizers had become a mainstay in VA and psychiatric hospitals, elderly homes, prisons, and other institutions. One study of the drug profiles of psychiatric patients found that, on average, 10 percent of patients on VA wards received more than their recommended allotment, and on wards where understaffing and inadequate training were acute, 40 percent of patients

received excessive amounts. In nursing homes, the excessive use of tranquilizers was considered so rampant that the president of the National Council of Senior Citizens implored Congress to investigate this "forced pacification program." See "Tightening the Lid on Legal Drugs," *Science News*, June 14, 1975; and J. Maurice Rogers, "Drug Abuse: Just What the Doctor Ordered," *Psychology Today* 5 (Sept. 1971): 18.

10. Parry, "Use of Psychotropic Drugs," 799–809. The poor and the less wealthy were no less likely to use chemical agents, but they were more likely to favor proprietary drugs such as alcohol for "escape drinking," over prescription agents. These studies included an important investigation of national patterns of tranquilizer use, the first of its kind, published in 1973 in the *Archives of General Psychiatry*. Cosponsored by the National Institute of Mental Health, the Social Research Group, and the Institute for Research in Social Behavior, the national study drew from a series of studies launched in 1966. H. Parry et al., "National Patterns of Psychotherapeutic Drug Use," *Archives of General Psychiatry* 28 (June 1973): 769–783. The newer data confirmed Parry's earlier findings on women and tranquilizers. For an excellent overview of prescribing and utilization studies in the 1960s and 1970s, see Mickey S. Smith, *A Social History of Minor Tranquilizers: The Quest for Small Comfort in the Age of Anxiety* (New York: Pharmaceutical Products Press, 1985), 37–63. Parry, "Patterns of Psychotropic Drug Use," *Journal of Drug Issues* 1 (1971): 269–273.

11. David Musto, *The American Disease: Origins of Narcotic Control* (New Haven, CT: Yale University Press, 1973); Jim Hogshire, *Pills-A-Go-Go: A Fiendish Investigation into Pill Marketing, Art, History & Consumption* (Los Angeles: Feral House, 1999), 180; Philip Jenkins, *Synthetic Panics: The Symbolic Politics of Designer Drugs* (New York: New York University Press, 1999). Stephen R. Kandall, *Substance and Shadow: Women and Addiction in the United States* (Cambridge: Harvard University Press, 1999), 14–27. Jason Szabo, *Incurable and Intolerable: Chronic Disease and Slow Death in Nineteenth-Century France* (Piscataway, NJ: Rutgers University Press, 2009), chap. 7; *Merck's 1899 Manual of the Materia Medica* (1899; New York: Merck, 1999); Matt Clark et al., "Drugs and Psychiatry: A New Era," *Newsweek*, Nov. 12, 1979, 101.

12. S. Nassir Ghaemi, *Polypharmacy in Psychiatry* (New York: Marcel Dekker, 2002), 319–320; David Healy, *The Creation of Psychopharmacology* (Cambridge: Harvard University Press, 2002), 354; Tom Ban, personal communication to author, Mar. 10, 2008.

13. David T. Courtwright, *Dark Paradise: A History of Opiate Addiction in America Before 1940* (Cambridge: Harvard University Press, 1982), 168–169. Courtwright, *Forces of Habit: Drugs and the Making of the Modern World* (Cambridge: Harvard University Press, 2001), 89; Pauline Maier et al., *Inventing America: A History of the United States* (New York: Norton, 2003), 2:958. On the political and cultural discrediting of LSD and the medical implications of its stigmatization, see Erika Dyck, "Flashback: Psychiatric Experimentation with LSD in Historical Perspective," *Canadian Journal of Psychiatry* 50 (June 2005): 381–387. "Jane Fonda Accused of Smuggling," *New York Times*, Nov. 4, 1970, 52.

14. Barbara W. Wyden, "A Child on Drugs," *New York Times*, Aug. 20, 1967, SM63.

15. Tragically, the young girl died. "Greenwich Girl, 11, Dies After Inhaling a Frosting Spray," *New York Times*, Oct. 4, 1967, 35. Byron Porterfield, "Narcotics Seized in Raid on East Hampton Party," *New York Times*, Aug. 26, 1965, 1.

16. "Drug Culture: Take a Look at Your Office," *Business Week*, Aug. 15, 1970, 83; Herzberg, "The Pill You Love," 86–88. "Health Talk: The Uppers and Downers of Middle-Class Prescription-Drug Addicts," *Washington Post*, Sept. 14, 1979, A1. J. Anthony Lukas, "Americans Are Found to Be Increasingly Oriented Toward Wide Variety of Drugs," *New York Times*, Jan. 8, 1969, 1; "Greenwich Girl," 35; Martin Arnold, "The Drug Scene: A

Growing Number of America's Elite Are Quietly 'Turning On,'" *New York Times*, Jan. 10, 1968, 26.

17. Quoted in Susan Lynn Speaker, "Too Many Pills: Patients, Physicians, and the Myth of Overmedication in America, 1955–1980" (Ph.D. diss., University of Pennsylvania, 1992), 47. Herzberg, "The Pill You Love," 86. Richard Nixon, remarks to the American Medical Association's House of Delegates Meeting in Atlantic City, New Jersey, June 22, 1971, in John T. Woolley and Gerhard Peters, The American Presidency Project, www .presidency.ucsb.edu/ws/index.php?pid=3051 (accessed Apr. 27, 2008).

18. "Condemnation of drug abuse has been primarily directed against hippies and narcotics addicts," Leonard S. Brahen, director of medical research and education in the Nassau County Department of Drug and Alcohol Addiction, told participants at the 1972 meeting of the New York State Medical Society. "We now recognize that the abuse of mood changing drugs is more extensive, involving people in all socioeconomic classes." Leonard S. Brahen, "Housewife Drug Abuse," *Journal of Drug Education* 3 (Spring 1973): 13.

19. "Connecticut Finds Excessive Drug Use," *New York Times*, Mar. 18, 1964, 43; Victor Cohn, "Women's Drug Dependency Called an Epidemic," *Washington Post*, Apr. 12, 1978, A2. Brahen, "Housewife Drug Abuse," 13.

20. Morris Chafetz and Patrick Young, "The Complete Book of Women and Pills," *Good Housekeeping*, Apr. 1979, 73–76; Carl D. Chambers and Dodi Schultz, "Housewives and the Drug Habit," *Ladies Home Journal*, Dec. 1971; "Danger Ahead! Valium: The Pill You Love Can Turn on You," *Vogue*, Feb. 1975, 152–153. Chambers and Schultz, "Women and Drugs," 191.

21. Letter of Aug. 2, 1977, Manufacturers Files, AF14–324, Hoffman-La Roche, FDA History Office.

22. Gerald L. Klerman, "Drugs and Social Values," *International Journal of the Addictions* 5 (June 1970): 316; 313–319; D. I. Manheimer et al., "Popular Attitudes and Beliefs About Tranquilizers," *American Journal of Psychiatry* 130 (1973): 1246–1253; F. Kraupl Taylor, "The Damnation of Benzodiazepines," *British Journal of Psychiatry* 154 (1989): 697–704; Yolles, quoted in B. I. Koerner, "The Father of Mother's Little Helpers," *U.S. News and World Report*, Dec. 27, 1999, 58.

23. Maya Pines, "Case Focuses on Behavioral Therapy," *New York Times*, May 12, 1982, D20; Jenny Hope, "End of Valium the 'Little Helper,'" *Daily Mail*, Jan. 20, 2002. Lisa Callhan, Connie Mayer, and Henry J. Steadman, "Insanity Defense in the United States–Post-Hinkley," *Mental Health and Physical Disability Report* 11, no. 1 (Feb. 1987): 54–59; "U.S. Moves to Curb Insanity Defense," *New York Times*, July 20, 1982.

24. Susan Speaker, "From 'Happiness Pills' to National Nightmare: Changing Cultural Assessments of Minor Tranquilizers in America, 1955–1980," *Journal of the History of Medicine and Allied Sciences* 52 (1997): 338–376; Speaker, "Too Many Pills"; Harvey Wasserman, "Ralph Nader," in *The Reader's Companion to American History*, ed. Eric Foner and John A. Garraty (Boston: Houghton Mifflin, 1991), 768–769; David Bollier, *Citizen Action and Other Big Ideas: A History of Ralph Nader and the Modern Consumer Movement* (Washington, DC: Center for Study of Responsive Law, 1989).

25. Sara Evans, *Personal Politics: The Roots of Women's Liberation in the Civil Rights Movement and the New Left* (New York: Vintage, 1979); Susan Brownmiller, *In Our Time: Memoir of a Revolution* (New York: Delta, 1999); Sandra Morgan, *Into our Hands: The Women's Health Movement in the United States, 1969–1990* (New Brunswick, NJ: Rutgers University Press, 2002); Elizabeth Siegel Watkins, *The Estrogen Elixir: A History of Hormone Replacement Therapy in America* (Baltimore: Johns Hopkins University Press, 2007), 112–114; Wendy Kline,

"'Please Include This in Your Book': Readers Respond to *Our Bodies, Ourselves*," *Bulletin of the History of Medicine* 79 (Spring 2005): 81–110; Christabelle Sethna, "The Evolution of the Birth Control Handbook: From Student Peer-Education Manual to Feminist Self-empowerment Text, 1968–1975," *Canadian Bulletin of the History of Medicine* 23 (2006): 89–118.

26. Andrea Tone, *Devices and Desires: A History of Contraceptives in America* (New York: Hill & Wang, 2001), 244–249; Judith A. Houck, "What Do These Women Want? Feminist Responses to Feminine Forever, 1963–1980," *Bulletin of the History of Medicine* 77 (Spring 2003): 117–118.

27. Tone, *Devices and Desires*, 249–250.

28. Tone, *Devices and Desires*, 249–250.

29. Kline, "'Please Include This," 81–110; Houck, "What Do These Women Want?" 103–109. Watkins, *Estrogen Elixir*, 116–117; Barbara Seaman, *The Greatest Experiment Ever Performed on Women: Exploding the Estrogen Myth* (New York: Hyperion, 2003), 37–39, 43–44, 212–213; "About NWHN," *National Women's Heath Network: A Voice for Women, A Network For Change*, www.nwhn.org/about (accessed Aug. 4, 2007); Norma Swenson, "Women's Health Movement," in *The Readers' Guide to U.S. Women's History*, ed. Wilman Mankiller et al. (Boston: Houghton Mifflin, 1998), 648.

30. Tone, *Devices and Desires*, 261–280.

31. Aug. 1970 letter to FDA, Manufacturers Files, AF14–324, Hoffman-La Roche, FDA History Office.

32. One mother wrote Ann Landers about her twenty-seven-year-old son, whose attachment to drugs seemed to be outweighed only by his apathy: he "lives at home and refuses to work." He smokes cigarettes, takes methadone, and the "doctors have given him prescriptions for Valium plus a lot of other stuff." This wasn't the mother's image of what having a grown-up son would mean. "Why must aged parents be forced to keep a son who is in such terrible shape and makes their life a living hell?" she demanded. Ann counseled the miserable mom to send him for treatment at a drug addiction clinic. Ann Landers column, *Washington Post*, Nov. 7, 1975, B7. On the importance of celebrity illness testimonials to popular understandings of medicine, see Barron H. Lemur, *When Illness Goes Public: Celebrity Patients and How We Look at Medicine* (Baltimore: Johns Hopkins University Press, 2006).

33. Ford, quoted in Clark, Gosnell, and Whitmore, "Prisoner of Pills," 77.

34. Jennifer Steinhauer, "Back in View, a First Lady with Her Own Legacy," *New York Times*, Dec. 31, 2006, www.nytimes.com/2006/12/31/us/31betty.html?scp=1&sq=Betty+Ford+%2B+Jennifer+Steinhauer&st=nyt (accessed Apr. 27, 2008); Neely Tucker, "Betty Ford, Again Putting On a Brave Face," *Washington Post*, Dec. 29, 2006.

35. Betty Ford with Chris Chase, *The Times of My Life* (New York: Harper & Row/Reader's Digest Association, 1978), 282, 285–286; Clark, Gosnell, and Whitmore, "Prisoner of Pills," 77.

36. Betty Ford with Chris Chase, *Betty: A Glad Awakening* (New York: Doubleday, 1987), 41.

37. Ford, *Glad Awakening*, 45–49; Ford, *Times of My Life*, 280–283, 286, 290–292. Muriel Nellis, "Accidental Drug Addiction," *Harper's Bazaar*, Aug. 1978, 34.

38. Barbara Gordon, *I'm Dancing As Fast As I Can* (New York: Harper & Row, 1979), 4–8, 11, 16, 184; Gordon, "In Her Own Words: Addicted to Valium," *People*, June 18, 1979, 91–92, 97–98; Gordon, interview by Andrea Tone, July 19, 2006, New York City.

39. Gordon, *Dancing*, 34, 36, 50–51.

40. Gordon, *Dancing*, 85, 90, 94, 184.

41. Gordon, interview by Tone.

42. Gordon, interview by Tone. Gordon, quoted in "In Her Own Words," 91–92, 97–98.

43. Gordon, interview by Tone.

44. Gordon, "In Her Own Words," 91–92, 97–98; Gordon, interview by Tone.

45. Richard Hughes and Robert Brewin, *The Tranquilizing of America: Pill Popping and the American Way of Life* (New York: Harcourt, Brace, Jovanovich, 1979), 61.

46. Hughes and Brewin, *Tranquilizing of America*, 9.

47. Cowan, cited in Hughes and Brewin, *Tranquilizing of America*, 64. "Valium Addictive, Navy Doctors Warns," *L.A. Herald*, Sept. 11, 1979.

48. On the gendering of depression and other psychiatric disorders, see Elizabeth Lunbeck, *The Psychiatric Persuasion: Knowledge, Gender, and Power in Modern America* (Princeton, NJ: Princeton University Press, 1994); Laura Hirshbein, "Science, Gender, and the Emergence of Depression in American Psychiatry, 1952–1980," *Journal of the History of Medicine and Allied Sciences* 61 (Apr. 2006): 187–216; Ilina Singh, "Not Just Naughty: 50 Years of Stimulant Drug Advertising," in *Medicating Modern America; Prescription Drugs in History*, ed. Andrea Tone and Elizabeth Siegel Watkins (New York: New York University Press, 2007), 131–155; Jonathan Metzl, *Prozac on the Couch: Prescribing Gender in the Era of Wonder Drugs* (Durham, NC: Duke University Press 2003). In 1970, 92.4 percent of general physicians and 93.8 percent of obstetrician-gynecologists were male. See Kline, "Please Include This," 85–86. Penelope McMillan, "Women and Tranquilizers," *Ladies Home Journal*, Nov. 1976, 164; Clark, Gosnell, Whitmore, "Prisoner of Pills," 77.

49. Letter of Mar. 21, 1963, Manufacturers Files, AF14–324, Hoffman-La Roche, FDA History Office.

50. William Nolen, "Tired? Nervous? Here's a Pill," *McCall's*, Apr. 1973, 16, 18, 22. *New York Times*, Mar. 30, 1976, 18; "A Small Fix for America's Drug Habit," *New York Times*, July 17, 1980, 18. Ford, *Times of My Life*, 307. Letter to the FDA, Manufacturers Files, AF14–324, Hoffman-La Roche, FDA History Office. Hughes and Brewin, *Tranquilizing America*, 65. Kline, quoted in Gilbert Cant, "Valiumania," *New York Times Magazine*, Feb. 1, 1976, 40–41. Linda Murray, "Why Users of Valium, Librium Aren't So Tranquil," *Chicago Daily News*, Feb. 4, 1976.

51. Ruth Cooperstock, "Sex Differences in Psychotropic Drug Use," *Social Science Medicine* 12 (July 1978): 179–186; Ruth Cooperstock and Henry L. Lennard, "Some Social Meanings of Tranquilizer Use," *Sociology of Health and Illness* 14 (Dec. 1979): 331–347; "Non-Working Wives Over 34 Are Biggest Users of Tranquilizers, Research Shows," n.d., Manufacturers Files, AF14–324, Hoffman-La Roche, FDA History Office; Bart, quoted in McMillan, "Women and Tranquilizers," 165. Cooperstock (1928–1985) was a medical sociologist whose pioneering research in women and pharmaceuticals was internationally acclaimed. Appointed to the Addiction Research Foundation in Toronto in 1966, she received a joint appointment in the Department of Behavioral Science in the Faculty of Medicine at the University of Toronto in 1981. *Remembering Ruth Cooperstock: Women and Pharmaceuticals Twenty Years Later* (Toronto: Women and Health Protection, 2006), 1.

52. Barbara Gibson testimony, *Women's Dependency on Prescription Drugs*, 47.

53. Rogers, "Drug Abuse—Just What the Doctor Ordered," 16–24. Roland Berg, "The Over-Medicated Woman," *McCall's*, Sept. 1971, 109–111. Kennedy, quoted in *The Use and Misuse of Benzodiazepines: Hearing Before the Subcommittee on Health and Scientific Research of the Committee on Labor and Human Resources*, United States Senate, Ninety-sixth Congress (Washington, DC: Government Printing Office, Sept. 10, 1979).

54. K. Robert Keiser and Woodrow Jones Jr., "Do the American Medical Association's Campaign Contributions Influence Health Care Legislation?" *Medical Care* 24 (Aug. 1986):

761–766; Adam Clymer, "Spending on 1982 Congress Races Was a Record $314 Million," *New York Times,* Jan. 11, 1983, B11; Warren Weaver Jr., "Special Interests Spend $60 Million," *New York Times,* Nov. 7, 1982, A27; Paul Starr, *The Social Transformation of American Medicine* (New York: Basic, 1984); Gabriel Kolko, *The Triumph of Conservatism* (New York: Free Press, 1977); Andrea Tone, *The Business of Benevolence: Industrial Paternalism in Progressive America* (Ithaca, NY: Cornell University Press, 1997); Alice Kessler-Harris, *In Pursuit of Equity: Women, Men, and the Quest for Economic Citizenship in 20th Century America* (Oxford: Oxford University Press, 2001); Szabo, *Intolerable and Incurable*; Harry Marks, *The Progress of Experiment: Science and Therapeutic Reform in the United States, 1900–1990* (Cambridge: Cambridge University Press, 1997).

55. A student at the University of Texas wrote a livid letter to Senator Lloyd Bentsen. Like Barbara Gordon's psychiatrist, his mother's physician had failed to warn her of the side effects of abrupt withdrawal. His mother had suffered incalculable grief. "Her mental well-being has been completely destroyed," he raged. "No doctor or psychiatrist has been able to help because all of them are incompetent bastards." An Illinois man who had experienced the anguish of withdrawal hadn't known the cause of his symptoms (he had consulted six doctors "but yet they won't tell me what is wrong") until he watched the Kennedy hearings. "If it wasn't for that hearing," he insisted, "I'd still be wondering what is wrong with me. . . . Now I know." Letter of Sept. 29, 1979 to Tom Corcoran, Manufacturers Files, AF14–324, Hoffman-La Roche, FDA History Office. *Claudette Caughell and Donald Caughell, wife and husband, Appellants, v. Group Health Cooperative of Puget Sound; Robert Sherry, M.D., and Jane Doe Sherry and the marital community thereof; and Hoffman–La Roche, Inc., Respondents,* 124 Wn. 2d 217; 876 P.2d 898; 1994 Wash. LEXIS 453. *Barbara Muney Libertelli, Plaintiff, against Hoffman–La Roche, Inc. and Medical Economics Co., Division of Litton Industries, Inc., Defendants,* 1981 U.S. Dist. LEXIS 11049. The court ruled in favor of the defendants, Hoffman-La Roche and Medical Economics.

CHAPTER 9

1. Robert Reinhold, "U.S. Wins Agreement on Warning to Doctors on Use of Tranquilizers," *New York Times,* July 11, 1980, A1.

2. Mickey S. Smith, *A Social History of Minor Tranquilizers: The Quest for Small Comfort in the Age of Anxiety* (New York: Pharmaceutical Products Press, 1985), 218–223. Phillip Lutz, "New Rules Cut Use of Tranquilizers," *New York Times,* Mar. 18, 1990, 12LI, 1; Michael S. Wilkes and Miriam Shuchman, "Pitching Doctors: Drug Companies' Ties to Physicians Are Often a Prescription for Expensive but Poor Treatment," *New York Times,* Nov. 5, 1989, SM88; L. Fraser and L. Davis, "Drug Law Backfires," *Health* 6 (Apr. 1992): 12; Michael de-Courcy Hinds, "Consumer's World: Anxiety Rises As New York Limits Tranquilizer Prescriptions," *New York Times,* Jan. 21, 1989, 35. The law exempted certain patients from the one-month limit. Those with panic disorders, convulsive disorders, narcolepsy, and pain associated with incurable diseases were allowed an initial three-month supply.

3. *The People of the State of Illinois v. Leslie Audi,* 392 N.E. 2d 248. *Rufus C. Cockrell v. State,* 392 So. 2d 541.

4. Philip M. Boffey, "Worldwide Use of Valium Draws New Scrutiny," *New York Times,* Oct. 13, 1981, C1; Alex Baenninger et al., *Good Chemistry: The Life and Legacy of Valium Inventor Leo Sternbach* (New York: McGraw Hill, 2004), 106; F. Kraupl Taylor, "The Damnation of Benzodiazepines," *British Journal of Psychiatry* 154 (1989): 697–704. BBC, *That's Life!* June 12, 1983, May 13, 1984; Ron Lacey and Shaun Woodward, *That's Life! Survey on*

Tranquillisers: With a Foreword by Esther Rantzen (London: British Broadcasting Corporation/MIND, National Association for Mental Health, 1985); Charles Medawar, *Power and Dependence: Social Audit on the Safety of Medicines* (London: Social Audit Limited, 1992); Medawar, interview by Andrea Tone, London, 2004; Malcolm Lader, interview by Andrea Tone, Paris 2004. The U.K. experience is well chronicled in Medawar's *Power and Dependence;* media, medical, and activist reports have also been catalogued and are available for review at www.benzo.org.uk. I am grateful to Andy Bell at BBC for helping me track down the *That's Life* broadcasts and a hard copy of the *That's Life* survey, and to Charles Medawar for his insightful and engaging analysis of U.K. regulatory developments and other matters.

5. Irwin Lerner, "How Americans Use Their Minor Tranquilizers," *New York Times,* Aug. 1, 1980, A22.

6. The ad campaign began in 1981. Ad cited in Smith, *Small Comfort,* 211. The FDA considered the ads misleading in their denial of the drug's habit-forming potential, and the acting branch chief for the Division of Drug Advertising and Labeling contacted Roche to revise the wording of the ads to disclose the probability of dependence. Letter from acting branch chief, Division of Drug Advertising and Labeling, Bureau of Drugs, to Drug Regulatory Affairs, Hoffman-La Roche Inc., July 10, 1981, Manufacturers Files, 14–324, Hoffman-La Roche, FDA History Office.

7. Stephen Epstein, "Activism, Drug Regulation, and the Politics of Therapeutic Evaluation in the AIDS Era: A Case Study of ddC and the 'Surrogate Markers' Debate," *Social Studies of Science* 27 (1997): 691–726; Andrea Tone, *Controlling Reproduction: An American History* (Wilmington, DE: Scholarly Resources, 1997).

8. Letter to Senator Gaylord Nelson, June 6, 1975, Manufacturers Files, AF14–324, Hoffman-La Roche, FDA History Office.

9. Letter to Representative Tom Foley, June 6, 1975, Manufacturers Files, AF 14–324, Hoffman-La Roche, FDA History Office; Letter to Senator Henry Jackson, June 6, 1975, Manufacturers Files, AF14–324, Hoffman-La Roche, FDA History Office.

10. Letter to FDA, July 1975, Manufacturers Files, AF14–324, Hoffman-La Roche, FDA History Office. Letter to FDA, Feb. 1975, Manufacturers Files, AF14–324, Hoffman-La Roche, FDA History Office. Letter to Congressman Donald Clancy, June 6, 1975, Manufacturers Files, AF14–324, Hoffman-La Roche, FDA History Office. Letter to the FDA, n.d., circa 1979, Manufacturers Files, AF14–324, Hoffman-La Roche, FDA History Office.

11. Letter to Honorable Lowell P. Weicker [1975], Manufacturers Files, AF14–324, Hoffman-La Roche, FDA History Office. Letter to Congressman John H. Dent, Apr. 25, 1975, Manufacturers Files, AF 14–324, Hoffman-La Roche, FDA History Office. Letter to Congressman Beard, Sept. 27, 1976, Manufacturers Files, 14–324, Hoffman-La Roche, FDA History Office.

12. Ironside, quoted in Elizabeth Heathcoate, "V is for Valium," *London Independent,* Nov. 23, 2003.

13. "Abuses Charged in Ads for Drugs," *New York Times,* Jan. 23, 1960, 4. Andrea Tone, "Heinz Lehmann: There at the Revolution," *Collegium International Neuro-Psychopharmacologicum Newsletter,* Mar. 2004, 16–17.

14. Wilkes and Schuchman, "Pitching Doctors," SM88; Alex Baenninger et al., *Good Chemistry,* 107; Fraser and Davis, "Drug Law Backfires," 12; Hinds, "Consumer's World," 35; Lutz, "New Rules," 12LI, 1.

15. Carl Salzman, *Benzodiazepine Dependence, Toxicity, and Abuse: A Task Force Report of the American Psychiatric Association* (Washington, DC: American Psychiatric Association, 1990), 52; C. Heather Ashton, "Benzodiazepine Abuse," in *Drink, Drugs, and Dependence: From Sci-*

ence to Clinical Practice, ed. Woody Caan and Jackie de Belleroche (London: Routledge, 2002), 197–212; *State of Tennessee v. Kenneth Allen Sisco,* 2000 Tenn. Crim App. Lexis 853, Oct. 30, 2000. Ronald Kotulak, "Addiction Fears Rise About Xanax," *Chicago Tribune,* Oct. 21, 2002; "Gov. Jeb Bush's Daughter Arrested in Xanax Prescription Fraud," benzo.org.uk, www.benzo.org.uk/msnbc2.htm (accessed Sept. 22, 2007).

16. C. Heather Ashton, *Benzodiazepines: How They Work and How to Withdraw,* Table 1, www.benzo.org.uk/manual (accessed Sept. 23, 2007).

17. "High Anxiety," *Consumer Reports Magazine* 58 (Jan. 1993): 19–24; "3 Drug Companies Get License to Sell Valium Equivalents," *New York Times,* Sept. 5, 1985, A20; "Valium, by Any Other Name," *New York Times,* Sept. 8, 1985, E24.

18. "High Anxiety," 19–24; Allen Frances et al., "The Classification of Panic Disorders: From Freud to DSM-IV," *Journal of Psychiatric Research* 27 (1993): suppl. 1, pp. 3–10; David Sheehan, "Angles on Panic," interview by David Healy in *The Psychopharmacologists,* ed. David Healy (London: Arnold, 2000), 3:479–484.

19. "High Anxiety," 19–24; "Three Drug Companies Get License to Sell Valium Equivalents," A20; Jackie Orr, *Panic Diaries: A Genealogy of Panic Disorder* (Durham, NC: Duke University Press, 2006), 223, 251–254. Panic disorder had been cleaved, along with general anxiety disorder, from DSM-I and II's more vague "anxiety neurosis." Frances et al., "Classification of Panic Disorders," 3–10; Peter R. Breggin, *Toxic Psychiatry: Why Therapy, Empathy, and Love Must Replace the Drugs, Electroshock, and Biochemical Theories of the "New Psychiatry"* (New York: St. Martin's, 1994), 251–253, 346–355.

20. "High Anxiety," 19–24; Edward Shorter and Peter Tyrer, "Separation of Anxiety and Depressive Disorders: Blind Alley in Psychopharmacology and Classification of Disease," *British Medical Journal,* July 19, 2003, 158; Kotulak, "Addiction Fears Rise About Xanax"; "Xanax Often Abused for Easy High," benzo.org.uk, www.benzo.org.uk/msnbc1.htm (accessed Sept. 22, 2007).

21. Dr. Dan Angres, quoted in Kotulak, "Addiction Fears Rise," 19–24; Ashton, *Benzodiazepines: How They Work and How to Withdraw,* Table 1; Salzman, *Benzodiazepine Dependence,* 36; Conrad M. Swartz, "Benzo Backbite," *Psychiatric Times,* Nov. 1, 2003, 8.

22. National Institute of Mental Health, "The Numbers Count: Mental Disorders in America," 2001, www.nimh.nih.gov/publicat/numbers.cfm (accessed Feb. 9, 2005); The Numbers Count: Mental Disorders in America, 2006 (rev.), www.nimh.nih.gov/publicat/numbers.cfm (accessed Sept. 7, 2007). The increase in the apparent prevalence of anxiety disorders between the two "counts" raises concerns about the facticity of diagnostic claims and symptom reportage. Anxiety Disorders Association of America, "Statistics and Facts About Anxiety Disorders," www.adaa.org/AboutADAA/PressRoom/Stats & Facts.asp (accessed Oct. 3, 2007); P. E. Greenberg et al., "The Economic Burden of Anxiety Disorders in the 1990s," *Journal of Clinical Psychiatry* 60 (July 1999): 427–435; R. L. DuPont et al., "Economic Costs of Anxiety Disorders," *Anxiety* 2 (1996): 167–172.

23. Salzman, *Benzodiazepine Dependence,* 12–13; E. H. Uhlenhuth et al., "Anxiety Disorders: Prevalence and Treatment," *Current Medical Research and Opinion* 8 (1984): supplement 8, 37–46; Eberhard H. Uhlenhuth et al., "Risks and Benefits of Long-Term Benzodiazepine Use," *Journal of Clinical Psychopharmacology* 8 (June 1988): 161–167; G. D. Mellinger, M. B. Balter, E. H. Uhlenhuth, "Prevalence and Correlates of the Long-term Regular Use of Anxiolytics," *JAMA* 251 (1984): 375–379; Jerrold F. Rosenbaum, "Benzodiazepines: Revisiting Clinical Issues in Treating Anxiety Disorders," *Primary Health Companion to the Journal of Clinical Psychiatry* 7 (2005): 23–30. Uhlenhuth et al., "Risks and Benefits of Long-Term Benzodiazepine Use," 161–167.

24. "Elizabeth Rasche Gonzalez, "Where Are All the Tranquilizer Junkies?" *Journal of the American Medical Association,* May 20, 1983, 2603–2604. Salzman, *Benzodiazepine Dependence,* 1, 55–59; Carl Salzman, "The APA Task Force Report on Benzodiazepine Dependence, Toxicity, and Abuse," editorial, *American Journal of Psychiatry* 148 (Feb. 1991): 151–152. "Report of the World Psychiatric Association, Task Force on Sedative Hypnotics," *European Psychiatry* 8 (1993): 45–49; Baenninger et al., *Good Chemistry,* 109. Leo H. Hollister et al., "Long-term Use of Diazepam," *JAMA,* Oct. 2, 1981, 1568–1570; Uhlenhuth et al., "Risks and Benefits," 161–167; J. H. Taaley, "But What If a Patient Gets Hooked? Fallacies About Long-Term Use of Benzodiazepines," *Postgrad Med* 87 (1990): 187–203; Mitchell B. Balter et al., "International Study of Expert Judgment on Therapeutic Use of Benzodiazepines and Other Psychotherapeutic Medications: Current Concerns," *Human Psychopharmacology* 8 (1993): 253–261; Linda Little, "Some Concerns About the Abuse of Benzodiazepines Unwarranted," *Clinical Psychiatry News,* Mar. 1, 2006, 31; Jay M. Pomerantz, "Risk Versus Benefit of Benzodiazepines," *Psychiatric Times,* Aug. 1, 2007, 4.

25. S. M. Linsen, F. G. Zitman, and M. H. M. Breteler, "Defining Benzodiazepine Dependence: The Confusion Persists," *European Psychiatry* 10 (1995): 306–311. Pomerantz, "Risk Versus Benefit," 4.

26. Edward Shorter and Peter Tyrer, "Separation of Anxiety and Depressive Disorders: Blind Alley in Psychopharmacology and Classification of Disease," 158–160; P. Tyrer, "The Case for Cothymia: Mixed Anxiety and Depression in a Single Disorder," *British Journal of Psychiatry* 179 (2001): 191–193; Hans-Jurgen Moller, "Anxiety Associated with Comorbid Depression," *Journal of Clinical Psychiatry* 63 (2002): suppl. 14, 22; Michael B. First, "Mutually Exclusive Versus Co-Occurring Diagnostic Categories: The Challenge of Diagnostic Comorbidity," *Psychopathology* 38, no. 4 (2005): 206–210. Stephen M. Stahl, "Mergers and Acquisitions Among Psychotropics: Antidepressant Takeover of Anxiety May Now Be Complete," *Journal of Clinical Psychiatry* 60, no. 5 (May 1999): 282–283; American Psychiatric Association, "Practice Guidelines for the Treatment of Patients with Panic Disorder," *American Journal Psychiatry* 155 (1988): suppl., 1–34; Greg Critser, *Generation RX: How Prescription Drugs Are Altering American Lives, Minds, and Bodies* (Boston: Houghton Mifflin, 2005), 66.

27. In DSM-III, social phobia was defined as a circumscribed fear of performance situations. It was characterized as follows: A persistent, irrational fear of, and compelling desire to avoid, a situation in which the individual is exposed to possible scrutiny by others and fears that he or she may act in a way that will be humiliating or embarrassing. Significant distress because of the disturbance and recognition by the individual that his or her fear is excessive or unreasonable not due to another mental disorder, such as major depression or avoidant personality disorder. American Psychiatric Association, *Diagnostic and Statistical Manual of Mental Disorders,* 3rd ed. [DSM-III] (Washington, DC: American Psychiatric Association, 1980), 228. Also see Stephanie Lloyd, "An Anxious Society: The French Importation of Social Phobia and the Appearance of a New Model of the Self" (Ph.D. diss., McGill University, 2006). Rosario B. Hidalgo, Stewart D. Barnett, and Jonathan R.T. Davison, "Social Anxiety Disorder in Review: Two Decades of Progress," *International Journal of Neuropsychopharmacology* 4 (2001): 279–298; Critser, *Generation Rx,* 66. The reference counts can be found in Shankar Vedantam, "Selling an Illness Helps Pharmaceutical Giant Peddle Its Pill," *Washington Post Service,* July 17, 2001, 2–3; Conrad M. Schwartz, "Benzo Backbite, Clinical Controversies," *Psychiatric Times,* Nov. 1, 2003, 8; Christopher Lane, "Shy on Drugs," *New York Times,* Sept. 21, 2007; Suein L. Hwang, "Workplace Stress? Pills Are No Panacea," *Wall Street Journal;* reprinted in *Atlanta Journal-Constitution,* Sept. 29, 2002, LB15; Anne McIlroy, "High Anxiety," *Globe and Mail,* Sept. 20, 2003; Hidalgo et al., "High Anxiety," 279–298.

28. Vedantam, "Selling an Illness"; McIlroy, "High Anxiety"; Ray Moynihan and Alan Cassels, *Selling Sickness: How the World's Biggest Pharmaceutical Companies Are Turning Us All Into Patients* (Vancouver: Greystone, 2005), 120–124. Barry Brand, quoted in Vedantam, "Selling an Illness." Moynihan and Cassels, *Selling Sickness*, 122; Vedantam, "Selling an Illness"; Lane, "Shy on Drugs"; McIlroy, "High Anxiety"; Steven G. Morgan, "Direct-to-Consumer Advertising and Expenditures on Prescription Drugs: A Comparison of Experiences in the States and Canada," *Open Medicine* 1 (2007): 37–45. Distraught executive Paxil ad, *American Journal of Psychiatry* 156 (Oct. 1999). "Empowered by Paxil Ad," *American Journal of Psychiatry* 158 (July 2001). For a trenchant analysis of the SAD campaign, see Lane, *Shyness*, 116–138. On the gendering of ads for psychiatric medications, see Jonathan Metzl, *Prozac on the Couch: Prescribing Gender in the Era of Wonder Drugs* (Durham, NC: Duke University Press, 2001). Andrea Tone and Elizabeth Siegel Watkins, introduction to *Medicating Modern America: Prescription Drugs in History* (New York: New York University Press, 2007), 1–14. The 1997 FDA Modernization Act loosened several FDA restrictions, including those governing the direct advertising of prescription drugs to consumers. See Jennifer Fishman, "Manufacturing Desire: The Commodification of Female Sexual Dysfunction," *Social Studies of Science* 34 (Apr 2004): 199.

29. "Social Anxiety Disorder: Miami Dolphin Ricky Williams," *Talk Today*, www .usatoday.com/community/chat/2002-10-22-williams.htm (accessed Oct. 7, 2007); Moynihan and Cassels, *Selling Sickness*, 119–138. "Wannstedt 'Shocked Again' at News," July 30, 2004, http://sports.espn.go.com/nfl/news/story?id=1848492 (accessed Mar. 25, 2008).

30. For current indications, see www.gsk.com/products/prescription_medicines/us/paxil.htm. *Anxious Moments* (Les Production Rivard and GlaxoSmithKlein, no date given), distributed at the annual meeting of the Canadian Psychiatric Association in Halifax, Nova Scotia, 2003. VHS films include *Coming Out of Hiding: Overcoming S.A.D.* and *Out from Under the Cloud: Overcoming Generalized Anxiety Disorder.*

31. The critical literature on the topic of overmedicalization is vast and includes Peter Conrad, *The Medicalization of Society: On the Transformation of Human Conditions into Treatable Disorders* (Baltimore: Johns Hopkins University Press, 2007); Charles Barber, *Comfortably Numb: How Psychiatry Is Medicating a Nation* (New York: Pantheon, 2008); Allan V. Horwitz and Jerome Wakefield, *The Loss of Sadness: How Psychiatry Transformed Normal Sorrow into Depressive Disorder* (New York: Oxford University Press, 2007); Moynihan and Cassels, *Selling Sickness;* David Healy, *Let Them Eat Prozac: The Unhealthy Relationship Between the Pharmaceutical Industry and Depression* (New York: New York University Press, 2004); Critser, *Generation RX;* Lane, *Shyness;* Ray Moynihan, Iona Heath, and David Henry, "Selling Sickness: The Pharmaceutical Industry and Disease Mongering," *British Medical Journal* 324 (2002): 886–901; Peter Conrad and Valerie Leiter, "Medicalization, Markets, and Consumers," *Journal of Health and Social Behavior* 45 (2004): 158–176. Angell, quoted in Vedantam, "Selling an Illness," 2. The film *A New Epidemic* was viewed at www.youtube.com (accessed Mar. 17, 2007). Peter Kramer, *Listening to Prozac* (New York: Penguin, 1994), 15; Jonathan M. Metzl, "Selling Sanity Through Gender," *Ms.*, Fall 2003, 42–45; Jacquelyn N. Zita, *Body Talk: Philosophical Reflections on Sex and Gender* (New York: Columbia University Press, 1998); Fishman, "Manufacturing Desire," 193. As bioethicist Carl Elliott has suggested, "The way to sell drugs is to sell psychiatric illness. If you are Paxil and you are the only manufacturer who had the drug for social anxiety disorder, it's in your interest to broaden the category as far as possible and make the borders as fuzzy as possible." Elliott, quoted in Vedantam, "Selling an Illness," 2.

32. Neil Rector of Toronto's Center for Addiction and Mental Health, quoted in McIlroy, "High Anxiety." Stein, quoted in Vedantam, "Selling an Illness," 2.

33. This point has been raised by Rex Cowdry, medical director of the National Alliance for the Mentally Ill, a patient advocacy group. See Vedantam, "Selling an Illness," 2. www.adaa.org/GettingHelp/AboutAnxietyDisorders.asp (accessed Mar. 30, 2008). Ross, quoted in Vedantam, "Selling an Illness," 3.

34. Stephen M. Stahl, "Don't Ask, Don't Tell, but Benzodiazepines Are Still the Leading Treatment for Anxiety Disorders," *Journal of Clinical Psychiatry* 63 (Sept. 2002): 756–757. In some patients they don't work at all; as many as 40 percent of patients with panic attacks, for instance, do not respond to SSRIs or other antidepressants. Baenninger et al., *Good Chemistry*, 97. If dependence is gauged by the severity and experience of discontinuation symptoms, it is clear that many SSRIs share a similar problem with benzodiazepines. For instance, Paxil (paroxetine), the SSRI most frequently prescribed as an anxiolytic, can cause severe withdrawal reactions that range from mild, transient headaches to nausea, insomnia, tremors, muscle pain, vertigo, and electric "zap" sensations in the brain. GSK's own clinical trial revealed that between 25 and 62 percent of patients experienced withdrawal symptoms. Instead of disclosing this information to consumers and doctors, however, the company initially suppressed it. Only in December 2001 did GSK incorporate a precautionary statement about withdrawal reactions in its packet insert, by which time millions of prescriptions had been sold. To date, insurance companies, patients, and pharmacies have filed more than 5,000 lawsuits in the United States and 2,500 in Britain (where the drug is sold under the brand name Seroxat) against GSK for Paxil addiction. To avoid withdrawal symptoms, long-term users of Paxil are generally advised to adopt the same tapering strategy recommended to benzodiazepine users, taking increasingly smaller doses over an extended period of time. Lane, *Shyness*, 139–149; Gardiner Harris, "Spitzer Sues a Drug Maker, Saying It Hid Negative Data," *New York Times,* June 3, 2004, A1; "Drug Maker Withheld Paxil Study Data: ABC News Uncovers Documents Unknown to Regulators and Many Doctors," Dec. 9, 2004, http://abcnews.go/com (accessed Oct. 12, 2007); transcript of ABC *Prime Time Live,* Dec. 9, 2004. "Anti-Depressant Addiction Warning, BBC News World Edition, June 11, 2001, http://news.bbc.co.uk/2/hi/health (accessed Oct. 12, 2007). The BBC program *Panorama* released an exposé of the hazards of Seroxat in Oct. 2004. I am grateful to Andy Bell at BBC for sharing details of the making of this program with me. A transcript can be found at http://news.bbc.co.uk/nol/shared/spl/hi/programmes/panorama/transcripts/takenontrust (accessed Oct. 12, 2007). Trial data and the medical letter for adult use of Paxil can be found on the company's website: www.gsk.com/media/paroxetine_adult.htm (accessed Oct. 12, 2007). Patients suffering from Paxil addiction can consult numerous websites, support groups, and books for counsel and advice. In addition, as part of an out of court settlement of a fraud case instigated by New York Attorney General Eliot Spitzer, the company has recently posted on its website summaries of recent clinical trials. Linda Little, "Some Concerns About the Abuse of Benzodiazepines Unwarranted," *Clinical Psychiatry News,* Mar. 1, 2006.

35. Mitchell B. Balter, Jerome Levine, and Dean I. Manheimer, "Cross-National Study of the Extent of Anti-Anxiety/Sedative Drug Use," *New England Journal of Medicine,* Apr. 4, 1974, 769–774. In addition to offering this evidence before government investigations, Clark defended the company's activities in the United States in newspapers and journal editorials. See, for instance, "Is the Abuse of Valium Exaggerated?" *Resident and Staff Physician,* Nov. 1979.

36. Heathcoate, "V is for Valium." Balter et al., "Cross-National Study," 769–774; William A. Nolen, "Tranquilizers: Their Use and Abuse," *McCall's,* May 1976, 94; Philip M. Boffey,

"Worldwide Use of Valium Draws New Scrutiny," *New York Times*, Oct. 13, 1981, C1. Rajaa Lagnaoui et al., "Patterns and Correlates of Benzodiazepine Use in the French General Population," *European Journal of Clinical Pharmacology* 60 (2004): 523–529; J. Lecadet et al., "Médicaments psychotropes: Consommations et pratiques de prescription en France métropolitaine. I Données nationales, 2000," *Revue médicale de l'assurance maladie* 34 (2003): 75–85. Also see J. P. Lepine and I. Gasquet, "Psychotropic Drug Use in France, Changes Over Time and Comparison with Other European Countries," *Bulletin de l'Académie nationale de médicine* 190 (June 2006): 1139–1144; Maurice M. Ohayon and Malcolm H. Lader, "Use of Psychotropic Medication in the General Population of France, Germany, Italy, and the United Kingdom," *Journal of Clinical Psychiatry* 63 (Sept. 2002): 817–825; A. Pélissolo et al., "Troubles anxieux et dépressifs chez 4,425 patients consommateurs de benzodiazepines au long cours en médecine générale," *Encephale* 33 (Jan.-Feb. 2007): 32–38. This finding takes on dramatic meaning when considered against the size of the French pharmaceutical market. With the French spending over US\$32 billion on drugs in 2006 (a disproportionately large number on psychotropic medications), France has the third largest pharmaceutical market in the world, second only to Japan (with sales of \$56.9 billion) and the United States (\$276.1 billion). Both public and private pharmaceutical expenditures have more than doubled in France in the past ten years and vastly exceed those in other European countries, such as Germany and England. While patients in Germany consult doctors more frequently, the disparity in drug use is largely explained by the liberalism with which French physicians prescribe medications; 90 percent of doctors' visits conclude with a script. Benzodiazepines are widely prescribed; public expenditures in France for the drugs are more than double what they are in Germany, even though the reimbursement allowance is about the same in both countries. Clinical guidelines in France recommend that the period for which benzodiazepines be prescribed be limited to four weeks for insomnia and twelve for anxiety. In practice, French doctors roundly ignore these recommendations. And they do so with impunity, because there is little regulation of doctors' prescribing behavior or restrictions on repeat prescribing. As one study of high benzodiazepine prevalence rates concluded, strategies to limit benzodiazepine use in France have proven "quite ineffective. . . . Instructions are not followed. Perhaps more forcible methods are needed than just information." "Top 10 Pharmaceutical Markets Worldwide, Sept. 2006," IMS Health Canada, www.imshealthcanada.com (accessed Sept. 13, 2007); Luc Nguyen-Kim et al., "Les politiques de prise en charge des médicaments en Allemagne, Angleterre et France," *Institut de Recherche et Documentation en Économie de la Santé* 99 (Oct. 2005); Sandrine Blanchard, "La France, championne d'Europe en prescription de médicaments," *Le Monde*, Oct. 18, 2005; "Des habitudes qui creusent les dépenses," *Le Monde*, Oct. 19, 2005. I am grateful to George Weisz for bringing these articles to my attention. The quotation is from Lagnaoui et al., "Patterns and Correlates of Benzodiazepine Use," 523–529.

37. Lynn Payer, *Medicine and Culture: Varieties of Treatment in the United States, England, West Germany, and France* (New York: Holt, 1988). See, for instance, Illana Lowy and George Weisz, "French Hormones: Progestins and Therapeutic Variation in France," *Social Science and Medicine* 60 (2005): 2609–2622; George Weisz, *Divide and Conquer: A Comparative History of Medical Specialization* (Oxford: Oxford University Press, 2006). Karl Rickels, interview by David Healy, 1998; transcript in author's possession.

38. Laurence J. Kirmayer, "Psychopharmacology in a Globalizing World: The Use of Antidepressants in Japan," *Transcultural Psychiatry* 39 (2002): 295–322. Takahashi, quoted in Kathryn Shulz, "Did Antidepressants Depress Japan?" *New York Times*, Aug. 22, 2004, 9. In her landmark ethnographic study of menopause, anthropologist Margaret Lock observed

how women's discussions of symptoms in Japan and North America were culturally mediated. While Japanese women complained of irritability and insomnia, North American women were more likely to discuss depression as problems. Different ways of framing biological experience—what gets recognized as disorderly or transgressive—generated different cultural understandings of what menopause meant as well as divergent treatment modalities. See Margaret Lock, *Encounters with Aging: Mythologies of Menopause in Japan and North America* (Berkeley: University of California Press, 1993); Margaret Lock and Patricia Kaufert, "Menopause, Local Biologies, and Cultures of Aging," *American Journal of Human Biology* 13 (July-Aug. 2001): 494–504. As psychiatrist and historian David Healy has argued, "despite medical reforms and a growing acceptance that benzodiazepines should not be prescribed for hypertension, ulcers, or similar conditions," Japanese patients and physicians continued to use them to treat what they regard as psychosomatic ailments. Healy, *Let Them Eat Prozac,* 7.

39. Toshi-Hiro Kobayakawa, interview by David Healy, in *The Psychopharamologists III: Interviews with David Healy,* ed. David Healy (New York: Oxford University Press), 285–287.

40. Kleinman, quoted in Schulz, "Did Antidepressants Depress Japan?" *New York Times,* Aug. 22, 2004, 9.

41. Draft of Summary Report of Workshop on Incapacitating Agents, July 31, 1986, International Archives of Neuro-Psychopharmacology, Vanderbilt University.

42. Antony Barnett, "US Plans to Strike Enemy with Valium: Pentagon Scientists Aim for Future Battlefield Victories with the Aid of Tranquillising Drugs and GM Bugs," *London Observer,* May 26, 2002; "Dexmedetomidine," http://dexmedetomidine.com (accessed Nov. 1, 2007).

43. Daniel G. Dupont, "Storm Before the Calm," *Scientific American* 288 (Feb. 2003): 17–19.

44. "Preparedness & Response," Homeland Security, www.dhs.gov/xprepresp (accessed Apr. 2, 2008). Homeland Security, www.dhs.gov/xlibrary/assets/grants_audit_uasitransit.pdf (accessed Apr. 2, 2008).

45. Abby Goodnough, "Post–9/11 Pain Found to Linger in Young Minds," *New York Times,* May 2, 2002, A1, A24. Sandro Galea, Jennifer Ahern, Heidi Resnick, Dean Kilpatrick, Michael Bucuvalas, Joel Gold, and David Vlahov, "Psychological Sequelae of the Sept. 11 Terrorist Attacks in New York City," *New England Journal of Medicine,* Mar. 28, 2002, 982–988. Based on their survey of 1,009 adults in the Manhattan area, the authors argued that "severe lasting psychological effects are generally seen after disaster causing extensive loss of life, property damage, and widespread financial strain and after disasters that are intentionally caused." These elements were all present in the Sept. 11 attacks, suggesting that the psychological sequelae in New York City are substantial and will be long-lasting.

46. Mark A. Schuster et al., "A National Survey of Stress Reactions after the Sept. 11, 2001, Terrorist Attacks," *New England Journal of Medicine,* Nov. 15, 2001, 1507–1513; R. Yehuda et al., "Pathological Responses to Terrorism," *Neuropsychopharmacology* 30 (2006): 1793–1805; Yuval Neira et al., eds., *9/11: Mental Health in the Wake of Terrorist Attacks* (New York: Cambridge University Press, 2006). For an insightful set of historical analyses on the metamorphosis of trauma and the impact of 9/11 on understandings of PTSD, see Allan Young, "Commentary," *Journal of Nervous and Mental Disease* 195 (Dec. 2007): 1031–1032; and Allan Young, "PTSD of the Virtual Kind—Trauma and Resilience in Post 9/11 America," in *Trauma and Memory: Reading, Healing, and Making Law,* ed. Nadav Davidovitch and Michal Alberstein (Palo Alto: Stanford University Press, 2007), 21–48.

47. Christine Gorman, "The Science of Anxiety," *Newsweek*, June 10, 2002, 46–54.

48. IMS Health Data, National Disease & Therapeutic Index, Diagnosis Visits, 2002–2006.

49. Karen Springen, "Taking the Worry Cure," *Newsweek*, Feb. 24, 2003, 52.

TABLE 1   Top 10 Drugs Prescribed for Anxiety States, 2006

Drug	Number of Prescriptions Dispensed (in thousands)
1. Alprazolam (Xanax)*	20,208
2. Lorazepam (Ativan)*	9,316
3. Clonazepam (Klonopin)*	5,902
4. Paroxetine HCL (Paxil)	4,923
5. Lexapro	3,616
6. Diazepam (Valium)*	3,064
7. Zoloft	2,757
8. Sertraline HCL (Zoloft)	2,228
9. Effexor XR	2,219
10. Citalopram HBR (Celexa)	2,086
Total, Top 10	56,319

*=benzodiazepine

Benzodiazepine total: 38,490 (68 percent of total Top 10)

Antidepressant total: 17,829 (32 percent of total Top 10)

Source: IMS Health Data

50. As Jerilyn Ross, president of the Anxiety Disorders Association of America, put it in 2002, "If mental health is the stepchild of the health-care system, then anxiety is the stepchild of the stepchild." Ross quoted in Gorman, "Science of Anxiety," 48. In one day, nurses staffing the booth screened about one hundred shoppers. Anne Marie Owens, "Psychiatric Analysis Comes to the Local Shopping Mall: Brisk Business at Anxiety Disorder Kiosk," *National Post*, May 10, 2004.

51. "Benzodiazepines: Revisiting Clinical Issues in Treating Anxiety Disorders," *Primary Care Companion Journal Clinical Psychiatry* 7 (2005): 23–28. The price survey, carried out by Theresa Howard at McGill University on Mar. 29, 2008, surveyed prices of generic Valium, generic Paxil, and name-brand Paxil at three retail pharmacies in Ballston Spa, New York, Fort Lauderdale, Florida, and Denver, Colorado. The results of Howard's survey, which compared prices at different doses, and was conducted over the telephone, is in the author's possession.

52. On Hilton's use of Xanax, see www.usmagazine.com/paris_hilton_sent_back_to Hollywood_jail, and www.associatedcontent.com/article/280795/paris_hilton_and_xanax_addiction.html (accessed Apr. 3, 2008); on Anna Nicole Smith, see http/abcnews.go.com/Health/story?id=2982406&page=1, and www.usmagazine.com/anna_nicole_smith_6 (accessed Apr. 3, 2008); on Heath Ledger, see http://abcnews.go.com/Health/Story?id=4251620&page=1 (accessed Apr. 3, 2008), and James Barron with Al Baker and Sewell Clannon reporting, "Medical Examiner Rules Ledger's Death Accidental," *New York Times*, Feb. 7, 2008, 3. In 2000, Pharmacia and Upjohn merged with Monsanto and Searle to create Pharmacia. In 2003 Pharmacia and Pfizer merged to create a unified company, Pfizer. "Quick Facts about Xanax XR," www.xanaxxr.com/quick/index.asp (accessed Oct. 5, 2007). Also see Xanax XR ad in *Medizine: Health Living*, second quarter 2004, 48d–48g.

53. "Cardinal Health's Zydis Drug Delivery Technology Used to Develop Quick-Dissolve Klonopin Wafers CIV," PR Newswire, New York, Sept. 30, 2003, 1. Hoffman-La Roche distributed the drug and Solvay Pharmaceuticals marketed it. The product was brought to market using Cardinal Health's patented Zydis quick-dissolve drug delivery technology. Klonopin Wafers promotion packet, "Therapy Designed with Patients in Mind"; Rapitab technology promotion packet. I am grateful to Leonore Tiefer for sharing these pamphlets and detailing samples with me. Also see "Cardinal Health's Zydis Drug Delivery Technology Used to Develop Quick-Dissolve Klonopin Wafers CIV," 1.

54. On the social meanings of medical marketing and consumer choice, also see Andrea Tone, "From Naughty Goods to Nicole Miller," *Culture, Medicine, and Psychiatry* 30 (June 2006): 249–267.

INDEX

Page locators in bold indicate photographs or illustrations.